The Word of WISDOM

The Word of Wisdom

Principle With Promise

By Mildred Nelson Smith

Herald Publishing House, Independence, Missouri

COPYRIGHT © 1977
Herald Publishing House
Independence, Missouri

All rights in this book are reserved. No part of the text may be reproduced in any form without written permission of the publishers, except brief quotations used in connection with reviews in magazines or newspapers.

Library of Congress Cataloging in Publication Data

Smith, Mildred Nelson,
   The Word of Wisdom.

   Bibliography: p.
   1. Nutrition. 2. Hygiene. 3. Smith, Joseph, 1805-1844. 4. Mormons and Mormonism. I. Title.
BX8643.D5S57   613.2   76-46311
ISBN 0-8309-0175-2

Printed in the United States of America

Dedication

To Lauree, whose suffering sparked my search for understanding.

CONTENTS

Preface 9
1. Scope and Setting of the Word of Wisdom 15
2. The Herbs Ordained for Man 32
3. Fruits That Provide Vitamin C 45
4. Cereals, the Staff of Life 57
5. Meats to Be Shared 98
6. Milk, a Repository of Nutrients 129
7. Weight Control 140
8. Well Born Children 174
9. Well Fed Infants 183
10. Alcohol 199
11. Tobacco 218
12. Hot Drinks and Strong Drinks 233
13. Some Problem Areas in Modern Nutrition Practice, Part I—Misinformation 246
14. Some Problem Areas in Modern Nutrition Practice, Part II—Methods of Food Production 260
15. Some Problem Areas in Modern Nutrition Practice, Part III—Additives 267
16. Other Elements of Good Health 295
Epilogue—A Statement on Nutrition 309

PREFACE

An experience with pellagra took me from a career as a general home economist back to university to study nutrition. It was what I learned about pellagra that gave me the key to the relationship of the Word of Wisdom to modern knowledge of the science of nutrition.

In the early days of World War II I worked in the southern part of the United States of America. My usually efficient and competent secretary, whose work load had been extended by loss of other personnel to the war effort, suddenly began to leave her work undone. Usually quiet and reserved, she became extremely talkative and self-assertive. Usually poised and courageous, she became highly agitated and fearful. Usually careful of property, she became destructive. Doctors to whom she was taken said she was drunk or drugged, and she was locked in a basement room of a community hospital to recover.

Instead of recovering, she grew steadily worse. Finally we obtained an appointment with a specialist in nervous disorders in St. Louis, Missouri. When he appeared at his office door to invite her in, my secretary-friend threw her shoes at him. He dodged the shoes, and without inviting her inside said, "Take her away and get her some food! I've seen dozens like her!"

While her parents took her back to the car I stayed to inquire, "Where shall we take her?" and "Will she ever be well?" To the first question he replied that there was only one place in the state of Missouri where her need would be recognized and she would receive proper treatment. To that hospital he referred us. To the second question he replied a bit heatedly,

"Of course she will be well! But the state you've got her in, it will take six months!"

It was four months later, instead of the six the specialist had predicted, that we were notified to come for my friend. We took from the hospital a well, normal, healthy young woman. She became the receptionist at the hospital neighboring the one in which she had been locked in a basement room. From there she entered Graceland College, graduated with honors, taught school, worked as a government employee, and finally met a young man whom she wished to marry.

Before making wedding plans the couple wrote to the hospital in which my secretary had received treatment to inquire whether there was any reason why they should not marry and have children. The response was that there was none. As long as she remained well fed, there would be no recurrence of her illness. That was in the 1940s, and in all the years that have intervened she has given much in service to her family, church, and community.

Lauree was an atypical pellagrin. Her problem was not easily recognized because she did not have the typical rash ("gloved hands") on her hands and feet which usually precedes the mental abberations of pellagrins. Proper treatment was not immediately available because niacin, the nutrient needed to prevent or cure pellagra, had only recently been discovered and its use in the treatment of mental illness associated with pellagra was little known.

When the specialist told us to get her some food and she would get well, I knew I had to know more about food and how to prevent such tragedies as would have occurred had we not found a physician who could help. Immediately I began to make arrangements to do graduate study.

I had been at Iowa State University only a few months when I attended a conference of Far West Stake at St. Joseph, Missouri, at which the Spirit of God ministered abundantly. During one of the services the Lord spoke to us through Apostle Oakman, telling us that the time would come when, though he desired to protect us, we could not expect that blessing unless we were obedient to the Word of Wisdom. He said other things that I have forgotten, but they reminded me of what I was learning at the university.

With great excitement I turned to Section 86 of the Doctrine and Covenants and began to make comparisons of the instructions given there with that which I was learning in my graduate work. I was especially intrigued, and am to this day, by the statement that "all grain is good for the food of man... nevertheless, wheat for man, and corn for the ox...."

Pellagra has always followed corn-eating people. The Italians began to succumb to the disease after corn was introduced from the Americas. It was they who named it "pellagra" or "rough skin" from the rash that usually signals the presence of the disease. A centuries-old manuscript, quoted in *Borden's Review of Nutrition Research* (December 1946, page 1) describes it thus:

> If you should traverse the hills of Brianza and Canavese, you would most likely meet some pitiable wrecks of humanity, with eyes fixed and glassy, with pale and sallow faces and arms scarred as by a burn or a large wound. You would see them advancing with trembling head and staggering gait like persons intoxicated or indeed, as though impelled by an invisible force, now falling on one side, now getting up and running in a straight line like a dog after its quarry and now again falling and uttering a senseless laugh or sob which pierces the heart.... Such are the pellagrins.

Not at this time, nor for centuries later, did those who observed the pellagrins know the cause of their distress. When it became apparent that the disease was associated with the use of corn as a major portion of the diet, it was thought that there was a toxin or infectious agent in corn that caused the disease with its 3 d's (dermatitis, diarrhea, and dementia) causing the feet and hands to be covered with the terrible rash and the mental capacities to be so devastated. It was between 1915 and the early 1920s that Dr. Joseph Goldberg of the U.S.A. Public Health Service determined that there was no poison involved but rather a nutritional deficiency that could be corrected by the use of milk, yeast, meats, and vegetables even if corn was still eaten. He also noted that people who had wheat as their major food did not develop the disease.

In the late 1930s niacin was discovered to be the vitamin that could prevent or cure the disease. This knowledge left investigators puzzled, because some of the foods that were effective in curing pellagra contained very little niacin. Then it was found that tryptophan, one of the amino acids contained abundantly in milk, for example, was a precursor of niacin in the body. If there was a good supply of tryptophan, the body could make all the niacin it needed.

I was particularly excited about all of this because when we learned about niacin and tryptophan, we found that while corn is severely deficient in both, wheat is well supplied with both nutrients. We learned this fact less than four decades ago. The Lord knew it all of the time and communicated the knowledge to us in his instruction that, although all grain is good for man (corn does not contain a dangerous toxin or bacterial agent of disease), wheat was made especially to fill the needs of man and corn to fill the needs of cattle.

Why can cows use corn as their principal item of diet without getting pellagra and man cannot? Cows have more than one stomach. The first one, the rumen, is a veritable factory of amino acids. As soon as the food enters it, bacteria resident there attack and prepare it for further digestion. When it is finally digested, needed nutrients have been manufactured from corn or even roughage eaten.

But man is made differently. He has no rumen, and his niacin or tryptophan must be preformed for him. We know it now. The Lord knew it always, and more than a century before science found the answer to such physical and mental ills as pellagra, he caused his prophet to advise us to eat in the way that would protect us from one of the most dread and then prevalent of nutritional diseases.

Recognizing this specific instance of the validity of the Lord's instruction in the Word of Wisdom, I set about to discover the relationship of his other instructions to more recent scientific discoveries. It is a thrilling quest which now I want to share with you.

Although much remains to be learned, there is abundant evidence of the validity of the Lord's counsel. If we interpret it according to his intent, we can trust it, and indeed need to use it to judge all the confusing array of information that constantly bombards us from scientists who are trying to learn the truth and from pseudoscientists and opportunists who want to make a quick dollar from our gullibility.

If we are to benefit by the instructions, however, we must know what God meant—not interpret it according to our prejudices, the half-truths we have read from some poorly informed but enthusiastic faddist, nor even the partial information of those who are carefully learning the facts. The instruction of the Lord to us (Doctrine and Covenants 90:4-5) is that "truth is knowledge of things as they are, and as they were, and as they are to come" and "All truth is independent in that sphere in which God has placed it, to act for itself, as all intelligence also, otherwise there is no existence."

What we believe about the Word of Wisdom does not change its instruction to us; and if we want to receive the blessings it promises, we must learn what God really said in it and live by the truth it teaches. It is something like taking a trip. If I am in Chicago, planning to go to San Francisco, but accidentally board a plane destined for New York, no matter how confident I am that that plane will get me to San Francisco I am going to be disappointed. The only way to get to San Francisco is to get off the east-bound plane and take another headed west. So it is with all truth. What we believe about it will not change things as they really are or were or are to come. If we want to live abundantly, we must learn the truth and align our lives with it.

Unfortunately, scientific knowledge concerning the functioning of our bodies, while vast, is still far from complete. Only recently are the facts concerning the use of tobacco becoming known—too late to save the millions of lives that have been damaged or terminated by its use. Only now are we beginning to learn some of the adverse effects of alcohol, caffeine, and other drugs on the organs and functions of our bodies and those of our children. Diets recently thought to be therapeutic are now discovered to have increased the severity of diseases they were designed to ameliorate and to have made the patients vulnerable to others. Good doctors disagree concerning quantities of nutrients needed and their use in the treatment of disease. Some people are allergic to foods generally known to be healthful.

As new knowledge becomes apparent, one thing is certain. The instruction of the Lord is no idle discipline, but a revelation of the "order and will of God in the temporal salvation of all . . ." as he declared (introduction to Doctrine and Covenants 86). I claim no monopoly on its interpretation. I have, however, spent a third of a century studying it, seeking to understand and to help others understand those scientific discoveries related to it, especially in the field of nutrition, and attempting to implement it in the life of our family. I have sought to learn as the Lord instructed (Doctrine and Covenants 85:36) "by study and also by faith." I hope the experience and the data I have to offer will be helpful in our mutual progress toward greater understanding and implementation of the truth of this "principle with promise" from the Lord.

My especial thanks go to our son, Howard Alan Smith, who read the manuscript and gave invaluable help from a journalist's point of view; to my brother, Norman M. Nelson, M.D., who read the chapters on alcohol, tobacco, and caffeine and made valuable suggestions; to Irene Landsberg, who gave me the benefit of her research into the status of nutrition information and interest during the 1830s; to Dr. Frederick R. Troeh, professor of agronomy, Iowa State University who read the chapter on methods of food production and made valuable suggestions; to those who read the manuscript at the request of the First Presidency; and to members of my family and church community who were patient while I took time out to write the book.

CHAPTER 1

Scope and Setting of the Word of Wisdom

To be a member of Christ's body has always challenged man (generic) to achieve some measure of perfection. Many have mistakenly assumed that what is termed "spiritual" perfection is all that is involved in effective participation in the Master's way. Modern revelation has taught us that this is not true. It is the "spirit and the body that is the soul of man."[1]

We should have known when the Master taught his early followers that their bodies were the temples of their God, not to be defiled, that he had in mind abundant life for the whole man—not just his spirit. But the early instruction was often misunderstood. It was regarded as a sort of discipline for the spirit rather than a principle of life meant to bring health and joy and the possibility of effective participation in the work the Master has called his people to accomplish. To make certain there was no need for continued misunderstanding, God spoke in 1833 to modern man through his prophet, Joseph Smith, giving a "Word of Wisdom," the text of which follows with the prophet's preface:

A word of wisdom for the benefit of the council of high priests, assembled in Kirtland, and the church; and also, the Saints in Zion. To be sent greeting, not by commandment, or constraint, but by revelation and the word of wisdom; showing forth the order and will of God in the temporal salvation of all Saints in the last days. Given for a principle, with promise; adapted to the capacity of the weak, and the weakest of all Saints, who are or can be called Saints.

1a. Behold, verily thus saith the Lord unto you, In consequence of evils and designs which do and will exist in the hearts of conspiring men in the last days, I have warned you, and forewarn you, by giving unto you this word of wisdom by revelation,

b. that inasmuch as any man drinketh wine or strong drink among you, behold, it is not good, neither meet in the sight of your Father, only in assembling yourselves together, to offer up your sacraments before him.

c. And behold, this should be wine; yea, pure wine of the grape of the vine, of your own make. And again, strong drinks are not for the belly, but for the washing of your bodies.

15

d. And again, tobacco is not for the body, neither for the belly, and is not good for man, but is an herb for bruises, and all sick cattle, to be used with judgment and skill.

c. And again, hot drinks are not for the body or belly.

2a. And again, verily I say unto you, All wholesome herbs hath God ordained for the constitution, nature, and use of man, every herb in the season thereof, and every fruit in the season thereof. All these to be used with prudence and thanksgiving.

b. Yea, flesh also, of beasts and of the fowls of the air, I, the Lord, hath ordained for the use of man, with thanksgiving. Nevertheless, they are to be used sparingly; and it is pleasing unto me that they should not be used only in times of winter, or of cold, or famine.

c. All grain is ordained for the use of man and of beasts, to be the staff of life, not only for man, but for the beasts of the field, and the fowls of the heaven, and all wild animals that run or creep on the earth; and these hath God made for the use of man only in times of famine and excess of hunger.

3a. All grain is good for the food of man, as also the fruit of the vine, that which yieldeth fruit, whether in the ground or above the ground.

b. Nevertheless, wheat for man, and corn for the ox, and oats for the horse, and rye for the fowls, and for swine, and for all beasts of the field, and barley for all useful animals, and for mild drinks, as also other grain.

c. And all Saints who remember to keep and do these sayings, walking in obedience to the commandments, shall receive health in their navel, and marrow to their bones, and shall find wisdom and great treasures of knowledge, even hidden treasures;

d. and shall run and not be weary, and shall walk and not faint; and I, the Lord, give unto them a promise that the destroying angel shall pass by them, as the children of Israel, and not slay them. Amen.[2]

It is God's will, then, that members of the body of Christ should be healthy. Our testimony of the Christ should be vibrant, authoritative. The efficacy of his message in calling us to life and love and happiness must be apparent in us if we are to witness truly of him. To make sure that we know of the possibilities and of the way in which they may be achieved, God shared his intelligence with us in this "principle with promise" revealing "the order and will of God" for us. For those who follow his instructions, he promises health of body and mind of superlative quality.

Definition of Health

When the World Health Organization of the United Nations Economic and Social Council defined "health" it was not content with the usual definitions. Rather this world organization defined health as "a state of complete physical, mental and social well-being and not merely the absence of disease or infirmity." What is more, it dared to set the attainment of such a state by all peoples as the objective toward which it now operated.

So, too, the Lord is not content with the usual concept of health. His definition was early embodied in the pronouncement of his Son, "I am come that they might have life, and that they might have it more abundantly."[3] Physical implications of this definition are more specifically stated now in the promise of "health to their navel and marrow to their bones," wisdom and treasures of knowledge, ability to run and not be weary, walk and not faint, and the ability to avoid epidemic death to those who follow the instructions, walking in obedience to the commandments.

The implications of such a delineation of the possibilities entice us to a closer investigation of the promises and the means by which they may be claimed. With the assurance of God to form the foundation of our faith, we may well set our standards high and move confidently toward their accomplishment.

Scope of the Scriptural Instruction on Health

The Word of Wisdom itself instructs us concerning those things that are to be taken into the body. Eat a wholesome diet. Eat it with prudence and thanksgiving. Avoid the use of tobacco, alcohol, strong drinks, and hot drinks. Follow these instructions while obeying all the commandments of the Savior. The health that results will please both us and the Father.

The injunction to walk in obedience to the commandments reminds us that there are other scriptural instructions concerning the achievement of maximum good health. The activities in which we engage, the rest and recreation which we take, our attitudes toward God, toward others, and toward life in general, the state of cleanliness in which we move all help to determine the degree of health that we may achieve.

God's concern that we live healthfully is evidenced by his repeated instructions to us concerning those areas of our lives:

See that you love one another; cease to be covetous; learn to impart one to another as the gospel requires; cease to be idle; cease to be unclean; cease to find fault one with another; cease to sleep longer than is needful; retire to thy bed early, that ye may not be weary; arise early, that your bodies and your minds may be invigorated; and above all things, clothe yourselves with the bonds of charity, as with a mantle, which is the bond of perfectness and peace; pray always.[4]

Again in modern revelation he directs:

> Be clean, be frugal, cease to complain of pain and sickness and distress of body; take sleep in the hours set apart by God for the rebuilding and strengthening of the body and mind;...retire early and...rise early that vigor of mind and body should be retained.[5]

Christ did not stop with instructing us in the ways of health. He was so interested in our well-being that he empowered those whom he called and ordained with the same healing power which he possessed. With it they minister to our mental, spiritual, and physical needs when circumstances beyond our control or our own failure to respond intelligently to our environment jeopardize our health.

A sound body with all parts functioning effectively, a mind alert and serene, a spirit that responds positively to the nature of God—these constitute health. As in all things, so in health; Christ is our example. Not once is it recorded that he was ill. Much of the time of his ministry was given to the restoration of health to others. His amazing capacity to withstand hunger, strenuous activity, and even the punishment meted out by his tormentors testify to a physically superb body. His reactions toward life, his persecutors, his heavenly Father, and all men certify that in him there was mental and spiritual perfection.

Not by Commandment or Constraint

Because Christ made us and wants us to be able to accomplish all that he had called us to do in the establishment of his kingdom on the earth, he spoke about health early in the history of the Restoration to all who had pledged themselves or would ever pledge themselves to the tasks of that kingdom. Because he has made our bodies our stewardship, he gave the revelation as an expression of love and concern—not by commandment or constraint.

In fact, if that part of the Word of Wisdom which deals with the use of food had been presented as a commandment, the church would have been obliged to reject it as a revelation from God. Already Christ had taught his people that "there is nothing from without, that entering into a man can defile him, *which is food* [italics mine]; but the things which come out of him; those are they that defile a man, that proceedeth forth out of the heart."[6] And Paul, who had been taught by the Spirit, wrote, "But meat commendeth us not to God; for neither, if we eat, are we the better; neither, if we eat not, are we the worse."[7] And Paul questioned, "For if I by grace be a partaker, why am I evil spoken of for that for which I gave thanks?"[8]

Paul also gave us the key to understanding how God expects us to use food, however. In the first letter to the Corinthian saints, Paul speaks of the freedom that Christians have since Christ fulfilled the law of Moses and ended the food taboos of that law. He says, "Wherefore, if meat make my brother to offend, I will eat no flesh while the world standeth, lest I make my brother to offend."[9] And in Chapter 10 of that letter he affirms,

> All things are not lawful for me, for all things are not expedient; all things are not lawful, for all things edify not. Let not man seek therefore his own, but every man another's good.... For the earth is the Lord's, and the fullness thereof.... Whether therefore ye eat, or drink, or whatsoever ye do, do all to the glory of God.

Status of the Word of Wisdom

The Word of Wisdom, then, is a "principle with promise." To follow its instructions is to respond to the love of God intelligently. While ignoring them will not catapult us into hell, it will leave us without the possibility of such physical, mental, and spiritual blessings as a loving heavenly Father wishes us to enjoy. Ignoring them will deprive us of spiritual blessings, not as punishment but because without physical and mental health we cannot accomplish all that God has called us into the kingdom to do. Thus we delay the establishment of love and peace and health for all mankind, and we miss the joy of maximum active participation in the great work of the Father.

God spoke of those who respond to his instructions by abiding by the laws of the universe of which they are a part as intelligent beings cleaving (adhering to or being faithful) to intelligence. Of those who attempt to avoid abiding by such instructions, he said they "are not justified."[10]

Some Evidence of Response

Intelligent response to the concern of the Master for our welfare becomes apparent. Healthy people are beautiful people. Perhaps by standards of glamour they may not have completely regular features or proportions, but their eyes are bright, their hair shines, and their skin is clear. They stand erect and walk with graceful stride. They can work hard or play hard. They know the real joy of living. They awaken rested and filled with anticipation. They meet the challenges of each day happily with clean, keen minds. They sleep peacefully without artificial aids.

Healthy persons are likely to be successful. They make a good impression on others. They learn well, make good use of available time, are dependable and good stewards.

To obtain or maintain good health, we must be free of conditions that impair or destroy our response to intelligence, our peace of mind, or life itself. To do this, we must know how a healthy person looks, feels, reacts; know the rules that govern or produce health; and follow the rules.

We have glimpsed briefly our goal in terms of beauty of body and spirit, energy, endurance, mental achievement, and social adjustment. We cannot examine or state all the requirements for the achievement of this goal. To do so would require that we review the entire gospel of Jesus Christ, for the whole gospel is directed toward creating those attitudes and actions that bring about right relations between us and our associates and God. The entire gospel is, then, concerned with the development of healthy personalities. To examine all of the pertinent facts would require lengthy texts. Many have been written and they may be consulted for specific information. In this book we will examine chiefly those areas that seem most closely allied with the Word of Wisdom itself.

Word of Wisdom—a Modern Food Plan

Of primary significance to the achievement of the excellent health spoken of by the Lord is the proper use of food. In another revelation, the Lord referred to it this way: "Unto every kingdom is given a law; and unto every law there are certain bounds also, and conditions.... That which is governed by law, is also preserved by law, and perfected and sanctified by the same."[11] Without food there is no life. To have abundant good health we must make intelligent use of food resources available.

Functions of Food

Every food is composed of nutrients, each with a specific set of functions. Foods that promote growth and repair tissues are called proteins. Others provide energy to permit these tissues to function and heat to keep them warm and alive. These are fats and carbohydrates. Still others regulate body processes and determine the extent of growth, repair, and activity that takes place. These include the vitamins, minerals, and water. (Technically water may qualify as a mineral, but we will treat it separately.)

Although each nutrient has specific functions, no one really occurs alone in nature or acts alone in the body. Proteins always have fats and carbohydrates with them in natural foods. Carbohydrates, even very nearly pure ones such as honey, carry some proteins with them and often fats. Fats never occur completely alone. And each of these basic nutrients carries with it some of the vitamins and minerals with which it works when it occurs naturally in foods. Even the driest food is part water. Wheat flour is about one-eighth water, and soda crackers baked from it retain about a four percent moisture content.

Team Concept of Nutrient Usage

In the body these nutrients form a well-trained, highly efficient team if they are permitted to do so. Proteins cannot build tissue without vitamins any more effectively than a pitcher can play ball with no one else on the ball diamond. Fats cannot burn to produce energy and heat without carbohydrates and certain vitamins any better than a batter can score without a pitched ball. Vitamins are like a coach without a team if they are not accompanied into the body by other nutrients with which they work and whose activity they direct. If any members of the team are missing or in short supply, food performs much like a ball club without a pitcher, with a blind catcher, a first baseman with a broken arm, or some other handicap, depending on the severity of the omission. Herein lies the danger of using many of the highly refined foods to which we have become accustomed. Often the team is broken up or completely devastated by the refinement.

On the other hand, an excess of one nutrient often handicaps the team. An excess of carbohydrates may drain the supply of B vitamins necessary for their metabolism. An excess of thiamin is likely to trigger a deficiency of other B vitamins not present in such generous amounts, much as two pitchers operating simultaneously on the same mound are likely to confuse the batter and render insufficient the bravest efforts of the most agile catcher. Herein lies one danger of overuse of dietary supplements.

On a ball team, each player not only plays his own position but performs many tasks. A pitcher not only throws the ball for the batter but catches the ball returned to him, throws it to the basemen so they can tag the runners, and in many leagues takes his turn at bat and runs the bases. So also every nutrient has a variety of functions on the team on which it serves, and every food a variety of nutrients with which to serve.

Just as one player on a ball diamond cannot play the game alone, so no one nutrient or even one food can accomplish all metabolic tasks alone. A pitcher who throws the ball toward the plate at which there is no batter and behind which there is no catcher just throws the ball away, wasting his effort. Similarly, persons who take huge amounts of vitamin A, for example, expecting it to make their hair shine are wasting their efforts if no protein is present to make the hair grow, fats to lubricate the follicles from which it grows, carbohydrates for the body to use in metabolizing the fats, vitamins B for the body to use in metabolizing the carbohydrates, vitamin E to keep the fats from becoming rancid and the vitamin A from being destroyed prematurely, vitamin C to permit the development of collagen so the tissues in which the hair stands may be strong, iron to transport oxygen to the cells so they can use the other nutrients, and so on.

When we say, therefore, that vitamin A is needed for beautiful hair, we are not saying that vitamin A alone can produce it. We are simply saying that the production of beautiful hair is one of the tasks in which vitamin A plays a prominent part. As with a ball game, although we know each player has a number of functions to perform, it is easier to understand the game if we know for what specific tasks each is responsible. Likewise it is easier for us to follow the best food practices if we understand some of their significance in providing health. To know what may happen to us if we do not eat vegetables may well be the factor that helps us decide to eat vegetables, even though we may not like them very well at first.

The laws that govern food production and use are minutely complex and bafflingly intricate. If we insist on peeling our potatoes, draining the liquid from our cooked vegetables down the sink, using unenriched white flour, and eating large quantities of sweets, we are likely to get into trouble. On the other hand, if we try to make up for our unwise practices by going on a crash diet or by taking quantities of vitamins and minerals as supplements, the results may be entirely unsatisfactory and tremendously expensive.

A Guide to Increased Understanding

Fortunately for us, the One who gave the laws concerning foods has also communicated the guidelines for our observance of them. He knows that only as we are obedient to those laws are we preserved and protected by them. Knowing that we could not be obedient without a dependable guide, He gave that guide in the Scriptures.

At the time the Word of Wisdom was given, nutrition as a science was hardly in its infancy. Some association had been noted between the prevention or cure of scurvy and the use of certain foods. In fact, James Lind had discovered that the use of lime or lemon juice or sauerkraut would prevent or cure the disease as early as 1747 (published 1753). It was not until forty-eight years later, after his death and the deaths of an estimated 200,000 victims of scurvy among the British sailors, however, that the British Admiralty began the distribution of the juices or sauerkraut to the sailors. The disease was eliminated where the foods were employed, and the British sailors were dubbed "limeys," but there was no knowledge of what it was in the foods that prevented or cured the disease.[12]

There was interest in foods from a religious point of view in the early nineteenth century. The Shakers were certain that it was sinful to eat meat or to marry. It was in response to the prophet's inquiry concerning these beliefs that the clear instruction of Doctrine and Covenants 49 was given two years earlier than the Word of Wisdom. To forbid the people to eat meat or to marry was not the Lord's purpose.

Vegetarianism was being advocated in the early 1830s by the Reverend Dr. William Miller who fathered the Adventist movement and by the Presbyterian reformer, the Reverend Sylvester Graham.[13] Reverend Graham believed that restricted use of meat and milk assisted in the cure of intemperate use of alcohol. His presently known published works began with a "Discourse on the Sober and Temperate Life" in 1832 and culminated in the *Graham Lectures on Human Life* in 1839. *A Treatise on Bread and Bread Baking* was published in 1837. His insistence on the use of all of the wheat instead of the more popular white flour resulted in his name being used to designate many whole wheat products.[14] (Today, the term "graham" means that wheat bran is used in the manufacture of a product but not necessarily that it is whole grain.)

On the other hand, there was Dr. Martin Payne, an active diet reformer who insisted that the proper diet consisted of meat, potatoes, milk, tea, and coffee. Dr. Payne believed that fruits and vegetables caused cholera. Many agreed with him. In 1830 the *New York Mirror* published the information that fresh fruits and vegetables should be forbidden to all, but especially to children. Later the *Chicago Journal* condemned the city council of that municipality for making Chicago the only large city not attempting to control cholera by forbidding the sale of fruits and vegetables. And Edward Hitchcock, clergyman, geologist, and president of Amherst College in Massachusetts, questioned the use of fruits, believing that salads and carrots were permissible only if eaten sparingly, that radishes were hard on the stomach, and that peas and beans were definitely unwholesome.[15]

During the decade that followed the advent of the Word of Wisdom, it was discovered that food was not one universal principle but contained proteins, fats, and carbohydrates, all of which were needed by man. At the turn of the century following, the best nutritional knowledge available indicated that a proper balance of these three nutrients was the essential factor in a good diet. The information was published in a U.S.A. Department of Agriculture bulletin in 1897, but the idea was discarded when it was found that mice fed such a diet died.[16]

Nearly six decades after God spoke through the prophet, Dr. Christiaan Eijkman learned that brown rice prevented or cured the dread beriberi of his chickens and of the Japanese navy while white rice promoted the disease. It was a long time after the discovery, however, that he began to believe that it was a nutrient that made the difference. Like those investigating pellagra, he was certain that there must be bacteria in white rice that caused the disease.[17]

It was nearly eighty years after the revelation that Casmir Funk coined the word that attempted to describe the minute but essential nutrients being discovered without which laboratory animals sickened and died. In 1912 he called them "vitamines" because he mistakenly thought them to be related to the nitrogenous foods already known to be necessary for life. Later their true nature became apparent and the spelling was changed to "vitamin."[18]

A whole century after the Word of Wisdom was given, the place of vitamins in nutrition was so tenuous that in 1932 a pharmaceutical firm offered an award of $15,000 to the investigator who, among other things, would determine the clinical value of vitamin A (if any) in human medicine.

Modern Pronouncement of Fact

Now, more than 140 years after the instruction was given, over fifty vitamins, minerals, and other nutrients necessary to life have been identified. Prodigious amounts of nutritional information have been assembled. And the Word of Wisdom is continually validated.

During World War II it became apparent that there was need for better eating practices in the U.S.A. if people were to be physically and mentally fit to meet the rigors of war. Scientists involved in nutrition research were asked to devise a simple food plan by which persons could check their eating habits. If they were eating what was listed in the plan daily, they could be reasonably certain that they were getting the foods that present knowledge indicated would be most apt to result in healthful living.

Although that plan has undergone minor revisions since its inception and has been adapted for use in many nations, the chief categories of essential foods remain the same. And these categories are amazingly similar to those the Lord recommended more than a century before the "Basic Seven" (now "Basic Four" in the U.S.A.)[19] were prescribed. A comparison of the instructions of this modern food plan with those shared by the Lord shows these parallels:

1. Section 86:2 recommends the use of all wholesome herbs (seed plants which do not develop woody persistent tissue but are more or less soft and succulent, especially the foliage and stems, according to *Webster's Dictionary*). The basic food plan designates a dark green or yellow vegetable at least every other day.

2. Section 86 advises that God has similarly designed fruits for the human diet. The modern food plan recommends the daily use of citrus or other fruits and vegetables containing vitamin C.

3. Section 86:3 informs us that "the fruit of the vine, that which yieldeth fruit whether in the ground or above the ground" is also to be used for food. The basic foods include "other vegetables and fruits."

4. Section 86 recommends the inclusion of flesh foods "of beasts and of fowls" in the diet sparingly, with thanksgiving and at designated times and under specified circumstances. Modern food plans call for two servings of a high protein food daily, and include in the list meats, poultry, fish, eggs, cheese, dry beans and peas, nuts, and combinations of proteins. Only recently have there been cautions against eating excessive amounts of meats (see chapters on cereals and meats) from both a physical and social point of view.

5. Grain, especially wheat, is designated as the staff of life in the Word of Wisdom. Modern food plans call for four servings of whole grain, enriched, or restored breads, flours, or cereals daily, and wheat is the most widely used of all the cereals grown.

In our comparison, we have checked every group of the modern food plan except milk. (In the Basic Seven there was a spot for butter or a substitute. This has been dropped as more fats are included in prepared foods and more vitamin A is included in enrichment processes.)

The fact that milk is not specifically mentioned in Section 86 does not mean that the Lord meant us to ignore it as a food. Surely he did not have to tell us that he meant for us to use milk, since he made it for our first food. Then, throughout the Scriptures, when the Lord spoke of lands in which his people would be most prosperous and happy, he designated them as lands "flowing with milk and honey." Joseph Smith, as other prophets before him, had so described the Lord's choice lands.

It is interesting, too, that the prophet Isaiah spoke of a time to come when all who were left in the land would eat butter and honey, and the butter would be available from the abundance of the milk that the cows and sheep would produce.[20] This might refer either to butter as we know it or to curdled milk, but the making of butter was not unknown. One of the proverbs uses a metaphor, "Surely the churning of milk bringeth forth butter."[21]

As a sidelight, it is interesting to note that the modern food plan places honey among those high energy foods that may be eaten in addition to the basic foods but not in place of them. The Scriptures agree. Section 86 omits honey, and in spite of its frequent mention with milk and butter, the author of Proverbs warns us, "It is not good to eat much honey."[22] No such advice to limit the use of milk is given. Only those who continue to use milk as their only food to the exclusion of other essential dietary items are spoken of as immature and unwise in the metaphor used by the apostle Paul concerning the "milk" of the gospel.[23] With this designation, modern nutrition heartily agrees. It, too, insists upon a variety of essential foods for the developing body.

For over a century before science stated it, the message of the Restoration has held for the world the plan most likely to result in maximum good health for its adherents. Any people with the faith and insight to adopt it as a way of life will enjoy a superior degree of health, vitality, and increased capacity for achieving worthwhile goals.

Areas of Significance

The promises of the Lord to those who do adopt the Word of Wisdom way of life point up some areas of particular significance. Children fortunate enough to come into the world through parents who have responded intelligently to the advice of the Lord will have "health to their navels" (will be well born). The vital processes of life will continue normally, as is indicated by the promise of "marrow to their bones," if they continue that intelligent response. Mental processes will be enhanced as is indicated by the "wisdom and great treasures of knowledge, even hidden treasures" available to them. Vast reserves of energy and efficiently operating musculature that permit them to "run and not be weary, to walk and not faint" are possible. And the way can be a veritable preserver of life in times of epidemics of fatal disease, likened by the Lord to the passage of the angel of death over the children of Israel while the Egyptians were killed. This has become apparent already, for example, in the knowledge that the elimination of tobacco protects from the deaths associated with its use.

The efficacy of the Word of Wisdom way in affecting all of these areas of life affirmatively has been verified repeatedly since the Master inspired his prophet to speak to us of it. The way by which we may claim the benefits here described requires only our intelligent response to our environment.

The Lord anticipated our lack of understanding and faith in this as in other matters and instructed, "As all have not faith, seek ye diligently and teach one another words of wisdom; seek learning even by study, and also by faith."[24] It is my intention to examine this document, revealed through the prophet so long ago, in terms of the best information available from the best books written on the subjects of nutrition and health. I hope that the quest will result in strengthened faith in the prophetic ministry and in intelligent acceptance of that ministry as a guide through the maze of scientific and pseudoscientific information by which we are constantly beseiged.

Definition of Terms—Dietary Standards

Throughout the text to follow two terms will be used repeatedly (frequently abbreviated to save space).

Minimum Daily Requirement (MDR): that amount of a nutrient known to be needed for life and the prevention of deficiency disease under the most ideal circumstances. Many labels on foods and food supplements (vitamins and minerals) have long listed ingredients according to Minimum Daily Requirements. Recent laws require that this practice be dropped in the U.S.A., but some countries still use MDR labeling.

Recommended Daily Dietary Allowance (RDA): the term used in the United States for the amount of a nutrient that is expected to reasonably cover the known nutritional need for that nutrient of practically all healthy people if taken daily. It is intended to cover individual differences in need but may not cover all those differences that are genetically induced. It does not take into account special needs that come from infection, metabolic disorder, chronic disease, or other abnormalities that require special dietary treatment. It is expected, however, that the recommended amount will provide a safe level of intake to allow for normal conditions of stress. It does not cover variations in nutrient content of food caused by losses due to poor food handling and preparation. The amounts specified are the amounts recommended to be taken into the body to maintain good health.[25] This is the definition that will be used here. Equivalent terms in other nations include Canada's "Canadian Dietary Standards," the United Nation's Food and Agricultural Organization (FAO), and World Health Organization (WHO) terms "Recommended" or "Safe Level of Intake." Standards for other nations tend to be lower than the U.S.A. Recommended Daily Dietary Allowances (RDAs).

Another term used in the U.S.A. for labeling purposes is "U.S. RDA." This is developed by the Food and Drug Administration from Recommended Daily Dietary Allowance listed in the National Research Council's charts of RDAs. All foods or food supplements in interstate trade that are labeled "enriched," "fortified," or have health claims must refer to the U.S. RDA instead of the MDR used formerly. U.S. RDAs presently in use are shown on the following page.

Dietary standards are subject to revision as newer knowledge indicates the advisability of change. In the U.S.A. such revisions are usually made at five-year intervals. U.S.A. recommendations decided on in 1973 and published in 1974 are used in this book as desirable intakes of nutrients unless it is otherwise stated.

Recommended Daily Dietary Allowances for energy are stated in terms of kilocalories (often written Calories with a capital *C*). This refers to the amount of heat required to raise the temperature of one kilogram of water from 15 to 16 degrees Celsius. When *calories* is written with a small *c* it refers to calories in general or may stand for the amount of heat necessary if one gram of water is substituted for the kilogram in the previous definition.[26]

Because Recommended Daily Dietary Allowances are set for some nutrients, there is a tendency to ascribe to each of these one specific function in the body. We have seen that this is not

U.S. RDAs for Vitamins and Minerals[27]

Nutrient	Unit of Measurement	0-12 Mo. Infants	Under 4 Years	Adults and Children 4 or more years	Pregnant or Lactating Women
Vitamin A	Inter. Units	1,500	2,500	5,000	8,000
Vitamin D	Inter. Units	400	400	400	400
Vitamin E	Inter. Units	5	10	30	30
Vitamin C	Milligrams	35	40	60	60
Folic Acid	Milligrams	0.1	0.2	0.4	0.8
Thiamin (B_1)	Milligrams	0.5	0.7	1.5	1.7
Riboflavin (B_2)	Milligrams	0.6	0.8	1.7	2.0
Niacin (B_3)	Milligrams	8	9	20	20
Vitamin B_6	Milligrams	0.4	0.7	2.0	2.5
Vitamin B_{12}	Micrograms	2	3	6	8
Biotin	Milligrams	0.15	0.15	0.30	0.30
Pantothenic Acid	Milligrams	3	5	10	10
Calcium	Grams	0.6	0.8	1.0	1.3
Iron	Milligrams	15	10	18	18
Phosphorus	Grams	0.5	0.8	1.0	1.3
Iodine	Micrograms	45	70	150	150
Magnesium	Milligrams	70	200	400	450
Zinc	Milligrams	5	8	15	15
Copper	Milligrams	0.6	1	2	2

1,000 micrograms (mcg) = 1 milligram (mg)
1,000 milligrams (mg) = 1 gram (g)
For comparison, 1 level teaspoon white sugar weighs about 4 grams.

---

the case, and it will be helpful to understand that the team concept of nutrient usage is fundamental in this book.

Keeping in mind this team concept, let us examine some of the reasons God spoke to the world as he did in giving us the Word of Wisdom with its related scriptures. Although its provisions are illuminated by modern research, much still remains to be learned. We know enough to make us confident that the instruction is valid, and that if we really want abundant health for all, we must follow it.

---

1. Doctrine and Covenants 85:4.
2. *Ibid.*, 86.
3. Holy Scriptures, John 10:10.
4. Doctrine and Covenants 85:38.
5. *Ibid.*, 119:9.
6. Holy Scriptures, Mark 7:15.
7. *Ibid.*, I Cor. 8:8.
8. *Ibid.*, I Cor. 10:30.
9. *Ibid.*, I Cor. 8:13.
10. Doctrine and Covenants 85:10.
11. *Ibid.*, 85:9, 8a.

12. Franklin C. Bing, "Nutrition Research and Education in the Age of Franklin," *Journal of the American Dietetics Association*, Vol. 68, No. 1, Jan. 1976, pp. 14-21. Also W. J. McCormick, *Journal of Applied Nutrition*, Vol. 15, 1962, p. 4. Comment from *The Summary*, Vol. 17, Dec. 1965, p. 22 (published by the Shute Foundation for Medical Research, London, Ontario).
13. *American Peoples Encyclopedia*, Spencer Press, Inc., Chicago, by name.
14. *Ibid.*
15. Unpublished information prepared by Irene Landsberg for presentation to Home Economics Association, Reorganized Church of Jesus Christ of Latter Day Saints. Used by permission.
16. L. Jean Bogert, George M. Briggs, Doris Howes Calloway, (all Ph.Ds.), *Nutrition and Physical Fitness*, 9th Edition, W. B. Saunders Co., Philadelphia, London, Toronto, 1973, p. 105.
17. *Ibid.*, pp. 117-119.
18. *Ibid.*, p. 106.
19. *Ibid.*, pp. 15-16.
20. Holy Scriptures, Isaiah 7:21-22.
21. *Ibid.*, Proverbs 30:33.
22. *Ibid.*, Proverbs 25:27.
23. *Ibid.*, Hebrews 5:12-13.
24. Doctrine and Covenants 85:36.
25. National Academy of Sciences, *Recommended Dietary Allowances*, Eighth Edition 1974, pp. 1-20.
26. National Academy of Sciences, *op. cit.*, p. 25.
27. Source of U.S. RDAs: For vitamins—Jane Heenan, "Myths of Vitamins," reprint from *FDA Consumer*, March 1974, DHEW Pub. No. (FDA) 74-2053; for minerals—G. Edward Damon, "A Primer in Dietary Minerals," reprint from *FDA Consumer*, Sept. 1974, DHEW Pub. No. (FDA) 75-2013.

CHAPTER 2

The Herbs Ordained for Man
(In the Season Thereof)

All wholesome herbs God hath ordained for the constitution, nature, and use of man, every herb in the season thereof.—Doctrine and Covenants 86:2a.

God made us. He also made the plants. He knows how each is constituted—of what each is made, what each requires to continue life, and how each can contribute to the welfare of the other. That he ordained *wholesome* herbs for our constitution, nature, and use indicates that he made some green, leafy plants to serve our need and equipped us by nature to utilize these foods and enjoy them.

Definition of Herbs

Herbs, by botanical definition, are the succulent flowering plants with stems that do not grow woody or persistent in growth. Some are good for food. Others are good for medicine, but in smaller amounts than would be used as food. Others are poisonous. These are not designed as food for us, and the Lord intends that we should distinguish between those that are wholesome and those that are not. Indeed, he pointed out one of the herbs that was not intended for our use when he warned that "tobacco is not for the body, neither for the belly, and is not good for man...."

Rhubarb, for example, is an herb that combines wholesomeness with danger.[1] It is one of the most deadly of plants if we eat the leaves or drink a tea made from them. The stems, however, are good for food if the stalk is cut about 1½ inches below the leaf to avoid getting excessive amounts of the deleterious substances from the leaves, especially oxalic acid.

Oleander, poinsettia, lily of the valley, and many other decorative and common garden plants are on the poisonous plant list maintained by public health services. It is wise to be informed of these.

The herbs that are wholesome, however, have a special place in the dietary. Included in the wholesome herb category are the following:

Green Leafy Vegetables	Cabbage
Parsley	Brussel sprouts
Kale	Lettuce
Collards	Mint
Mustard greens	Alfalfa
Turnip greens	Crotalaria
Beet greens	
Spinach	*Other Green Vegetables*
Chard	Broccoli (also leaves)
Endive	Cauliflower (also leaves)
Sorrel, Poke,	Celery (also leaves)
Dandelion, Lambsquarter,	Asparagus
Dock, and other	Chives
wild greens	Green onions
Chicory	Some peppers

While many plants are good for food, God is here instructing us that there is some special function or functions of these green ones that make them important to our diets. We are aware of some of these functions.

Vitamin A Value

We have known for several decades now that the carotene contained in green vegetables has vitamin A value in the human body. Vitamin A value also occurs in yellow vegetables and fruits, and vitamin A itself is found in whole milk, butter, liver, and foods to which it has been added for enrichment or fortification. Without the vegetables, however, it is difficult to obtain amounts recommended for good health.

To get a day's supply of vitamin A value for males in the

family, 5,000 International Units (1,000 Retinol Equivalents)*
from butter would require 1/3 of a pound (0.15 kg) supplying
nearly 1,100 Calories. A similar day's supply of the nutrient
from parsley, kale, spinach, or carrots may easily be had from a
two- to three-ounce (56-84 gram) serving with only 20 to 25
Calories.

Liver is the richest source of vitamin A that we know.
Many of the varieties in the markets average in the neighborhood
of 200,000 IU (40,000 RE) per pound (0.45 kg). A three-ounce
(84 g) serving of this potency will supply enough of the nutrient
to last males 7½ days and females 9⅓ days. Since vitamin A is
stored in the tissues, it would do just that.

Bear's liver, however, is so potent in vitamin A that a very
small portion may be toxic. Polar bear liver may contain as
much as 8,000,000 IU (1,600,000 RE) per pound (0.45 kg). If
eaten in the same quantities as other meats it can cause severe
illness. Artic explorers have suffered loss of hair, peeling skin,
severe headaches, vomiting, blurred vision, neuritis, bone pain,
and death from using it.[2]

Comparatively few people eat liver to supply their need for
vitamin A, however, and need to include wholesome herbs
regularly in the diet. When vitamin A stores are depleted,
manifestations of the deficiency can be tragic.

Because vitamin A is an integral part of some of the tissues
of the body, there can be no normal fetus developed without it.
Since it is a part of the rhodopsin of the visual purple of the
eyes, without it there can be no adaptation to light variations.
Even if the adaptation occurs but is slowed by an insufficient
amount of the vitamin, there is "night blindness," a condition that
is a nuisance when one enters a darkened room and a definite
accident hazard when one faces traffic at night.

Severe lack that persists causes dry, scaly eyelids, red, irritated
eyeballs, and finally keratomalacia (characterized by dry spots
on the cornea followed by death of the cells) and the disease
xeropthalmia,[3] which is currently the chief cause of blindness
among children of the developing countries of South America,
Asia, and Africa. Some 10,000 to 12,000 children of India alone

---

*Vitamin A terminology has been changed from International Units to Retinol Equivalents. One RE = five IU. Vitamin A exists as Retinol.

are reported blinded by the disease yearly.[4] The total may reach 100,000.

Vitamin A is an essential nutrient for one of the largest and most active organs of the body, the skin. Without sufficient A, it cannot develop into a smooth, soft, supple, clear, healthy organ that efficiently performs its functions of covering, protecting, lubricating, cooling, and eliminating wastes. Because a healthy skin, glistening hair, and sparkling eyes are such important factors in beauty, and vitamin A is so important to their wellbeing, it has been dubbed the "beauty vitamin."

Just as the outside of the body is covered with skin, so the inside is lined with "skin" called mucous membrane. The healthy functioning of this tissue likewise requires abundant supplies of vitamin A. If the membrane is functioning well, it stands guard against many agents that would cause disease. This is true of the respiratory tract, the digestive and excretory systems. Because of this association of healthy tissue with resistance to disease, vitamin A has gained a reputation as an aid to prevention of disease.

Vitamin A is essential for complete skeletal development. Hereditary genes determine the maximum height to which one may normally grow, but nutrition helps determine whether the potential is reached. Statistics show young people of the present generation, on the average, outgrow their parents. People of small stature in their native lands move to the United States and Canada, for instance, and produce children of much larger physique. In the nutritional and other health practices that bring this about, vitamin A plays a vital role.

Our interest in skeletal growth is not just to have tall people. The central nervous system is enclosed in skeletal structures and needs adequate skeletal development for its own best functioning.[5]

Important members on the team with vitamin A are fats, vitamin E, and zinc. Vitamin A is fat soluble and so is transported, utilized, and stored in conjunction with fats. Vitamin E protects both the fats and the A from oxidation and preserves them for their functions in the body. Without zinc, the vitamin A stored in the liver cannot be withdrawn for use. For this reason, when the diet is low in zinc, the body may respond as though it is low in vitamin A. Also on the team are such nutrients as riboflavin and calcium, with which the vitamin A works to prolong the prime of life.

Vitamin A, then, works on a team that does all this: (1) makes possible sight adaptation to light and dark, (2) prevents a form of blindness still prevalent in much of the world, (3) promotes maximum skeletal growth, allowing room for central nervous system development and permitting one to reach his/her growth potential, (4) promotes clear, soft, smooth, healthy, skin, shiny hair, and sparkling eyes, (5) stands guard against disease as it helps develop and maintain healthy mucous membrane in nose, throat, respiratory and digestive systems, (6) enters into the production of normal, healthy young, (7) helps prolong the prime of life.

Other Nutrients Supplied by Herbs

Because of their vitamin A values, green, leafy, and yellow foods are often spoken of interchangably. Now there are at least five reasons for specifying green and leafy in addition to yellow vegetables. The green and leafy ones have significantly superior amounts of (1) minerals that include calcium, iron, magnesium, zinc, phosphorus, copper, (2) folacin, (3) vitamin E, (4) vitamin C, and (5) vitamin K.

Although we have long been aware of minerals available in green leafy vegetables, it has not seemed terribly important to stress their use for this purpose. We have expected that iron would be supplied principally by meats aided by cereals and incidentally other foods; calcium would come from milk; and the other minerals would largely take care of themselves, except for iodine which would be provided by iodized salt.

Now, however, that we are more aware of the needs of those who do not have meat and milk available, when many are turning to vegetarian diets by choice as well as of necessity, and as other mineral needs are becoming apparent due to extensive consumption of highly refined dietaries, it is significant that green and leafy vegetables supply minerals. At least it is comforting to know that a 3½ ounce (100g) serving of parsley, garden weight, and a similar size serving of beef liver have almost the same amount of iron and that identical weights of kale and regular hamburger provide comparable amounts of the mineral. This size serving of green leafy vegetables may, if the vegetable is not one high in oxalic acid, also provide a significant amount of calcium—about half as much as an eight ounce (240 ml) serving of milk—along with phosphorus, magnesium, zinc, copper, and other minerals necessary to life.

Some herbs such as spinach, beet greens, and chard have some of their minerals bound to oxalic acid in such a way that they are not completely available for use, however, and a smaller proportion of the iron is absorbed from plant materials than from animal products. It is difficult to get the iron and calcium and other minerals needed, at least in Western cultures, without the use of at least milk and eggs.

Iodine is a special problem. In large areas of the world soils are deficient in the mineral, creating vast goiter belts—areas in which simple goiter occurs frequently unless iodine is supplied from some outside source. Because food supplies come from many areas of the world, those in the markets may or may not contain needed iodine. Sea foods and iodized salt are able to fill the need when other available foods cannot.

Folacin

Folacin is a term used for a number of substances showing folic acid activity, including pteroylglutamic acid, and has been known to be essential to life for many years. Other names by which it has been known before it was properly identified include vitamins Bc, M, U, citrovorum factor and *Lactobacillus casei* factor. It was first included in the U.S.A. National Research Council's Recommended Dietary Allowances in 1968.

In animal nutrition, folacin has been a critical factor in the production of healthy young. In studies in which the nutrient was omitted from the diet of healthy rats as early as the ninth day of pregnancy, the young ceased to develop. If it was left until the eleventh day, young were produced, but 95 percent of them were abnormal. There were fourteen known kinds of skeletal defects. Kidneys, lungs, and other internal organs were underdeveloped. Heart and blood vessels were malformed. Some had cataracts on their eyes. There were extreme brain deformities; some were born without heads, some with brains outside their skulls, some with brain cavities distended with fluid. Hormone glands were sometimes underdeveloped or missing. Sex development was abnormal. Anemias occurred frequently. There was extensive edema (swelling) of tissues, and other abnormalities existed.[6]

Although we do not experiment with human beings to see if the absence of folacin in the pregnant mother's diet produces the same kinds of abnormalities in children, human fetal damage has been ascribed to folate deficiency, and the nutrient is considered of special importance during pregnancy and lactation. The RDA of women is doubled during pregnancy.[7]

Unfortunately, many pregnant mothers, even in affluent countries, do not meet their RDAs, and it is believed that folacin deficiency is the most prevalent dietary deficiency of pregnant women in affluent countries.[8] Present studies indicate that teen-agers, and pregnant teen-agers in particular, have diets low in folacin because of their general neglect of fruits and vegetables in their diets. One study revealed most pregnant teen-agers with less than one third as much folacin as is recommended for safe delivery of their young.[9]

Other conditions of stress in which folacin needs are increased include alcoholism, liver disease, prematurity, and the taking of oral contraceptives. Its successful use in treatment of high cholesterol levels has been reported.

The most prevalent problem that develops with insufficient folacin is a macrocytic anemia. The marrow of the bones cannot generate hemoglobin without folacin. When the supply is inadequate, red blood cells are fewer in number, larger in size, and contain less hemoglobin than normal. Iron in the diet does not help.

Folacin has a particularly significant role to play with respect to vitamin B_{12}, which is necessary to prevent, cure, or prevent neurological damage from pernicious anemia. Folacin cannot prevent or cure the disease, but large amounts of it in the diet may mask the symptoms so well that a doctor may not correctly diagnose the disease until irreparable damage is done to the spinal column. It is for this reason that the U.S.A. Food and Drug Administration has restricted the amount of pure folic acid that may be sold without a prescription. If the need is filled for both the B_{12} and folacin, and there is no impairment of absorption of the B_{12}, no problem is known in taking fairly generous amounts of folacin. Food folacin is particularly safe since it is absorbed only one fourth as completely as pure folic acid.

There is a serious problem related to an imbalance of folacin and B_{12} occurring frequently among the new vegetarians. The vegetables, cereals, and fruits provide an abundance of folacin, but no B_{12}. If the new vegetarian has used animal products generously prior to conversion to the new way of life, there may be a supply of B_{12} in his/her tissues that may last three years or even more. When the supply is depleted, however, the presence of the folacin may mask the need for B_{12} until the spine is severely damaged. Early detection can lead to effective B_{12} therapy, but frequently this does not occur. The condition happens often and is known as "vegan back."[10]

For those who have earlier learned to class para-aminobenzoic acid among the vitamins, it is of interest to note that this compound does its work as a precursor of folacin and is no longer classed as a vitamin.

Knowledge about folacin content of foods is so new that there are conflicting data even in the best sources available. We do know that liver, yeast, and green leafy vegetables are good sources of the nutrient. Legumes, nuts, oranges, and whole wheat products supply fairly large amounts. Meats other than liver, root vegetables in general, many fruits, refined flour, sugar, and table fats are all poor sources or void of the substance all together. Milk makes a significant contribution to the diet except where the folacin has been destroyed by heat.[11]

Whole wheat bread provides a significant portion of folacin to the diet. White bread's contribution of folacin comes largely from its yeast, since 75 percent of the folacin is milled out of white flour and none is returned in enrichment to date. In addition about a third of the folacin bakes out of white bread; a much smaller proportion is lost from whole wheat. Toasting further affects the folacin content of white bread severely, while it affects that of whole wheat bread little.[12]

Folacin, like vitamin C, may be lost from foods by poor storage and high heat. Using properly refrigerated fruits and vegetables raw, or at least cooked only crisp-tender, is important.

Although data are still uncertain, one research team has suggested that a person who is not pregnant and not already folacin deficient should be able to get the recommended amount of the vitamin by including in his daily food supply 2 cups (480 ml) milk, 4 ounces (120 ml) fresh or frozen orange juice or 1 large banana, 4 slices whole wheat bread, 3½ ounces (100 g) leafy green vegetable eaten raw and 1 egg yolk. The importance of the leafy green vegetable is apparent when it is noted that it provides this proposed dietary with more than 30 percent of its folacin.[13]

Vitamin K

Vitamin K is necessary for the formation of prothrombin that permits blood to clot. Without it we would be like rats that have had a dose of warfarin and bleed to death when they get a slight injury. Newborn babes seem particularly susceptible to severe bleeding and are sometimes given an extra supply of vitamin K just after birth to assure them a supply sufficient to last until they have established an intestinal bacterial flora to produce needed amounts.

Once bacteria that produce the vitamin thrive in the intestines, there may be little danger of deficiency unless there is treatment with antibiotics that destroy the bacteria or some other problem develops increasing the need for the nutrient. For safety's sake, it is wise to have a dietary supply of the vitamin. This is easily accomplished, for vitamin K is produced by the action of light on plant tissues and is accumulated largely in the chloroplasts. All leafy green vegetables provide vitamin K. The outer leaves of such foods as cabbage are much richer in the nutrient than the inner leaves, as they are also richer in vitamins A, C, and E.

Like vitamins A, D, and E, vitamin K is fat soluble and is stored in the body. It can be toxic. The best way to get needed supplies is by eating green, leafy vegetables—the wholesome herbs.

Vitamin E

Although vitamin E is included in seed oils in greater concentration than in green vegetables, the amount provided by the herbs is significant and comes with a much smaller cost caloriewise. (See discussion of vitamin E in the chapter on cereals for further information.)

Vitamin C

Vitamin C and its place in the dietary will be discussed in the chapter to follow concerned with fruits for a special purpose.

It is interesting to note here that the vitamin C content of many green vegetables is higher than that found in most citrus fruits, tomatoes, and raw cabbage, the traditional sources of supply for most North Americans. Three-fourths cup of many cooked greens will easily fill the RDA for most women and men. Only half a cup of fresh, properly cooked broccoli or brussels sprouts will fill the RDA of even a pregnant or lactating woman. With proper care, these vegetables may offer even more vitamin C when eaten raw.

Raw vegetables and fruits not protected by natural food acids as those in citrus fruits and tomatoes contain an enzyme that readily destroys vitamin C when it is activated. Destruction accelerates when the foods are dried (or wilted), bruised or cut. If these non-acid foods, as most green leafy vegetables are, are to be frozen, many of them need to have the enzyme inactivated by blanching (boiling briefly then chilling quickly) if vitamin C is to be retained. Non-acid foods that are dried naturally or in a dehydrator generally have only a small proportion of the nutrient left. Acid foods such as oranges, rose hips, and tomatoes retain their vitamin C well in dehydration.

If green vegetables are cooked, special care must be taken to preserve the vitamin C. They need to be cooked quickly in as small an amount of water as possible. It even helps if the water has been previously boiled to remove air from it. Cooking should never be in a copper or iron kettle. Copper and iron catalyze the destruction of the vitamin. And soda should never be used. The lid should be left off to let the volatile acids escape, and the vegetable carefully tended until it is bright green from the redistribution of the chlorophyll. The cooking should be stopped before the bright color fades and the vegetable served immediately. (See chapter on fruits for further information on vitamin C and ways to preserve it in foods.)

Comparative Value of Green Vegetables

A comparison of the food values in one pound (0.45 kg) kale, one of the most nutritious of the green leafy vegetables, and that of some meats may help us appreciate how valuable these herbs are that the Lord instructed us to use. (The use of a pound of kale a day is not recommended for one person—this is only a comparison.) One pound (0.45 kg) of kale provides the following:

Nutrient	Amount	Comparison
Protein	23 grams	1/4 lb. (112 g) hamburger has 20.3 g. (kale's biological value is less than meat, and would need supplementation).
Calcium	964 mg.	More than 21 lb. (9.45 kg) hamburger. Equal to 3½ cups (0.84 liter) milk.
Iron	10.4 mg.	1 lb. (0.45 kg) sirloin steak has 10.5 mg.
Vitamin A value	39,000 IU (7.800 RE)	More than 433 lb. (195 kg) lean hamburger. Equals about 3/4 lb. (0.34 kg) pork liver.
Thiamin (B_1)	0.63 mg.	Equals 1.8 lb. (0.8 kg) regular hamburger.
Riboflavin (B_2)	0.94 mg.	Equals 1⅓ lb. (0.77 kg) reg. hamburger. Equals 2-1/5 cups (0.53 liter) milk.
Niacin (B_3)	8.0 mg.	Equals 6.4 oz. (182 g) reg. hamburger or steak.
Vitamin C	720.0 mg.	Muscle meats have no vitamin C. Equals 5 lb. (2.25 kg) beef liver. Equals 4⅓ lb. (1.95 kg) oranges.
Folacin*	316.0 mcg.	Muscle meats have little or no folacin. Equals about 1/4 lb. (0.11 kg) beef liver.

Vitamin E—Adequate data not available, but dark green, leafy vegetables are a good source. Meats are a poor source.

Vitamin B_{12}—Not contained in vegetables. Animal foods a good source.

It is apparent that except for protein, niacin, and vitamin B_{12}, kale is far richer in essential nutrients noted than an equal weight of beef, excluding liver. Few vegetables equal kale, but many surpass meats, weight for weight, in many essential nutrients. Since without adequate protein, niacin, and vitamin B_{12} life is not

---

*Folacin data are from L. Jean Bogert, *Nutrition and Physical Fitness*, 1973. Data are from 1961 research and may not reflect total folacin content.

possible, it is apparent that herbs are not adequate alone. They are extremely valuable, however, and it is wisdom to use them daily as the Lord and the science of nutrition suggests.

"In the Season Thereof"

The Lord spoke of "ordaining" herbs and fruits for the use of man, each "in the season thereof." Some have interpreted this to be an instruction to use foods just as they come from field and orchard and at no other time unless they can be kept without processing. Actually, the statement says nothing about when foods should be used—only about when the Lord provided them. Consistently through the Scriptures "season" has referred to the time in which the Lord has provided for our needs. Deuteronomy 28:12 speaks of the Lord giving rain "in his season." Job 5:26 tells of a shock of corn coming "in his season." Doctrine and Covenants 59:4 speaks of all things that come from the earth "in the season thereof."

That God did not mention it directly does not change the fact that fruits and vegetables are usually less expensive at the time of harvest (if one doesn't demand the first of the crop or wait until the produce is scarce) and are rarely more flavorful or more nutritious than when they are fresh. When foods are grown commercially, however, varieties often are chosen more for their harvest and shipping qualities than for flavor or nutrition. Tomatoes grown for canning, for example, may be much more tasty and have a higher vitamin C content than those grown for shipment that must ripen at one time for the pickers, be picked partially green, and remain firm during long transport. Green, leafy vegetables, broccoli, corn, and green beans that take days to reach the consumer's table may not retain as much of the labile (perishable) nutrients as their counterparts processed at the peak of their perfection and stored properly in freezers and cans.

The ideal is to eat foods, correctly prepared, straight from one's own properly fertilized and cared-for garden, but for most of the world's population in urban areas and in cold climates this is impossible. In general, correct freezing procedures preserve food most nearly as it comes from harvest, if it is kept at low enough temperatures on its journey to the table (zero degrees Fahrenheit—minus 18 degrees Celsius or below). Canned foods, because of the high heat treatment necessary to preserve them, are changed in texture, flavor, and nutritive content. Many of the lost nutrients are still in the liquid and may be served if the cook is clever and resourceful. Careless preparation of fresh or frozen foods can be as destructive of nutrients as canning. Drying, in general, is more destructive of nutrients such as vitamin C and folacin than other forms of preservation. Further losses of these and other vitamins occur during storage in air. Minerals and some vitamins are well retained. Commercial dehydration employing vacuum and freezing is less destructive of nutrients. Preservation by irradiation may prove effective in retaining fresh characteristics through long periods of storage but it is not yet generally available.[14]

God's challenge to us is to harvest the foods in the season in which he has provided them and to care for them in such a way that the nutrients they contain at harvest are available as much as possible at the time they are served. Each individual will need to determine which form of available food best fills his/her need.

1. Wilma Roberts James, *Know Your Poisonous Plants*, Naturegraph Publishers, Healdsburg, California, 1973; Rhubarb—p. 65; Oleander—p. 55; Poinsettia—p. 87; Lily of the Valley—p. 44. For more technical information see John M. Kingsbury, *Poisonous Plants of the United States and Canada*, Prentice-Hall, Inc., Englewood Cliffs, N.J., 1964; Rhubarb—pp. 230-231 (describes symptoms and death); Oleander and Lily of the Valley—p. 32 for names and pp. 264-265 for dangers; Poinsettia—pp. 188-189 (describes symptoms and notes death). Also "Tips for Your Home and Family," *Today's Health*, Aug., 1971, p. 69.
2. Eva D. Wilson, Katherine H. Fisher, Mary E. Fuqua, *Principles of Nutrition*, John Wiley and Sons, Inc., N.Y., London, Sydney, Toronto, Third Edition, 1975, p. 222. Also "Dangers of Eating Bear Meat," *Journal of the American Medical Association*, Vol. 220, 1972, p. 274, extracted in *Journal of the American Dietetics Association*, Vol. 62, No. 2, Feb., 1973, p. 203.
3. *Dorland's Illustrated Medical Dictionary*, 25th Edition, W.B. Saunders, Philadelphia, London, Toronto, 1974, Entries "Xerophthalmia" and "Keratomalacia."
4. C. L. Brooke and W. M. Corte, "Vitamin A Fortification of Tea," *Food Technology*, Feb., 1972, p. 50. Extracted in *Journal of the American Dietetics Association*, Vol. 61, Sept., 1972, p. 326.
5. Wilson, *et al., op. cit.*, p. 219.
6. Roger J. Williams, *Nutrition Against Disease*, Pitman Pub. Corp., N.Y., 1971, pp. 59-60, citing numerous studies reported in the *Journal of Nutrition, Proceedings of the Society for Experimental Biology and Medicine*, and *Nutrition Reviews* ("Folic Acid and Pregnancy I," *Nutrition Reviews*, Vol. 25, 1967, p. 325, and "Folic Acid and Pregnancy II," *Nutrition Reviews*, Vol. 26, 1968, p. 5).
7. National Academy of Sciences, *Recommended Dietary Allowances*, Eighth Edition, 1974, p. 74.
8. "Today's Health News," *Today's Health*, Nov. 1972, p. 8 (Reporting from *The Medical Letter*.)
9. Mildred S. Van de Mark, R.D., and Audrey Clever Wright, R.D., "Hemoglobin and Folate Levels of Pregnant Teen-Agers," *Journal of the American Dietetics Association*, Vol. 61, No. 5, Nov. 1972, pp. 511-515.
10. U. D. Register, Ph.D., R.D., and L. M. Sonnenberg, R.D., "Scientific and Practical Considerations of the Vegetarian Diet," *Journal of the American Dietetics Association*, Vol. 62, March 1973, p. 257. Also Darla Erhard, R.D., M.P.H., "The New Vegetarians," *Nutrition Today*, Vol. 8, No. 6, Nov./Dec., 1973, pp. 8-9.
11. Susan Butterfield and Doris Howes Calloway, Ph.D. (University of California, Berkeley), "Folacin in Wheat and Selected Foods," *Journal of the American Dietetics Association*, Vol. 60, No. 4, April 1972, pp. 310-314.
12. Faye M. Dong and Susan M. Pace, (U. of Calif., Berkeley), "Folate Distribution in Fruit Juices," *Journal of the American Dietetics Association*, Vol. 62, No. 2, Feb. 1973, p. 162. Also National Academy of Sciences, *op. cit.*, p. 71.
13. Butterfield and Calloway, *op. cit.*, p. 314.
14. Special Report, "The Effects of Food Processing on Nutritional Values," *Nutrition Reviews*, Vol. 33, No. 4, April 1975, p. 123.

CHAPTER 3

Fruits that Provide Vitamin C
(With a Subsection on Other Fruits and Vegetables)

...God hath ordained for the constitution, nature, and use of man...every fruit in the season thereof.—Doctrine 86:2a.

Fruits also were "ordained" for our use. Like herbs, they offer many nutrients necessary to life and health in forms that tempt us to consume them. Some of them perform an especial service in providing vitamin C in a form that will withstand comparatively long storage without serious deterioration.

Long before it had a name, vitamin C (ascorbic acid and related substances) was at work in every living creature. Many animals are able to form vitamin C from other food substances, but men, monkeys, guinea pigs, and a few other animals have to have the nutrient in their food. Without it oral tissues become cheesy and bleed easily. Teeth loosen. Joints become swollen and painful. Muscles ache. Hemorrhages that look like bruises occur just under the epidermis of the skin, in the joints, muscles, and intestines. Wounds refuse to heal, and death can ensue. Many died in countries characterized by winter and on extended sea voyages until protective measures were discovered and applied to prevent scurvy.

Vitamin C works on many teams, all of which are necessary to prevent scurvy which was once so prevalent and so devastating that medical men thought all disease must spring from it.[1] Scurvy was described as early as 1500 B.C. The nutrient was first isolated and named in the second decade of this century, almost a hundred years after God called attention to the fact that he had provided food which would prevent or cure the disease.

One of the basic tasks of vitamin C is to help build and maintain collagen,[2] the chief protein of skin, cartilage, bone, and connective

45

tissue. It forms about 30 percent of all the protein of our bodies. While vitamin C cannot form collagen without the other nutrients needed to form protein, it is apparent that without the vitamin our bodies can neither develop nor function properly.

Some of the functions of the nutrient teams of which vitamin C is an essential part are as follows:

1. Keep gums and oral tissues firm and healthy. Typical of scurvy are cheesy, bleeding gums. Teeth may loosen and fall out. Gangrene is possible.

2. Prevent muscle aches and pains, often mistaken for rheumatism or "growing pains," well known to those generations for whom oranges were a special treat at Christmas, grapefruit an oddity, and the fruit and vegetable supply of every winter was dependent on the contents of the root cellar and the jars of food preserved from the summer's harvest. Such ailments are much less familiar to those who have modern transportation and marketing of fresh foods and modern means of processing available foods.

3. Prevent easy rupturing of blood vessels. The first overt sign of scurvy in many adults is the appearance of petechiae (spots that look like tiny bruises where blood has escaped the vessels and effused into the skin).

4. Promote healing of wounds, lesions such as ulcers, and broken bones.

5. Protect against infections and bacterial toxins by stimulating white corpuscles to act against the invaders.

6. Aid in the absorption and utilization of calcium. Vitamin C is especially important for this purpose during pregnancy, lactation, early childhood, healing of fractured bones, and when calcium nutrition is most difficult to maintain in the elderly.

7. Influence the absorption of iron from the intestines, the deposition of iron in the liver, and the production of hemoglobin.

8. Affect the secretion of hormones by the adrenal cortex.

9. Detoxify some environmental poisons such as lead.

10. May affect the common cold desirably.

11. Function as an antioxidant in foods and tissues.

In spite of the essential nature of vitamin C, very little of it is stored in the tissues. It must be supplied regularly for body processes to be sustained optimally. It is water soluble, and any excess taken is promptly flushed from the system in perspiration, urine, and even breath moisture.

Amount of Vitamin C Required

Just how much vitamin C is needed daily is a matter of some controversy. Food standards of different nations vary drastically, and some respected scientists urge the use of many times the most generous RDA of any nation.

The absolute minimum daily intake of the nutrient necessary to prevent scurvy is set at 10 milligrams.[3] Just avoiding scurvy is not enough, however. Scurvy indicates nearly complete depletion of tissues. Britain has set twice that amount, 20 mg, as standard for an adult. Canada has trebled it with 30 mg as standard. This is also the standard adopted by the Food and Agricultural Organization of the United Nations for nonpregnant, nonlactating adults. The U.S.A. had set 55 mg for nonpregnant, nonlactating women and 60 mg for adult males in 1968, but reduced the RDA for all of these to 45 mg in the 1973 revision.

Studies based on the amount of vitamin C retained when the nutrient is fed indicate that the U.S.A. RDAs should be adequate to cover most individual variations in need and to allow for some stress. There may be some exceptions. It is apparent that smokers need almost twice as much C as nonsmokers to maintain the same concentration of the nutrient in their tissues.[4] Apparently they do not use more of it in body functions; they just cannot absorb as much from their food. Dr. R. J. Williams and others believe that schizophrenics metabolize more of the nutrient than others and so have need of greater supplies.[5]

Dr. Linus Pauling and others have proposed the use of massive doses of the vitamin to prevent or cure the common cold and to prevent or treat numerous other diseases.[6*] Even though he recognizes that the excess vitamin C passes through the body rapidly, Dr. Pauling believes that it does its work on the way through, much as penicillin.

Studies carried out in Canada and the USA have indicated that while persons taking large doses of the vitamin may have as many colds as others, their colds may be less severe. Some tests have indicated there may even be fewer colds. The way in which it may be helpful is still to be elucidated.

---

*See Linus Pauling, *Vitamin C and the Common Cold*, W. H. Freeman Co., San Francisco, 1970, and Irwin Stone, *The Healing Factor*, "Vitamin C" Against Disease, G and D Publishers, Inc., Division of Charter Communications, Inc., 1120 Ave. of the Americas, N.Y., N.Y., 1972.

One research team believes the combination of zinc and ascorbic acid may be effective against some viruses. Dr. Bruce Korant has reported that small amounts of zinc ascorbate inhibited the viruses that cause colds in his studies while ascorbic acid alone had no effect. Dr. Korant found commercial vitamin C tablets contained enough zinc to make a difference in his tests.[7]

While the use of large amounts of ascorbic acid does seem intriguing when urged by reputable scientists, there are many questions to be answered concerning the effect of massive doses before such recommendations should be accepted without reservation.

Large amounts of the vitamin have proved toxic to guinea pigs fed on low protein diets that included large amounts of cereal. Growth was retarded and the animals died young. On diets containing needed protein, adverse effects on growth and longevity were not found.[8]

There is indication that long-term use of large amounts of vitamin C may accustom the body to high dosages and so cause it to become scorbutic (develop scurvy) readily when it is necessary to return to "normal" amounts. This response has been demonstrated in adults and in babies born to mothers who used large amounts of the vitamin during pregnancy.[9]

With massive doses of vitamin C there is increased oxalate formation which favors the development of oxalate stones in kidneys and bladders. Dr. Linus Pauling notes the advisability of using sodium ascorbate instead of pure ascorbic acid or of otherwise neutralizing the acid if one is susceptible to kidney stone formation.[10]

In guinea pigs, one of the few animals other than man that cannot form its own vitamin C, massive doses of the vitamin have been noted to interfere with reproduction.[11] Studies are being initiated to determine whether it may affect human reproduction, but to date there is no information available in this vital area.

Massive doses of the vitamin when taken without food have a laxative effect which may pose problems especially for the elderly and very young. The presence of the nutrient in the urine may give false values for sugar and thus interfere with the management of diabetes. And other problems have been noted in animal experiments which may or may not be applicable to people.[12]

One finding which applies to people is that doses of vitamin C as small as 100 mg tend to destroy vitamin B_{12}. The effect of a 100 mg dose is minimal if the meal with which it is associated is high in B_{12}, but more than half the B_{12} may be destroyed if the meal is low in the nutrient. At dosages of 250 mg, about one-fourth the B_{12} of meals high in the nutrient may be destroyed and more than 80 percent of that in meals low in the nutrient; 500 mg vitamin C may destroy about half the B_{12} of high B_{12} meals and 95 percent of low B_{12} meals. The vitamin C does not have to be taken with the meal to be destructive.[13]

Our physician recommends that we limit our consumption of the vitamin to a maximum of 250 mg daily except for brief periods when it is being used as a medication at 1,000 to 4,000 mg levels.[14] Tissue saturation is obtained in most people at levels of 100 mg to 250 mg daily, and some studies indicate that no additional benefit is received from regular use of larger doses. Dr. Irwin Stone, originator of the vitamin C method of managing colds and other viral infections, contends that the failure to show benefit derives from inadequate dosage.[15]

If we accept the necessity of using extremely large amounts of the nutrient regularly, we will have to abandon the idea of getting needed amounts from foods. Even the acerola cherry, one of the foods most potent in vitamin C, would have to be eaten a pound a day or more to fill some recommendations.

If, on the other hand, we accept the RDAs of the World Health Organization's FAO and of the Western nations as being adequate except in situations including long-standing deficiencies, disease, traumatic stress, and possibly smoking, when larger amounts may be needed, perhaps medicinally, we can easily obtain required amounts from our food. A small orange, half a grapefruit, or a very small serving of broccoli, properly prepared, would each provide the entire American RDA for an adult. A dietary based on the daily food plan of science and of the Scriptures would easily double or treble the amount. Present knowledge indicates this may be the wisest choice to make for regular use, from both the standpoint of stewardship and health.

Vitamin C as Supplement

Ascorbic acid can be purchased quite cheaply in tablet or

crystalline form. It is effective as vitamin C—as effective as that from plants.[16] It is just vitamin C, however. Not one of the other members of the teams on which it works is present unless as a contaminant.

This is also true when fruit-flavored crystals with vitamin C added are substituted for real fruit. Orange-flavored crystals, for example, contain nothing nutritive except energy, largely from sugar, and vitamin C. Oranges, on the other hand, provide significant amounts of folacin, are good sources of vitamin B_1 needed to metabolize the natural sugar present, contribute niacin, vitamin A value, potassium, some protein, small amounts of other vitamins and minerals, and bioflavinoids, still thought by some to be of significance in the maintenance of health, plus the energy and vitamin C, and all at a cost often less than that of the crystals.

Imitation fruit drinks rarely contain as much vitamin C as the fruit they imitate if that fruit is known for its vitamin C. What it does contain is far less stable than that from real fruit.[17] It disappears rapidly in storage even under the best conditions. The real fruit has protective substances that keep the vitamin potent for days even under less than ideal conditions.

For maximum nutritive value, real fruit is preferable. Artificially flavored crystals or imitation fruit drinks are not an adequate substitute for the real thing just because they contain vitamin C. (There are fruit crystals of the real fruit that do contain other members of the teams on which vitamin C works.)

Food Sources Other Than Fruit

We have noted the excellent way in which green and leafy vegetables provide vitamin C when properly handled. Fresh potatoes also provide a significant amount of vitamin C when properly prepared. Unfortunately, modern dehydrated varieties are very low in the nutrient unless they are fortified with it. Fresh mashed potatoes contain only about half the vitamin C of the raw potatoes from which they are made if they are pared, boiled, and the water drained away. "Instant" potatoes have only about half the C of these fresh mashed ones. The nutrient content, including vitamin C, of fresh mashed potatoes may be increased substantially by boiling the potatoes in their well scrubbed skins in a small amount of water and mashing them, skin and all, in the cooking water. Dry milk may then be added to provide flavor and nutrition.

Other potato products also vary in vitamin C content. Baked in their skins, they lose little of the nutrient. French fried, they lose about half their potency. Potato chips retain only a very small portion of their original ascorbic acid, but used in the quantity in which they are consumed, they provide a significant amount to the diet. Frozen mashed or hash brown potatoes compare with dehydrated forms with C content (about one-fourth that of the fresh potato).

Fruits Rich in Vitamin C

Some of the fruits on which the people of the world depend for certain supplies of vitamin C include oranges, grapefruit, lemons, kumquats, tangerines, strawberries, cantaloupe, papaya, lichi (lychees), mangos, guava, lilikoi (passion fruit), and tomatoes. The camu-camu berry of Peru ranks with the acerola cherry as highly potent in the nutrient. Rose hips are used by many native populations and are becoming increasingly popular as the basic ingredient of a non-stimulating warm drink that does not require a lot of sweetening. Studies completed at the University of Alberta, Canada, indicate that three average rose hips have vitamin C equal to that of a medium orange.

Most fruits rich in vitamin C are delightful to eat raw. In this form, none of the nutrient is lost to cooking procedures. They are also created with built-in systems that preserve much of their potency during cooking and storage procedures that would destroy much of the vitamin in other foods. Eighty to ninety percent of the ascorbic acid of oranges, tomatoes, and rose hips survives freezing, canning, and drying.

Even the skins of citrus fruits are excellent sources of vitamin C and other nutrients, and may often be used as food. Orange skins are often eaten plain or ground, mixed with cranberries or other fruit and served as a relish or in fruit-flavored gelatin as a salad or dessert. Lemon peel sliced thin and cooked with dried fruit gives a delightful flavor while it adds vitamin C to the resultant dessert or breakfast dish. Grated, the rinds give added interest to puddings and toppings. Fruitcakes, sweet breads, and marmalades all are characterized by their presence.

Conserving Vitamin C in Foods

While some of the fruits are equipped to preserve vitamin C, poor handling can be destructive of the nutrient. And there are many foods, as we have seen, that have little protection for the nutrient. Here are some helps for retaining the maximum C content of food:

1. Protect from wilting by using proper storage containers and refrigeration. Commercial aids include waxing and control of gases in the environment.

2. Prepare for serving just before serving time. Refrigerate promptly and continuously until serving time.

3. Dip cut fruits in salt or vinegar water or add tart fruit juice, ascorbic acid (vitamin C), citric acid, or another antioxidant.

4. Keep leftover foods tightly covered in a container that just fits the amount of food to be stored. Eliminating air reduces destruction.

5. Do not use soda. To keep tomato soup from curdling and still retain the vitamin, pour hot tomatoes slowly into hot white sauce and serve immediately.

6. Do not use copper or iron kettles for vitamin C foods.

7. Cook vegetables only until they are crisp tender and brilliantly colored.

8. Cook with skins on when possible.

9. Cut into small pieces only if all liquid is to be served as in soup.

10. Never soak or cook in more water than will be served. If any food must be drained, keep the liquid for soup, gravy, or beverage and *use* it all. (Dr. Henry C. Sherman suggests that we may feed our sinks better than our stomachs.) Draining canned foods results in the loss of half or more of the water soluble vitamins along with varying amounts of minerals and other nutrients.

11. Eliminate air during cooking when possible. Boil the water before adding the food. Cover non-green foods such as potatoes with a tight fitting lid. Pressure cooking eliminates air and shortens cooking time for some foods.

12. Cool foods quickly if they are to be stored or frozen. It is better to cool and reheat than to keep them warm over a long period of time. Vitamin C is preserved and bacterial count is kept at a minimum. (To be safe bacteriologically foods must

be kept below 40 °F (4.5 °C) or above 140 °F (60 °C).

13. Store frozen foods at zero degrees Fahrenheit (-18 degrees Celsius) or lower. At this low temperature, vitamin C is stable for years. At higher temperatures it is lost rapidly. Alternate freezing and thawing is especially destructive of the nutrient. Purchase frozen foods only from those stores that never allow their foods to thaw, and keep a thermometer in home freezers.

14. Follow accepted procedures as described in government bulletins or authentic cookbooks when canning or freezing foods. Some foods must be blanched to stop enzyme action if vitamin C is to be preserved. Many retain more C when canned by water bath than open kettle. Nonacid foods *must* be canned under pressure to be safe from botulism. If *nonacid foods* are canned without pressure, they should be boiled for 10 to 15 minutes before they are tasted or served. Boiling will not destroy the botulin organism but will inactivate the toxin that it forms. This is not designed to preserve food value but to preserve life!

Vitamin C, an Antioxidant in Foods

Ascorbic acid and its related substances that serve as antioxidants in nature's food supply also serve a practical purpose in the preparation and preservation of foods. Added to fruits that tend to darken quickly after they are peeled or cut it retards the oxidation that is responsible for the darkening. Crystalline ascorbic acid is usually available for home use, generally in a mixture with some sort of simple sugar and citric acid. Salad making and home preservation of peaches, apples, and bananas benefit from its use.

For commercial use, sorbic (erythorbic) acid, which has about five percent as much vitamin C activity as pure ascorbic acid, is often used in drying fruits and in keeping flour and cereal products and convenience foods fresh.[18] When antioxidants with vitamin C value are used, they add food value but with the expectation that some of the added value will be used up in protecting the food. Antioxidants do their work by taking up oxygen that would otherwise affect the food adversely.

Variations in Vitamin C Content of Foods

Fruits and vegetables vary in their vitamin C content according to the variety grown, the climatic conditions under which they are grown, and the stage of maturity at which they are harvested. The plant uses air, water, and sunshine to manufacture the nutrient. Soil determines how well the plant can grow but not the amount of vitamin produced in equal amounts of fruit. Some varieties contain many times the vitamin content of other varieties of the same species. Those fruits and vegetables grown in the sun have larger amounts than those grown in the shade. Those harvested while slightly immature may carry more than those allowed to mature. There is a stage called "fully ripe" just before fruits achieve full color at which time the C content is at a maximum. Citrus fruits, tomatoes, acerola cherries and many other fruits retain this maximum well.[19]

Finally

While vitamin C is available in many foods, daily use of one of the fruits with a certain supply is recommended. Used fresh or processed, they are valuable and may safely be used generously. It is their generous use that has made scurvy a rarity in developed countries and favorably affected health in general.

Scurvy is still frequently a part of the misery of less fortunate people, however. Prisoners of war in Southeast Asia suffered from it extensively.[20] And recent studies show a surprisingly large number of native people in developed areas consuming amounts that are at best marginal.[21]

It is God's intent that no person be poorly nourished in this as other nutrients. He ordained these special fruits for our use. We will benefit by using them regularly.

Other Fruits and Vegetables

....the fruit of the vine, that which yieldeth fruit, whether in the ground or above the ground.—Doctrine and Covenants 86:3a.

In addition to the two groups of foods just considered, herbs and special fruits, there are many fruits and vegetables that just supply a little of a lot of nutrients needed for maximum health. Dietary plans call them "other fruits and vegetables." They fill the chinks of the diet. No one nutrient or set of nutrients predominates, as far as we know, but the total effect of generous use of these foods is to add materially to our body's store of vitamins, minerals, protein, fiber, energy, pectin, and other substances needed for good health.

To more completely understand what the Lord had in mind when he designated "fruit of the vine" as good for man, we need to know that the botanical definition of fruit is not limited to the sweet, fleshy products of plants that contain seeds. Any product of a plant is its fruit. If the product is edible and wholesome, it is included as food good for man.

Prepared for our use, then, are valuable tuberous foods such as the potato of Northern Europe and America and the taro of the South Seas; pod foods such as beans (frijoles) of many lands and various kinds of peas; peanuts; bulbs of onions, garlic, leeks, scallions; seed-bearing fruits that are not sweet such as okra, peppers, cucumbers, eggplant, breadfruit, pumpkins, squash, vegetable marrow; those fruits that are sweet but do not have a high concentration of vitamin C such as bananas, pears, most apples, grapes, star fruit, figs, dates, and many others including nuts of all sorts.

God also spoke of "that which yieldeth fruit." This would include roots of plants which contribute richly to our enjoyment and nutrition—carrots, beets, salsify, gobo (dock) of the Orient, jicama of Mexico and Central America, radishes, sweet potatoes, yams, rutabaga, manioc or casava (itself poisonous, but tapioca is made from it). There are also stems that are succulent and delightful to use as are celery, rhubarb, and asparagus.

As with vitamin C foods and the green leafy ones, proper storage and preparation help to determine whether we get maximum nutrition from these foods. Even though there is a much smaller portion of vitamin C in pineapple than there is in oranges, for example, to get the most value from pineapple we need to preserve that which is there. Here are some ways to assure that maximum value is received:

1. Use the skins when possible. This saves waste and adds nutrients. Potatoes, for example, have their most valuable mineral content concentrated just under the rough outside skin. Scouring the potato with a metal or nylon pot scraper will remove the dirt with the roughest of the outer skin leaving the nutrients in the food. Apples with the peel have 2½ times the vitamin E value of peeled apples, and pears with peel have five times the E value of those that are peeled.

2. Serve all of the water used in cooking.

3. Keep foods such as apples, peaches, potatoes, and beets a bit on the acid side to preserve color and nutrients. A bit of lemon juice or vinegar keeps apples and beets bright. A touch of these acids or cream of tartar may keep the flavones of potatoes from turning dark in hard water or even restore bright color to those that have darkened.

4. Store properly before preparing for cooking or serving.

5. Refrigerate properly after they have been prepared or cooked.

6. Consult government publications and reliable cookbooks for information about the care, preparation, and preservation of these foods. Learn to enjoy the tremendous bounty a loving Father has provided for pleasure and health![22]

---

1. L. Jean Bogert, George M. Briggs, Doris Howes Calloway, *Nutrition and Physical Fitness*, Ninth Edition, W. B. Saunders Co., Philadelphia and London, 1973, p. 172.
2. National Academy of Sciences, *Recommended Dietary Allowances*, 1974, p. 63. Also Roger J. Williams, *Nutrition Against Disease*, Pitman Pub. Corp., N.Y., 1971, p. 83.
3. Bogert, *et al.*, *op. cit.* p. 178. Also National Academy of Sciences, *op. cit.*, p. 64.
4. Omer Pelletier, Ph.D., "Cigarette Smoking and Vitamin C," *Nutrition Today*, Autumn, 1970, pp. 12-15.
5. Williams, *op. cit.*, pp. 155-156.
6. Dr. Linus Pauling, "For the Best of Health—how much vitamin C do you need?", *Executive Health*, Vol. 12, No. 3, Dec. 1975, with references.
7. "Today's Health News," *Today's Health*, Sept. 1974, p. 12.
8. I. B. Chatterjee, "Evolution and the Biosynthesis of Ascorbic Acid," *Science*, Vol. 182, Dec. 21, 1973, p. 1271. Abstracted in *Journal of the American Dietetics Association*, Vol. 64, No. 3, Mar. 1974, p. 340.
9. W. J. Rhead, and G. N. Schrauzer, "Risks of Long Term Ascorbic Acid Overdose," *Nutrition Reviews*, Vol. 29, 1971, p. 262.
10. Pauling, *op. cit.*
11. M. P. Lamden, Ph.D., "Dangers of Massive Vitamin C Intake," *New England Journal of Medicine*, Vol. 284, No. 6, 1971, p. 336.
12. *Ibid.*
13. Victor Herbert, M.D., Elizabeth Jacobs, M.D., "Destruction of Vitamin B_{12} by Ascorbic Acid," *JAMA*, (*Journal of the American Medical Association*) Vol. 230, Oct. 14, 1974, p. 241.
14. G. A. Veeman, "How Much Vitamin C Should I Take?", *Focus*, Vol. 10, No. 5, Community Health Services Association, Saskatoon, Saskatchewan, Canada, Sept./Oct. 1974.
15. Irving Stone, "Megadoses of Vitamin C," *Nutrition Today*, Vol. 10, No. 3, 1975, p. 35.
16. Linus Pauling, *Vitamin C and the Common Cold*, W. H. Freeman Co., San Francisco, 1970, p. 88.
17. Food and Drug Directorate (Canadian) *Dispatch*, "Vitamin C, the Nutritional Plus in Orange Drinks, Are You Getting It?", June, 1970.
18. Bogert, *et al.*, *op. cit.*, p. 179.
19. *Ibid.*, p. 180.
20. "The Story of Michael Benge, Betty Ann Olsen and Henry Blood" as told to the Editor of *Nutrition Today*, May/June 1973, pp. 9-10.
21. "Highlights from the Ten-State Nutrition Survey," official summary published by *Nutrition Today*, July/Aug. 1972, pp. 9-10. Also *Nutrition Canada, National Survey*, a report by Nutrition Canada to the Department of National Health and Welfare, 1973, p. 62.
22. Doctrine and Covenants 59:4-5.

CHAPTER 4

Cereals, the Staff of Life

All grain is ordained for the use of man and of beasts, to be the staff of life.... Nevertheless, wheat for man.—Doctrine and Covenants 86:2c, 3b.

Grains are of such importance that they have been designated as the staff of life by God and used as such by vast populations for centuries. Among the grains, wheat has been designated by God as the one specifically designed to meet human need. In practice, the Food and Agriculture Organization of the United Nations report, 1970, declared, "Wheat is the most widely cultivated food plant. It is eaten in various forms by more than a billion human beings, and makes a larger contribution to the calories and protein available to man than any other food." Current food plans specify that good diets will include at least four servings of whole grain, enriched, restored, or fortified cereal foods daily.

Grains are of special value in feeding all of the world healthfully. They provide vast quantities of essential nutrients at comparatively low cost in terms of land and resources. They are of such flavor and can be used in such a variety of ways that they are staple foods enjoyed indefinitely and demanded regularly. They are easily transported and safely stored for long periods of time. They are "ordained...to be the staff of life...for man."

Cereals Provide Protein to Alleviate World Hunger

Although often called starchy food by the uninformed, grains currently provide 70 percent or more of the protein of the world's dietary. In most areas they are the chief protein eaten, providing 90 percent or more of this essential nutrient available to many in the developing nations. Even in the U.S.A. until recently they were the source of as much protein as meat provided in spite of our propensity for eating huge quantities of the latter.

Food grains are primary sources of protein. When they are fed to animals, the products that result are secondary sources of the nutrient. These sources provide excellent food that is enjoyable but costly in terms of resources required for their production.

These costs vary with the efficiency with which an animal uses the primary foods. Finished beef, to which the North American population is accustomed, may require as much as 21 pounds (9.5 kg) of plant protein to produce one pound (0.45 kg) of meat protein. The average of all meats produced results in one pound of meat protein being formed for every eight to ten pounds (3.6 to 4.5 kg) of plant protein fed. Milk and egg production are more efficient—about five pounds plant protein produce one pound animal protein.[1]

Some of the plant protein converted into animal protein comes from grazing areas not suited to other forms of cultivation and from foods not suitable for human consumption. It is good stewardship to use these resources in the production of food. In developed countries, however, disproportionate amounts of food grains are also used to feed livestock. While in developing countries less than 10 percent of the grain is fed to animals, in the U.S.A. nearly 80 percent goes to livestock. Releasing some of these grains for human consumption could assist materially in solving the world's food problems. God anticipated this need in his instruction to make grains our staff of life and to eat meats sparingly. Those concerned with feeding the world continue to affirm the validity of the instruction.

From the early days of World War II, when Dr. Henry C. Sherman pointed out that if the U.S.A. would reduce its meat consumption to only that meat produced in areas not suitable for other cultivation we could easily feed another nation as large as ours with both being more healthfully fed, until today when the specter of hunger hangs heavy over much of the world, concerned specialists have been calling our attention to the need for reserving more food grains for human consumption. According to the *USDA Yearbook of Agriculture, 1969*, cutting the country's animal population by one-half would release enough grains for human consumption to meet the calorie deficit of the nonsocialist developing countries four times over. Frances Moore Lappe in her book, *Diet for a Small Planet*, 1971, reports that the dean of agriculture of Ohio State University has estimated that feeding animals only those foods not suitable for human consumption would increase the world's food supply by 35 percent—nearly enough to close the gap between protein supplies needed and those now available.[2]*

For food grains released for human consumption to be of real value in meeting human need, two inherent problems will have to be solved. One is the problem of distribution, both logistic and political; the other is the problem of protein quality.

Nature and Use of Proteins

The need for high quality protein in the diet is well established. Protein is the major constituent, except water, of muscles, brains, skin, hair, nails, tendons, the framework of bones, the hemoglobin and serum of blood, hormones and enzymes which regulate all body processes, and antibodies which make possible resistance to infection and immunity to disease. Protein helps maintain a balance between acids and bases and keeps the water content of tissues under control. It is essential for the production of milk for our young. Amounts not used for these purposes provide energy for our bodies. Without it there can be no growth and no repair of tissues.

Although the body can turn protein into fats and carbohydrates to fill part of our need for these substances, nothing can take the place of protein. The protein molecule is intricate, containing nitrogen as well as the carbon, hydrogen, and oxygen found in other energy producing foods, and frequently has additional essential nutrients such as sulfur and phosphorus attached. Minute amounts of protein can be synthesized in the body using non-protein nitrogen, but it is impossible for the human body to produce the essential amino acids that it needs.

All proteins are formed from amino acids, about twenty-two of which are known to exist naturally in tissues. Some of these the body can synthesize principally by tearing down proteins provided in foods and reforming them into the acids needed. Adults apparently cannot synthesize eight of them, however, and they must be provided in food. Infants need nine. These

---

*See also *Overcoming World Hunger*, a symposium edited by Clifford M. Hardin, published by Prentice Hall, 1969 and Dr. Wallace Aykroyd, *Conquest of Famine*, Chatto and Windus Ltd. (England), Reader's Digest Press (U.S.A.), 1975 (Dr. Aykroyd was director of the Nutrition Division of the United Nations' FAO from 1946 to 1960.)

"essential amino acids," for adults are isoleucine, leucine, lysine, methionine, phenylalanine, threonine, tryptophan, and valine. Infants also need histidine preformed for them. These essential amino acids should comprise about 20 percent of the protein of the adult diet, 35 percent of the diet of an infant.

Significantly, all of the essential amino acids must be present at one time for the body to use them efficiently. Only those that can be matched together to form a pattern that the body needs can be used as protein. The rest are torn apart and reformed into carbohydrates or fats to be used for energy or stored as fat. The nitrogen containing fraction becomes a waste product that the kidneys must eliminate. The process is rather like a game of English scrabble. It is necessary to draw vowels and consonants that can be formed into words in order to play. Those that cannot be matched have to be discarded. They even become a liability when they must be deducted from the final score. Likewise, excessive waste products of protein metabolism may become damaging to kidneys and other portions of the body.

On the other hand, if there are not enough amino acids present to supply the need, the body has to tear down its own tissues to get the essential ones. If this process continues long enough to deplete body tissues, disease occurs—anemias, infections, and edema (swelling) as water collects in wasted tissues. The distended stomachs of the victims of kwashiorkor or starvation reflect this condition.

For the body to use essential amino acids most efficiently it must have them in proportions close to that of eggs, the most nearly perfectly utilized protein known. Even eggs are not perfectly used. On a scale of one to 100 percent perfect utilization of protein set by the Food and Agriculture Organization of the United Nations, food proteins are rated as follows:[3]

Food Protein	*Percent Utilized*	*Food Protein*	*Percent Utilized*
Eggs	94	Brown Rice	70
Milk	82	White Rice	63
Fish	81	Whole wheat	59
Beef	73	White Flour	51
Meats (Av.)	67	Soybeans.	60 (Tofu rates higher)
		Other beans	40 to 60

These scores for single foods are not necessarily the scores for a meal. When eaten in a meal, the amino acids form a pool from which the body can select those it needs. When foods are combined that complement each other's supply of essential amino acids, the value of all of them may be enhanced.[4] In fact, the average mixed diet of the U.S.A. is considered to have a biological value approximating 70 percent in spite of the fact that much of the protein comes from cereals, legumes, and meats that are used less efficiently than that.[5]

In general, animal proteins have been thought of as having all of the essential amino acids and so have been termed "complete" proteins. Plants have been considered more likely to be short in at least one essential and thus have been termed "incomplete" proteins. Some plant proteins, however, are as "complete" as some animal proteins, as noted in the chart above, and at least one animal protein is very "incomplete." Gelatin is an animal protein almost entirely void of either tryptophan or lysine, both of which are essential for human life.

When it was learned that a small amount of a "complete" protein could be combined with a large amount of an "incomplete" one or that two "incomplete" ones, each of which supplied that which the other lacked, could be served together to form meals of high quality, the discovery was called nutrition's greatest contribution to suffering humanity. The knowledge makes it possible to use the resources of the world to feed its people.

Because it is designated as especially for man, wheat is a good example. It has all of the essential amino acids. In fact, adults (except pregnant and lactating women) can eat enough of it to get all of the protein they need. Since it does have lysine in short supply, however, to eat enough to get the needed lysine would be to waste many of the other essential acids.

If, however, wheat is eaten with beans or milk, the resultant pool of amino acids is of very high quality. In the first combination beans provide the lysine for the wheat, the wheat provides the sulfur containing acids that the beans lack, and the value of the protein of the meal goes well into the range of animal protein. With milk and wheat, the total protein value approaches that of milk.

Trying to combine protein foods to get a maximum of essential amino acids could be a real problem for the menu planner.

Fortunately, to be absolutely specific is not necessary, and we have already incorporated many good combinations into our eating patterns. We often eat bread or cereals with milk, tortillas, corn bread or Boston Brown bread with beans, potatoes with eggs or cheese, cauliflower, broccoli or asparagus with cheese sauce, spinach with eggs, vegetables with rice, mushrooms in casserole with vegetables and some animal protein, all of which provide total protein of excellent quality.

Those fortunate enough to have milk available can make good use of all vegetable protein in every meal simply by using milk as a beverage or in some other form regularly, at least at every meal in which there is not a supply of eggs, fish, or meat. Those who have their intake of animal foods restricted, voluntarily or by necessity, might want to consult a source that treats the subject more completely than this book does. (Mrs. Lappe's *Diet for a Small Planet* may be helpful.)

Milk Compared with Meat as a Complement to Wheat

Long before the protein needs of the body were understood, bread and milk were regular components of many dietaries. Now, since we know that amino acids of the two foods combine to provide excellent protein nutrition at moderate cost and each supplies nutrients the other lacks, we understand the value of the combination.

Meat also supplies needed amino acids, but it generally costs more than milk, and meat's nutritional composition is so similar to wheat's that it duplicates many of the nutrients provided by wheat instead of adding other needed nutrients to the diet as milk does. Meat supplies iron. So does wheat. Meat contains B vitamins—thiamin, niacin, pyridoxine, riboflavin, folacin, B_{12}, and others. Wheat has them all except B_{12}, with more of the B_6 group and falacin, calorie for calorie, than any meat but liver and more B_1 than any but liver and pork, which are exceptionally rich in the substance. Meat has more niacin than wheat, but both are good sources of the vitamin.

Either milk or meat can supply the vitamin B_{12} not found in wheat. Both milk and meat need the magnesium that wheat can supply for nutritional balance.

Both wheat and meat have so little riboflavin that they need another source, as milk, to augment their supply. Both are extremely low in calcium content. Milk is an excellent source of the nutrient.

It is particularly important that a rich source of calcium accompany cereals in the dietary. Cereals, especially wheat and oats, contain phytin which may combine with minerals, principally with calcium and magnesium, in the food, making them unavailable to the body. A good supply of calcium assures enough calcium for the phytin and the body. Since there is only a limited amount of phytin present, it can combine with only a limited amount of mineral. The calcium and magnesium that are left over are free for nutritional use provided other members of the team are present.* Milk provides the calcium and frequently the vitamin D needed to balance the diet when cereals are eaten. Meat is no help at all (unless it is liver, which offers some vitamin D).

The chart, "Whole Wheat Bread and Milk Compared with Meats" which follows indicates graphically the low cost and high nutritive value of bread and milk when compared with meat. Data for the chart are taken from *Agriculture Handbook #8, Composition of Foods*, except for vitamin B_6 data which are from *Home Economics Research Report No. 36, USDA*. Other sources give variable data, especially for hamburger. Canadian Department of National Health and Welfare publications give the Calories of ¼ pound (112 g) hamburger as 364 instead of the U.S.A. 304, the protein content as 18.2 grams instead of the U.S.A. 20.3, and the iron content as 2.6 grams instead of the U.S.A. 3.0. The cost ratio is that of early 1975 Canadian prices for T-bone steak, regular grind hamburger, commercial whole wheat bread, and milk reconstituted from dry milk. Fluid skim milk would increase the cost of the bread and milk to about half the cost of the hamburger.

---

*Until recently the use of whole wheat bread by the children of Dublin during the last war and the use of whole wheat chapatis by East Indian people had been blamed for high incidence of rickets among the populations. Recent investigation has indicated that those Indians who have adequate supplies of vitamin D available do not suffer from negative calcium balance even when eating large amounts of chapatis. Many do not have sufficient of the vitamin, however, because of their dark skin and their custom of wearing clothing that shields them from the sun." Data are not available on the supplies of vitamin D or calcium to the children of Dublin, but the fact that one reason the law requiring the use of the whole grain was changed was that many were sifting out the bran from their flour and wasting it indicates that it was not whole grain that was at fault. Further discussion of phytin follows under availability of iron.

WHOLE WHEAT BREAD AND MILK COMPARED WITH MEATS
Percent highest RDA for nonpregnant, nonlactating adults

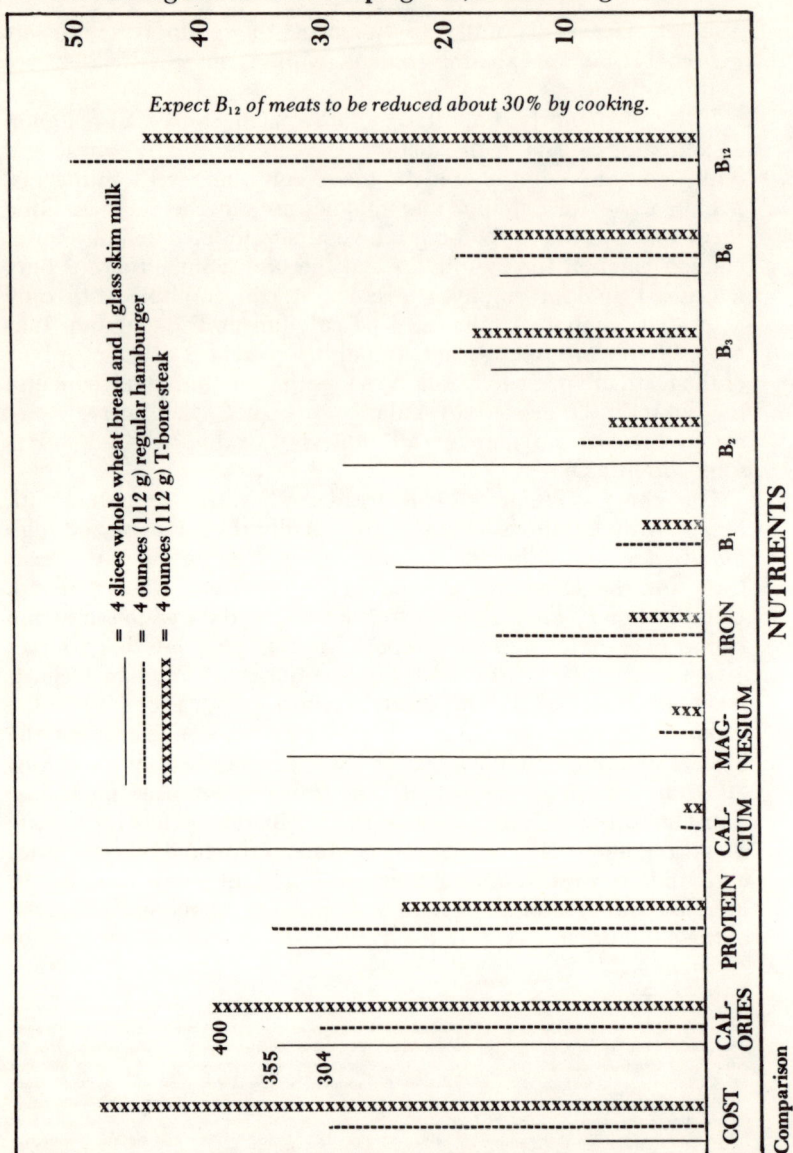

Expect B_{12} of meats to be reduced about 30% by cooking.

Legend:
- —— = 4 slices whole wheat bread and 1 glass skim milk
- - - - = 4 ounces (112 g) regular hamburger
- xxxxxxxxxx = 4 ounces (112 g) T-bone steak

NUTRIENTS: COST, CALORIES, PROTEIN, CALCIUM, MAGNESIUM, IRON, B_1, B_2, B_3, B_6, B_{12}

Calories: 400, 355, 304

Comparison

Although the data are only approximations as are all food table data, and the costs will vary, it is easy to see that the nutritive value of whole wheat bread and milk is comparable to meats in many areas and far exceeds it in others, while the cost is only a fraction of the cost of the meats. If meat is too expensive an item for the food budget, then whole wheat bread and milk may be served instead, with the net result nutritionally favorable in at least four ways:

1. The protein of the bread and milk will be as valuable or more so than the meats, and there may be more of it in a portion of equal Calories.

2. The bread and milk provides one fourth to one half of the calcium, magnesium, thiamin, and riboflavin recommended for the most demanding reference adults* except those who are pregnant or lactating. The meat has only traces of calcium or magnesium, and vitamins B_1 and B_2 are present in amounts one tenth or less of the RDAs of the same adults.

3. Although not shown on the chart, bread and milk are very low in saturated fatty acids, even when whole milk is used. Meats provide large amounts of saturated fatty acids. If whole milk was used with the bread in the chart, there would be about 4.5 grams of the saturated fat present compared with 12 grams in the hamburger and 19 grams in the steak.

4. The whole wheat bread provides fiber needed to prevent or ameliorate problems that frequently develop in the digestive tract when refined foods are used. It also helps the body successfully handle cholesterol provided by other foods.

Value of Fiber in the Diet

Until recently fiber was thought by many to be a useless, indigestible irritant. Now it is known to be an essential of every good diet. In fact, Denis P. Burkitt, M.D., of the Medical Research Council, London, England, has stated:

> ...even if only half of what the evidence suggests is true, then routinely adding fiber to our diet may turn out to be as important a preventive health measure as not smoking—or perhaps more important. Moreover there is absolutely no indication that replacing white bread with wholemeal bread, and adding reasonable amounts of cereal fiber to what we now eat could do any harm at all.

---

*Adults of size and ages specified in RDA charts.

Dr. Burkitt expresses the belief that in investigating the relationship between the use of refined carbohydrate and disease there has been "pointed the way to understanding and possibly preventing many of the commonest diseases of the Western world today."[7]

Some of the diseases thought to be related to the lack of fiber in the diet include:

1. Constipation—now treated by more than 700 over-the-counter laxatives sold in drugstores, supermarkets, and "health food" stores plus an estimated one percent of the medical prescriptions in countries in which refined foods are extensively used. The *Medical Letter on Drugs and Therapeutics*[8] has advised readers of the significant problems caused by every type of laxative on the market, concluding that only dietary fiber from whole grains, fruits, and vegetables is really safe, causes no adverse effects, is cheap, available, and contraindicated (should not be used) only if there has been narrowing of the bowel by adhesions or other abnormalities.

If whole grains are not used regularly, bran in some form should be used routinely by most people. As the fiber passes through the digestive tract it absorbs water, forming a bulky, soft mass that is easily eliminated, taking with it bile acids and other wastes that cause difficulties if they remain in the lower digestive tract for prolonged periods of time.

2. Diverticulosis—an oddity in the nineteenth century which now affects nearly one third of all Westerners over fifty years of age. For decades a low residue diet was thought to be the proper treatment for the disease, which is characterized by pockets (diverticula) formed in the walls of the colon which become inflamed and may abscess or even perforate. Now the use of large amounts of wheat bran is being found effective in bringing relief from suffering and healing to the tissues.[9] When fiber is absent, small, hard stools form. In an effort to expel them, the colon builds up a large amount of pressure, and divides itself into segments intended to move the feces along toward the anus. The combination of segmentation, hard feces, and pressure forces the feces into the walls of the colon forming the pockets or diverticula, it is believed.

3. Colitis—irritated bowels with diarrhea not caused by specific bacteria.[10] As Dr. Burkitt indicates, "... adding fiber to diet

seems to normalize bowel function in some very basic way."

4. Cancer of the colon and rectum—endemic in areas in which there is a small amount of fiber in the diet coupled with a high concentration of refined carbohydrates and hard animal fats, especially beef.

While further studies are needed to describe the specific relationship between this type of cancer and diet, Dr. Burkitt and others* point out that the bacteria of the colon-rectum of one on a low fiber, high hard fat diet are capable of degrading bile acids in the feces to compounds that are potentially carcinogenic (able to produce cancer). Without fiber the resultant chemicals remain in contact with the tissues for a prolonged time.

While we await further information, it is recommended that all rectal bleeding should be checked immediately by a physician, and that consideration be given to including more fiber, fewer refined carbohydrates, and fewer hard fats in the diets of all those who have adopted the style of diet that is associated with the cancer.

5. Obesity—also endemic in areas in which refined carbohydrates and high fat diets prevail. Calories are concentrated in these foods, and without fiber to accompany them, a feeling of fullness may not be achieved until more calories have been consumed than are needed.

6. Diseases related to pressure built up in straining to evacuate hard feces—hemorrhoids, appendicitis, hiatus hernia (hernia of the esophagus), and varicose veins.

7. Other diseases believed to be related to a low fiber-high fat diet include diabetes, gall stones, coronary heart disease, and clotting in the deep veins.[11]

Journal of the American Dietetics Association authors noted above conclude that using unrefined carbohydrate foods as wholemeal bread, unpeeled potatoes, brown rice, and fruit might protect against manifestations of overnutrition and noninfective disorders of the digestive tract.

Certainly fiber is an essential ingredient of a healthful diet. With the use of whole grain cereals and fruits and vegetables

---

*See also Jerry E. Bishop, "Cancer vs. What You Eat," *Science Digest*, March 1974, pp. 10-14. Also "Diet, Intestinal Flora and Colon Cancer," *Nutrition Reviews*, Vol. 33, No. 5, May 1975, p. 136.

as the Lord has counseled, there should be no lack of it in our diets. Without them we are, as the Word of Wisdom implies, like the Egyptians of Moses' day—susceptible to the diseases that destroy life and health.

Other Nutrients Provided by Cereals: Iron and Copper

Closely allied with protein, keeping blood rich with hemoglobin and able to carry vital oxygen to all the tissues of the body are the minerals iron and copper (without which the iron cannot be utilized). Without them, there is nutritional anemia. Body cells cannot get oxygen and so cannot use foods available in the blood. Without well nourished cells, the victim of the disease lacks energy, becomes pale, tired, listless, is more susceptible to other diseases, has a poor appetite, loses weight, becomes irritable, and finally dies if the situation is not corrected.

Fortunately, death rarely occurs from this type of nutritional anemia in developed countries where medical services find and correct the situation. In developing nations, however, and among some of the new dietary cults, the situation may become extremely dangerous or fatal. In some areas the presence of parasites such as hookworm further complicates and intensifies the problem.

Even in affluent countries such as Canada and the U.S.A., recent surveys (1973 and 1972 respectively) have revealed a high incidence of iron deficiency anemia. Among young children, this has long been recognized as the most prevalent nutritional disease in these countries. The need for iron and copper is especially critical for children who are not fed human milk (see chapter on child feeding).

All through the period of growth, both boys and girls must have rich supplies of these minerals to remain healthy. Teen-age girls require more than most boys because they menstruate monthly with the loss of blood taking with it 0.6 to 1.0 mg iron daily. During the period of most rapid growth, however, the need is the same for both sexes.

Pregnant and lactating mothers have an especial need for large supplies of iron and copper. During both states, there should be enough of the minerals to supply the need of mother and child. The child should be born with a rich store of copper and enough iron to last for about six months when supplemented by mother's milk, and the mother should have sufficient of the minerals to allow her to quickly replace blood lost in childbirth. When menstruation recurs, the need for blood replacement is the same as for a teen-ager.

Until recent surveys indicated otherwise, men who were eating enough of a variety of foods to supply needed calories were presumed to be getting adequate supplies of iron in their diet to care for all their needs with the possible exception of blood loss through accident or blood bank offerings. Both U.S.A. and Canadian surveys have indicated, however, that men have extremely low stores of iron under present dietary conditions.

When there is blood loss by accident, donation, childbirth, or menstruation, to replace 500 ml (approximately one pint) of blood, the body needs 90 mg of iron. Copper needs are much less but essential. Fortunately, when there is increased need, the body responds with increased efficiency in absorbing dietary iron to fill the need quickly if iron rich foods or supplements are provided.

Normally we absorb, on the average, about 10 percent of the iron that we eat. Cereal grains, when eaten alone, may be absorbed at a rate of about 5 percent. In times of special need, "body wisdom"—as Dr. Roger Williams calls it—increases the rate of absorption, and it may be increased by the presence of other nutrients in a meal.

Vitamin C eaten with iron-containing foods increases iron absorption by transforming the chemical form in which iron often occurs (ferric, now called iron III) to a more easily absorbed form (ferrous, now called iron II). This characteristic is reason enough to include in every meal some fruit or vegetable containing vitamin C. The fact that ferrous iron is more readily absorbed is a consideration that should affect the selection of iron for enrichment or supplementation.

The presence of a number of amino acids also increases the amount of iron that is absorbed. For this reason it is wise to take iron in food, and the combination of cereals or vegetables with eggs, milk, meats, legumes, or other sources of these amino acids will enhance their value.

As with proteins, whole grains contribute vast supplies of iron and copper to the world's dietary. Milling these grains to make refined products, however, reduces the supply drastically. To make white flour from whole wheat, for example, removes three-fourths of the iron, 90 percent of the copper, and 30 percent of the lysine. In an effort to prevent iron deficiencies, the iron is returned to many milled products. To date, the copper is not returned, and rarely is the lysine.

Phytin and Availability of Minerals

Phytin of cereals can affect the availability of iron as it affects the availability of calcium and magnesium. Most of the phytin occurs naturally in combination with magnesium and calcium with much smaller amounts combined with iron. These phytates are not irretrievably lost, however.

Enzymes called phytases occur naturally in all cereals. Given an opportunity, they can break down the phytates into whatever mineral is involved and phytin. The phytin is further separated into phosphorus and inositol which the body needs. These enzymes work during food preparation. In yeast bread making, dough that is allowed to rise a total of three hours has about 60 percent of its phytates transformed into needed nutrients. Longer rising results in larger amounts of transformation. When cereals are puffed, about 70 percent of the phytates are broken down. When they are flaked, about one-third of the phytin is transformed into needed nutrients.[12]

If the body is well supplied with vitamin B_6, even those minerals that remain as phytates are not all lost. With adequate supplies of B_6, the body can metabolize not only some of the phytates but also some of the oxalates that likewise precipitate some of the minerals of fruits, vegetables, and beverages. Whole wheat provides vitamin B_6 generously. It is not yet a standard nutrient for enrichment except in Sweden, but is used in some cereal enrichment in the U.S.A.

Magnesium

Since 1968 the U.S.A. Recommended Dietary Allowances have included magnesium. Whole grains are proving one of the richest sources of the mineral available, although nuts and legumes are excellent sources and many vegetables and fruits contain significant amounts. Milk and meats have small portions of the mineral, but one slice of whole wheat bread offers as much as a whole quarter pound (112 g) of the best of the meats. Milled grains, with bran and germ removed, have lost more than 80 percent of their magnesium, and to date none is returned in enrichment.

We have known for years that magnesium was an essential ingredient of many animal diets. Without it, cattle develop neuromuscular problems that lead to convulsion and death. The lining membrane of their hearts and the large arteries calcify as do their muscles, diaphrams, spleens, and sometimes kidneys and livers.

It was not until 1960, however, that it became undeniably apparent that man also needs to be concerned about his supply of magnesium. Symptoms of magnesium deficiency are similar to those of calcium deficiency—mental depression, muscle weakness, dizziness, painful muscle cramps (tetany), convulsions, sometimes involving the feet and hands in slow, writhing motions that are difficult if not impossible to control. Symptoms usually occur when a malnourished person faces some stress such as a severe infection, loss of intestinal secretions through vomiting, diarrhea, or other disorder, or when there has been a long period of therapy during which fluids have been injected into the body. One who follows the food plan of his country and includes whole grains should not be short of the mineral unless there is some unusual need.

B Vitamins

Seeds of plants (whole grains among them) are the most important source of B vitamins in nature's storehouse. Like the minerals, they are concentrated in the germ with its adjacent scutellum and the bran, especially the aleurone layer—portions of the grain that are removed in milling processes that produce polished rice, white flour, farina, and the like. With the offal that is largely fed to animals goes seven eighths of the vitamin B_1 (thiamin), three-fourths of the B_2 (riboflavin), seven-eighths of the B_3 (niacin), three-fourths to 90 percent of the B_6 (pyridoxine), and four-fifths of the folacin.

Every calorie that is used for energy requires a whole battery of B vitamins to burn it up (metabolize it). If the B vitamins that are removed in processing are not returned in some form of enrichment, restoration, or fortification, the resultant food is impoverished to the point of providing large numbers of calories without nutrients needed for the body to use them. Disease results. Specific diseases are associated with lack of some of the vitamins, but we must remember that they all work on a team. Frequently when there is lack of one there is lack of others, except in controlled laboratory situations.

Thiamin (B_1)

Beriberi is the disease that results if the diet is low in B_1 (thiamin). In Shingalese, the term means "I can't." The disease was described before the birth of Christ; it still disables and kills large numbers of people who use polished rice as a major food. Until late in the last century it devastated the crews of sailing vessels in the Orient. Then a Japanese officer named Takaki persuaded authorities to replace some of the polished rice of the sailor's dietary with whole wheat bread and to increase the allowance of milk and vegetables. He did it to provide more protein for the men but inadvertently added enough B_1 to bring the men back from their voyages alive.

A Dutch physician named Eijkman is credited with the discovery that there is something in whole grain rice that cures or prevents the disease. The substance was isolated half a century later (1926). Its chemical identity was established in 1936 and it was named thiamine (now spelled thiamin).

For every 1,000 Calories eaten one needs about 0.5 mg vitamin B_1. If there is not enough B_1 to metabolize the Calories, the sheaths of the nerves deteriorate. Emotional disturbances appear often leading to severe anxiety hysteria. Nervous disorders develop rapidly, and the muscles served by the nerves become paralyzed and shrink. Reflexes disappear, appendages grow numb. Hearts become involved, and death ensues.

Classic studies conducted by Dr. Norman Jolliffe and his associates at Bellevue Hospital, New York, and by Dr. R. D. Williams and his associates at Mayo Clinic, Rochester, Minnesota, in 1939-1940 demonstrated some of the symptoms that accompany thiamin deprivation. Without thiamin their volunteers soon complained of fatigue, weakness, loss of appetite, pain in the stomach, tenderness, heaviness and pain in calf muscles, burning feet, shortness of breath, muscle cramps, and heart palpitation. Attitudes and behavior changed. The volunteers became irritable, depressed, quarrelsome, uncooperative, fearful, suspicious. They were suddenly very sensitive to noise and pain. They had poor memory and difficulty in concentrating. They forgot where they put objects, told the same stories over and over again, started on errands and forgot where they were going.

All of these symptoms responded to vitamin B_1. One set of the above researchers gave an injection of B_1 to half their patients whose personality and physical condition had been altered by lack of vitamin B_1. The other half they gave saline solution (salt water). No one knew which he/she was getting. Within thirty minutes to twenty hours, every one of those with evidence of thiamin deficiency disease who had received the B_1 responded with truly amazing changes in personality. They were transformed from timid, apprehensive, shrinking, fearful, depressed, unreasonable, uncooperative persons to smiling, pleasant, friendly, cooperative, happy people. Not one of those who received the salt water showed similar improvement.[13]

These results of controlled studies led early researchers to suggest that at least some "neurotic traits" in children—temper tantrums, sleep walking, bed wetting, nightmares, behavior problems—may reflect the lack of sufficient thiamin in their diets rather than perverseness or immaturity. Certainly the polyneuritis of alcoholism and of those whose diets contain excessive amounts of sweets are associated with deficiencies of B vitamins including vitamin B_1.

Vitamin B_1 is lost by milling, by cooking with high, dry heat and by discarding water in which food is prepared. To preserve it in food:

(1) Use whole grains or every fraction of the milled.

(2) Wash foods briefly. Soak or cook only in water to be served.

(3) Use drippings from meats. The meat itself loses half its B_1 or more when it is roasted, one third when broiled, and one sixth when fried. Some of the lost vitamin remains in the drippings. Chill and remove fat, if desired, before using the liquid.

(4) Bake and toast lightly. Toasting until brown destroys one fifth to one third of the B_1 of white bread, less in whole wheat.

(5) Do not add soda to vegetables or legumes. If they must be cooked in extremely hard water, tomato or lemon juice or

vinegar in cooking help preserve B_1.

(6) Keep soda content of quick breads, cakes, and cookies low. One half teaspoon (2½ ml) soda per cup (240 ml) of average sour milk produces gas equivalent to 2 tsp. (10 ml) baking powder and generally keeps batter slightly acid.[14]

Keeping a diet rich in vitamin B_1 is not difficult. If the dietary choice is for refined foods, however, including large amounts of concentrated sweets and alcoholic beverages that provide only calories, thiamin must be provided from other sources or there will be trouble. Long before beriberi could be diagnosed, the consequence of such poor choices will be manifest in distorted appetites, jittery nerves, low resistance to disease, muscles that tire easily and work painfully, and difficulties with digestion and elimination.

B_1 deficiencies begin a vicious cycle. We have no pep, so crave a quick energy lift. To get the lift, we take a sweet bottle of pop or a glass of liquor, thereby further depleting our supply of thiamin. So we grow fat but not healthy.

Niacin (B_3)

When there is specific need for niacin, the disease that results is pellagra. Of the early symptoms it is difficult to tell which are from lack of niacin, however, and which are associated with thiamin, riboflavin, or vitamin B_6 deficiency.

We have discussed many aspects of this disease of the three D's—dermatitis, diarrhea, and dementia—in the preface of this book. While the rough skin (dermatitis) gives the disease its name, the mental abberations are its most tragic manifestations, other than death. Ten thousand people were reported to have died of pellegra in the U.S.A. in 1915. Two years later there were over 200,000 cases of the disease reported in the southern U.S.A., and it was variously estimated that 10 to 50 percent of the mental patients of the area were victims of the disease.

The psychosis of pellagra is characterized by loss of memory; disorientation as to time, place, or identity; confusion or confabulation (incessant talking) associated with mania, depression, delirium, or delusions of persecution (paranoia).

The addition of niacin to milled corn products and the return of the nutrient to white flour and polished rice has reduced the scourge of pellagra in many areas of the world. The disease is still a serious problem in parts of Africa, India, Egypt, Portugal, Latin America, and Yugoslavia and does occur even in the affluent nations where it has become fashionable for those who should know better to scorn the notion that there is still nutritional disease.

I saw a severe case of pellagra in a hospital patient in a modern western Canadian city recently. The disease is rare enough in the area that the patient's physicians did not recognize even its typical manifestations. After a summer of illness characterized by the three D's, the patient received niacin therapy which resulted in prompt and complete relief.

It is recommended that we have 6.6 mg niacin or its equivalent in tryptophan (sixty milligrams tryptophan are equal to one milligram niacin) for every 1,000 Calories that we eat.[15] Whole wheat provides niacin value to care for its calorie needs more than twice over. A one pound loaf of whole wheat bread offers 1,100 Calories with 21 mg niacin value (13 mg niacin and 8 mg equivalent from tryptophan)—enough to care for over 3,000 Calories.

Other sources of niacin value include meats, milk, eggs, and yeast. Actually milk and eggs have little niacin but their tryptophan content is so high that it easily meets the need. (Note that while tryptophan will care for niacin needs, niacin cannot completely replace tryptophan. This essential amino acid is needed by men at a daily rate of about 500 mg and by women at about 320 mg per day.) Here are some niacin values in 1,000 Calories of foods and the dietary Calories those values would care for:

Food	Niacin Equivalents	Dietary Calories
1,000 Calories of whole wheat bread provides	19 mg—enough for	3,000
1,000 Calories of eggs provides	19 mg—enough for	3,000
1,000 Calories of skim milk provides	22 mg—enough for	3,000
1,000 Calories of whole milk provides	13 mg—enough for	2,000
1,000 Calories of regular hamburger provides	26 mg—enough for	4,000
1,000 Calories yeast (bakers or brewers) provides	158 mg—enough for	24,000

Some niacin is produced by bacteria in human intestines. Diets high in vegetables and low in meats encourage this synthesis.

For most of us it is not difficult to get all of the niacin value we need from food. Some people may have an abnormality that increases the need. At the present time there is experimentation with and controversy over the use of massive doses of niacin in the treatment of schizophrenia and the type of learning disabilities often grouped under the term "dyslexia" in which objects are not perceived in their normal order or placement.*

The possibility of adverse effects makes it imperative that large doses of niacin not be taken without adequate medical supervision. Some people react with gastrointestinal distress and/or a painful rash and itching to some forms of niacin. Kidneys and livers may be damaged by excessive amounts of it. The heart's rhythm and use of oxygen may be affected adversely, so that it should not be taken in quantity just before sustained physical activity. Uric acid may accumulate in the blood and other abnormalities may occur with large doses. Self-medication is not advised.[16]

Riboflavin (B_2)

Cereals are not naturally a rich source of riboflavin, although wheat does carry about 0.6 of the amount recommended for its own calories. They have been chosen as carriers of the nutrient in enrichment programs to help insure an adequate supply for those who cannot or choose not to drink milk or to eat milk products, vegetables, and organ meats that provide it generously. For that reason, enriched cereals are usually richer in B_2 than the comparable whole grain. In milling white flour from wheat, three fourths of the B_2 that grew there is removed. Unless the product is enriched or restored, it makes an almost negligible contribution to filling riboflavin needs. (See chapter on milk for information.)

Pyridoxine (B_6)

While vitamin B_6 was discovered along with niacin in the 1930s and has long been known to be essential to physical and mental

---
*The Medical Letter, Je.6, 1975, p. 50, reports it as effective in lowering cholesterol and triglyceride levels in blood.

health, it was not included in the RDA lists until 1968. The first dramatic demonstration of human need for the nutrient came two decades ago when a large number of babies became extremely irritable and suffered convulsions. Investigation revealed that they were all taking a formula which had inadvertently been deprived of its B_6 by what was thought to be an improved method of processing. When the infants were given the vitamin, improvement was noted within minutes and recovery was complete.[17]

Since that time, many infants with pyridoxine-dependent convulsions have been observed, and epileptiform seizures have been observed in every species of laboratory animal tested, including man. Other symptoms of B_6 deficiency include nervous disorders similar to those displayed with the lack of other B vitamins—irritability, depression, confusion, and dizziness. There may be nausea and vomiting (as frequently occurs during pregnancy), weight loss, and anemia that does not respond to iron therapy. This anemia occurs because the body cannot form red blood cells without sufficient B_6. A dermatitis that begins in the angles of the mouth, around the eyes, and in the eyebrows and spreads over the face, neck, breasts, and loins is characteristic of the deficiency. The tongue may swell and become irritated. Kidney stones sometimes appear. Infections develop rapidly and do not respond to usually effective antibiotics until needed B_6 is supplied.

Vitamin B_6 is involved in the metabolism of proteins, and our need for the vitamin is closely associated with the amount of protein consumed—especially if that protein is of animal origin, high in tryptophan.[18] The vitamin serves as a catalyst in the transformation of tryptophan into niacin. Without adequate supplies, the transformation is incomplete, and an abnormal substance called xanthurenic acid is excreted in the urine. Xanthurenic acid is often found in the urine of pregnant women or those taking oral contraceptives, of alcoholics, the aging, those on excessively high protein diets, and those receiving excessive radiation, signaling in every case a need for more vitamin B_6.

The pyridoxine group is involved in fatty acid metabolism. With adequate amounts of B_6, unsaturated fatty acids are spared while the body shows a preference for using the saturated ones. Only with B_6 present can the body manufacture arachidonic acid, which is essential to life. Although it is not entirely clear with man, with sufficient B_6, rhesus monkeys are able to dispose of large quantities of cholesterol. Without the B_6 they rapidly develop atherosclerosis, dental caries, sclerosis of the liver, nervous system disorders, and other symptoms.[19]

All total, vitamin B_6 serves as a coenzyme in over 40 body reactions.[20] In addition to the metabolism of proteins and fatty acids, it is necessary for the body to change glycogen (the form in which the body stores carbohydrates in liver and muscle) to glucose for the body's use as energy. It must be present for the body to produce hormones and antibodies, is essential for normal functioning of all nervous system tissue, is involved in red cell formation. In short, it is a nutrient of major significance for all who wish to live healthfully. It is water soluble, and very little is stored in the body. It is needed daily.

The U.S.A. National Research Council RDA for B_6 is set at 2.0 mg for women with an additional 0.5 mg in case of pregnancy. There is serious discussion among investigators as to whether this is enough. Dr. P. György, the man who discovered the vitamin, suggests that pregnant women and those taking oral contraceptives should have 30 mg a day.[21] Since he finds B_6 effective in preventing or treating common premenstrual edema (swelling) and the edema that often accompanies pregnancy and finds that acute rheumatism and osteoarthritis in their early stages benefit from doses of the vitamin, he recommends that the daily allowance should be set at 25 mg. This would be more than the usual American diet normally provides as far as we can presently determine. Additional amounts are needed for therapy. Anemias caused by deficiencies in the vitamin require up to 500 mg for control, and radiation sickness needs doses in the range of 100 mg for effective therapy.[22]

Food sources of vitamin B_6[23] include the whole grains, especially important because of the quantity of cereals eaten in the world, vegetables (especially the green leafy ones), nuts, legumes (especially peanuts and soybeans), sunflower seeds, liver, muscle meats, fish, milk, and yeast. Among the fruits, bananas and avacados rank high.

Unfortunately, the vitamin B_6 in meats is especially vulnerable to heat. Half their potency is frequently destroyed by cooking and canning procedures. Ham does retain its potency better than beef, and liver is so rich in the nutrient that it still has an excellent supply even with half its B_6 gone. Ham or liver will offer seven times the B_6 of an equal weight of hamburger when fully cooked.

A two-ounce (56 g) whole wheat bun will provide as much B_6 as the quarter pound (112 g) hamburger inside. And one cup (240 ml) milk, fresh, pasteurized, or reconstituted from dry milk, offers 2½ times the B_6 of the hamburger. The high heat used in the preparation of canned evaporated milk or of dry cereals destroys about half of the vitamin. The nutrient can also be destroyed by light, especially in nonacid solution.

Folacin (Folic Acid)

Already we have seen the importance of folacin in the propagation and maintenance of the human race (see chapter on herbs).[24] Wheat is not a rich source of the nutrient when compared with green leafy vegetables; but when it is combined with yeast in bread its contribution to the diet is significant. Four slices of whole wheat bread contributes about one fifth of the RDA for a nonpregnant adult. Butterfield and Calloway (Berkeley, California, researchers) believe that because wheat is a staple of even the affluent American diet, whether wheat supplies its share of folacin may determine whether the population is adequately supplied with the nutrient.[25]

Tocopherols—Vitamin E

Vitamin E is an antioxidant provided by nature to prevent natural fats and oils from becoming rancid. It is fat soluble so occurs in the fatty portions of foods and functions in the fatty tissues of the body. There it is associated with vitamin C, the mineral selenium, and other antioxidants helping the tissues use oxygen efficiently, preventing substances that would irritate or destroy cells from developing, protecting vitamin A. Every cell membrane contains essential fatty acids; every cell must have its antioxidants.

Vitamin E's most biologically active form is d-alpha-tocopherol. Other tocopherols, beta, gamma, etc., and tocotrienols have vitamin E activity in varying amounts usually expected to total about 20 percent of the vitamin E activity of the diet. RDAs are established in terms of International Units of d-alpha-tocopherol. One IU vitamin E is defined as the activity of 1 mg of dl-a-tocopheryl acetate. Forms of d-alpha-tocopherol vary in potency as follows:

Synthetic dl-alpha-tocopheryl acetate	1 mg = 1 IU
Synthetic dl-alpha-tocopherol (free)	1 mg = 1.1 IU
Natural d-alpha-tocopherol	1 mg = 1.49 IU
Natural d-alpha-tocopherol acetate	1 mg = 1.36 IU[26]

After years of controversy—probably due to overly enthusiastic claims by some of its advocates and stubborn reaction of its detractors—vitamin E in 1968 was placed on the list of essential nutrients for which RDAs are established. Although the allowances varied from a modest 5 IU for infants to 30 IU for adults, "average" diets in the U.S.A., Canada, and Britain failed to meet the standards. American consumption is estimated to average about 7.4 mg (11.1 IU) d-a-tocopherol daily, Canadian about 6.4 mg (9.6 IU), and British about 5 mg (7.5 IU). After publication of the 1968 RDAs there was demand to reduce them on the assumption that the populaces had adjusted to lower levels of consumption, and those levels should, therefore, be adequate. The 1974 RDAs for adult males and females were reduced to 15 IU and 12 IU respectively.

Following the International Symposium for Vitamin E held in Minneapolis, Minnesota, September 27-28, 1973, the symposium's organizer, M.K. Horwitt, Ph.D., Professor of Biochemistry, St. Louis School of Medicine, St. Louis, Missouri, and veteran vitamin E researcher, summarized the "Status of Human Requirements for Vitamin E."* He concluded: "In effect, the range of 10-30 mg of d-a-tocopherol formerly suggested as the adult requirement is reinforced and any table of vitamin E requirements should clearly demonstrate this range."

The research which prompted the 1968 RDAs, ranging up to 30 IU for adult males, indicated that the need for vitamin E increases with increased intake of polyunsaturated fatty acids (abbreviated PUFA), and continues as long as those polyunsaturates

---

*See *American Journal of Clinical Nutrition*, Vol. 27:1182, 1974.

are a part of the tissues.[27] The popularity of diets high in PUFA in an effort to avoid heart disease has increased intake of these fatty acids tremendously, and with the increase there has been a concommitant increase in need for vitamin E. Fortunately, the oils that provide the polyunsaturates also provide vitamin E. Unfortunately, however, they do not always contain enough vitamin E to balance their PUFA.

When the 1968 RDAs were established, it was generally accepted that for every gram of PUFA, one should have at least 0.6 mg vitamin E. (The 1973 standards reduced the accepted need to 0.4 mg E per gram PUFA largely on the assumption that what we are getting must be enough.) In one study that involved 19 food oils, only cottonseed oil had enough of the vitamin to balance its own PUFA, according to the 1968 standards. Corn oil, which is particularly popular as a source of PUFA, had 0.4 mg vitamin E per gram PUFA. Wheat germ oil may have as much as 2 to 3 mg E for every gram PUFA but is seldom used as a food oil.

It is difficult to predict how much vitamin E activity a specific oil or plant will have because potency varies with the variety planted, growing conditions (under warm growing conditions, more vitamin E is produced), and maturity at harvest. Many of the oils are then refined, bleached, deodorized, and stored with varying losses in each situation. Even oils that are not refined or heated lose potency with storage. During prolonged heating required to deodorize the oil, sizable losses occur. Since hydrogenization saturates some of the PUFA, the ratio of vitamin E to PUFA increases with this process that makes shortening and margarine of some oils.

If polyunsaturated fatty acids are taken into the body and allowed to oxidize in the tissues, as they will if there is no antioxidant as vitamin E, or selenium which can partially replace the E, chemical changes occur in nucleic acids, in enzymes, and in other proteins which destroy their function. Cellular and subcellular membranes are most often affected. Damage to these membranes reduces the energy that can be produced to sustain work or play, and reduces the body's ability to metabolize drugs and to protect itself from toxins. Sometimes the cell membranes rupture, enzymes enter, and severe damage results. Blood cells are especially vulnerable. In tissue, many cells die and colored ceroid substances typical of aging accumulate. Muscle damage that resembles muscular dystrophy appears. Animals develop true muscular dystrophy that responds to vitamin E therapy, but human muscular dystrophy has not been found to so respond.

Vitamin E needs of infants are particularly crucial. Vitamin E deficiency anemia is characterized by rupturing of the blood cells as the membranes disintegrate because there is not enough of the vitamin present to prevent excessive oxidation of the PUFA of the tissues. The administration of iron simply speeds the process of oxidation and so increases the severity of the disease. This type of anemia occurs most frequently in premature infants, in those whose mothers had diets high in polyunsaturates during pregnancy, in those with insufficient calories and protein, and in those fed formula high in polyunsaturates without vitamin E fortification.[28]

Persons who live in areas subject to photochemical smog may benefit from taking generous amounts of vitamin E. Nitrogen dioxide and ozone are the two smog components that do the most damage to lungs by causing oxidative changes in the PUFA of the cell membranes. Dr. L. L. Tappel, Professor of Nutrition, Food Science, and Technology, University of California, has reported that rats well supplied with vitamin E do not suffer lung damage in smog that is typical of those not so protected. He believes that human lungs respond similarly and recommends that persons living in smog areas use the 1968 RDAs, 20 to 30 IUs of the vitamin for adults. He believes, too, that therapeutic doses running 3 to 20 times those RDAs are safe.[29]

Other conditions for which vitamin E has been used therapeutically (as a medicine) by responsible physicians include heart and circulatory ills, problems concerned with child bearing, treatment of burns to prevent contracting and disfiguring scars, increasing stamina for athletic events, maintaining normal blood configuration in astronauts.[30] Some of these are still controversial as far as general medical acceptance is concerned. Further research will surely elucidate the areas of usefulness.

Vitamin E research is complicated by the fact that the nutrient is stored in body fat, and enough may be stored to prevent the development of deficiency disease during long periods without dietary supplies. Also, in animals, at least, diseases that do result from deficiency of the vitamin are often not curable or require long periods of very large doses of the nutrient to effect a cure. Just doubling the concentration of the vitamin in body tissues requires about ten times the RDA.

Present research leaves no doubt, however, that it is imperative that adequate amounts of the vitamin be consumed. It is apparent, too, that there are conditions of impaired fat absorption, interference with digestion, and possibly especially high requirement when the usual food supplies are not enough. In general, large supplements should be taken only under the supervision of a physician. Although it has not been shown to be toxic at high concentrations as have vitamins A, K, and D, it does accumulate in the tissues, and for those who have high blood pressure there may be dangers as indicated by the experience of physicians who do find vitamin E therapy efficacious for some diseases. A physician should be able to tailor the dose properly and to determine whether other forms of therapy are needed. Self-medication in any disease state can delay proper treatment and sometimes results in tragedy.

Vitamin E is a nutrient known to be essential to life and health which is removed from whole grains, leaving the refined product a poor source of the vitamin. Wheat loses about 90 percent of its d-alpha-tocopherol when it is milled into white flour. Those tocopherols that are left have much less vitamin E activity and rapidly disappear under many bleaching procedures and with storage. Chemical treatments given cake flours leave them essentially void of any tocopherols at all. Fortunately, treatment with bromate or vitamin C does not affect vitamin E values.[31]

Wheat is not rich in vitamin E, but the quantity in which it is used makes it important as a source of the nutrient. Much of its activity is concentrated in the germ.[32] In areas where the germ is milled out of even the "whole wheat" flour, as is allowed in Canada, the resultant flour is a very poor source of the nutrient. Whole wheat that is really whole retains its vitamin E very well through moderately long periods of storage if the flour is covered closely and kept in a dry, cool place. Milling techniques that keep the flour cool during grinding help extend the storage period during which there is little loss. Freezing and storage at zero degrees Fahrenheit (-18 Celsius) allows lengthy storage without loss.[33]

Some vegetables are proving to be a good source of vitamin E. Others, along with fruits and animal products, all contribute to our supply. While conclusive data are still scarce, it appears that, excluding some seeds, dark green, slow-growing leaves are richest in the nutrient. Care must be taken in harvesting and storing these greens, however, if it is to be preserved. Sunlight seems to destroy vitamin E, so leaves that are harvested early in the morning have more of the nutrient than those harvested later in the day. When the leaf is damaged, an enzyme is activated that destroys the E. The green needs to be eaten immediately after preparation if it is eaten raw. Boiling, baking, or frying destroys the enzyme, however, without disturbing the vitamin.[34]

Among other fruits and vegetables, the more mature produce is generally higher in vitamin E, and those fruits with peel are often 2½ to five times richer in the nutrient than their peeled counterparts. Some oily seeds such as soybeans, peanuts, and almonds are rich in vitamin E. Some other seeds such as oats, barley, rice, peas, and ordinary beans are low in the nutrient.

Here is a list of some representative foods with alpha-tocopherol values found in the literature on vitamins. Other tocopherols present in the foods might increase the actual vitamin E values. Gamma-tocopherol is thought to have about 20 percent of the biological value of d-alpha-tocopherol. And studies on larger samples may indicate the values should be changed:

ALPHA-TOCOPHEROL CONTENT OF 100 GRAMS (3½ OUNCES) FOOD

FOOD	mg	FOOD	mg
Seeds		**Vegetables and Fruits**	
Almonds	27.0	Green Leafy Veg.	1.0-10.0
Peanuts	7.0-10.0	Asparagus	1.8
Wheat	1.4	Other Veg.	0.1-1.0
Wheat Germ	13.0	Most Fruits	0.1-1.0
		Wild Blackberries	3.5

FOOD	mg	FOOD	mg
Oils		**Animal Foods**	
Coconut	0.5	Eggs	1.0
Corn	11.0	Milk	0.1
Cottonseed	39.0	Beef	1.0
Rapeseed	18.4	Codfish	1.2
Safflower	39.0	Liver	2.0
Soybean	10.0		
Sunflower	49.0	**Other Foods**	
Wheat Germ	133.0	Yeast	0.0
Butter	2.0		
Lard	1.2		
Margarine	10.0		
Veg. Shortening	10.0		

Americans get about two thirds of their vitamin E from seed oils. A significant portion of these are now served in the form of convenience foods such as frozen french fried potatoes or TV dinners. Unfortunately, prepared foods, especially fried ones, lose vitamin E during frozen storage. Dependence on these foods for vitamin E could result in low intake.

It is evident that nature provides the tocopherols in generous proportions in many foods, but we often trade them off for the types of foods to which we have become accustomed and for the convenience of having food prepared for us. Grains are milled to white flour; fruits are peeled; oils are processed in many ways and stored for long periods of time; foods are fried, then frozen; green vegetables are neglected; needs are increased by diets high in PUFA and by environments polluted by our carelessness. Fortunately, it is possible for most of us to obtain recommended amounts of the nutrient if we choose to use wisely what is available to us.

Effects of Milling and Bleaching

It is apparent that there is a vast difference between the amounts of nutrients grown in wheat and those that remain in white flour. Many think this difference is due to "bleaching," but in this they are largely mistaken. "Bleaching" is primarily a process designed to age the flour rapidly so it may be used for yeast bread baking sooner than would be desirable if it aged naturally. Those who lived in my generation or who attempt to use freshly milled whole wheat flour understand. Newly milled flour produces dough that is difficult to manage and dark, heavy bread.

As it ages, chemical changes occur in the flour that make the dough easy to handle and the loaf light. To wait while this occurs naturally requires long, inconvenient, and costly storage. Addition of a "bleaching" agent reduces the cost and produces a more nearly uniform product—one that can be guaranteed to give good results every time.

The major loss of nutrients occurs in milling to produce the *un*bleached flour. The germ and bran are removed, including the scutellum and aluerone layers in which most of the vitamins and minerals are concentrated. That which remains is largely carbohydrate and protein with the protein that is left being reduced in quality by the removal of one third of the lysine, the amino acid already in short supply in the wheat. Bleached or unbleached, the resultant white flour is poor food indeed. Unless it is enriched it does not qualify as a basic food in modern food plans.

Forms in Which Cereals Are Used

There have been large-scale efforts to popularize the use of whole grains in affluent countries, but they have not been highly successful except in homes in which the mother is well-educated. To date, less than 10 percent of the commercial bread baked in the U.S.A. is whole wheat largely because people choose to buy white bread. To provide protection for those who choose white flour products, programs of "enrichment," "fortification," and "restoration" have been instituted. All are designed to return some of the nutrients removed or to use the grain as a carrier for nutrients known to be in short supply. Always they fall short of duplicating the original food that was created to be the "staff of life."

Grain foods are marketed as:

(1) *Whole grain.* These are products that have the outer husks removed and are cleaned. If cleaned abrasively, a very small portion of the outer layer of cellulose containing negligible quantities of vitamins, minerals, and proteins may be discarded.

If washed, small quantities of vitamin B_1 may be dissolved, so that care should be exercised and repeated washings avoided. Because of the possibility of contamination with dirt or from insect or rodent contact, cleaning is essential in spite of minimal losses.

(2) *Whole wheat or graham flour.* Government standards vary. In the U.S.A. both terms apply to ground wheat, roller milled or stone ground, in which all of the ingredients of cleaned wheat must be present in the original proportions up to 90 percent of the original weight of the wheat. Roller ground is more likely than stone ground to have had the endosperm flour chemically aged before the parts are reassembled. Stone ground may also be so treated.

In Canada whole wheat flour must have 95 percent of the wheat, but the law does not specify that all parts must be there in their original proportions. (Only "Crushed Wheat" or "Coarse Ground Wheat" must have their constituents unaltered.) This allows millers to remove much of the germ, which is about two percent of the weight of the wheat, and still label the flour "100 percent Whole Wheat." Germ is removed from much of Canadian "whole wheat" flour to improve the baking quality and to increase shelf life (period the flour will remain fresh). When heat and moisture are used in milling, rancidity does become a problem. In Canada, "graham" flour may simply be white flour with bran added.

Stone ground wheat flour is usually really whole wheat, but the germ may also be at least partially removed from it. (Check with the miller if you really want to know.) Retail merchants, even "health food" personnel, are frequently poorly informed.

A long list of additives is allowed in whole wheat flour in both Canada and the U.S.A. (The list is available from the Food and Drug Administration of the U.S.A. and the Health Protection Branch of Canada's government.) It is usually available at the public library or Extension Service offices. If any of the products used artificially age the flour the label must read "bleached" or "maturing agent added." Others need not be listed.

(3) *Enriched.* In Canada and the U.S.A., this applies to grains, especially wheat, corn, rice, that have had substantial portions of their nutrients removed in processing and have had iron, vitamin B_1 (thiamin), B_2 (riboflavin), B_3 (niacin), and sometimes calcium added to the depleted food to prevent deficiency diseases

caused by inadequate supplies of these nutrients. Canada also allows vitamin D, and Sweden includes B_6.

Standards of enrichment are set by many governments, but enrichment is rarely compelled. In the U.S.A. federal standards must be met only if products are labeled "enriched" and pass into interstate commerce. Thirty of the fifty states and Puerto Rico have laws compelling enrichment, however. Newfoundland alone in Canada has compulsory enrichment. In other provinces, enrichment is voluntary, but if the term is applied the product must meet national standards.

At present most of the white flour sold in Canada and the U.S.A. is probably enriched, according to the Wheat Flour Institute of the U.S.A. and the Bakery Foods Foundation of Canada. Unbleached flour probably is not enriched. Cake flour is hardly ever enriched. Flours used in pastes as macaroni, spaghetti, and noodles frequently are not enriched. (Read the label.) The pastes and white rice must be more heavily enriched than other products if they are labeled "enriched" to assure that there will be significant amounts of the added nutrients after the food is prepared, unless they carry a warning not to drain or rinse and have no recipe that calls for rinsing or draining. Breakfast cereals, except farina and grits, may be "enriched" at will in the U.S.A. but must be limited to those nutrients allowed in flour in Canada.

An estimated 90 percent of bread sold in the U.S.A. and Canada is enriched, but only about 60 percent of the buns, rolls, crackers, and other breadstuff, including frozen bread doughs, are so treated. In Canada milk solids must be included in "enriched" bread. In the U.S.A. milk is frequently used because it provides a product with characteristics customers like, but it is not required.

Dark breads may not be of superior nutritive value. They may be made of all white flour, enriched or plain, with only caramel, molasses, or a little bran for coloring. If unenriched they are, like cakes, pastries, and pastes, of so little nutritional value that they cannot qualify as a basic food. Percentages of whole wheat flour in dark breads in the U.S.A. may run as low as 10 percent and rarely go higher than 45 percent unless labeled "100 percent" whole wheat. Ingredient lists may help determine how much is there. If "wheat flour" is listed first, there is less than half of the flour whole wheat. If the whole wheat comes after the milk solids, sugar, or yeast, there is little to darken the bread but coloring matter.

To meet federal standards in Canada, the percentage of "whole wheat" flour must appear on the label, or the label must say that the product is merely colored with a specified matter. Anything containing 60 percent or more whole wheat flour may be labeled "whole wheat." To get all of the wheat, it is necessary to purchase "100 percent" whole wheat. Bread labeled "100 percent Whole Wheat" may be low in wheat germ in Canada. In the U.S.A. whole wheat dough may have been kneaded with white flour and so contain a small amount that is not whole grain value.

Where essential nutrients are returned or added to grains, some of the more flagrant nutritional diseases prevalent only a third of a century ago have been reduced to infrequency. Pellagra is no longer rampant in the southern U.S.A. Beriberi is seldom seen in the developed countries. Simple iron anemias are thought to be reduced, although a simultaneous reduction in iron consumption from water pipes, cooking utensils, well water, and green vegetables has left an amazing number extant.

In an effort to eliminate some of these anemias and to insure better intake of vitamins B_1, B_2, and B_3, new high levels of enrichment were set beginning April 12, 1974, in the U.S.A. Iron levels are especially high. Bread labeled "enriched" by federal standards must now have 25 mg iron per pound (0.45 kg)—twice the maximum previously allowed—and white flour must contain 40 mg iron per pound (0.45 kg)—two and one half times the former maximum.

While such high levels of iron may be helpful to some who do not or cannot eat meats, eggs, green vegetables, and whole grain foods, some investigators see real danger in such large amounts of supplemental iron. Children are susceptible to iron poisoning.[35] Some persons have metabolic errors that allow abnormal absorption and storage of iron when an excess is present in their diets. Iron never works alone, and it does not cure all anemias. In fact, it may make some worse. Attention needs to be given to all the nutrients involved in modern anemias, and to problems concerned with the way the body absorbs and handles the iron it receives.[36]

If there are dangers from the new levels of iron enrichment, they may be avoided by simply using only whole grain products. If refined products are used, they should be enriched. There is more danger for most people in too little of the necessary nutrients used in enrichment than in too much iron. Caution should be used in giving supplemental iron to those, especially children, eating a large amount of the enriched products, however. Vitamin E and supplemental iron should not be taken at the same time. Increased oxidation destroys much of the vitamin E's value.

Levels of thiamin, riboflavin, and niacin have also been increased in the new standards. Charts now in use will reflect the old standards which are much too low. In these three vitamins and iron, products made with enriched white flour will probably exceed those made with whole grains. Here is how the whole grain, white unenriched, and white enriched flours and breads, by U.S.A. standards and by Canadian standards, compare in these four nutrients:

COMPARISON OF BREADS, WHOLE GRAIN, WHITE, AND WHITE ENRICHED

Type of Wheat Bread 1 lb (0.45 kg)	Thiamin mg	Riboflavin mg	Niacin mg	Iron mg
Whole Wheat	1.20	1.03	13.0	10.4
White Unenriched	.31	.04	5.0	3.2
White Enriched (Can.)	1.4-2.4	0.8-1.8	10.0-15	8.0-12.5
White Enriched (U.S.A.)	1.80	1.10	15.0	25.0

COMPARISON OF FLOURS, WHOLE GRAIN, WHITE, AND WHITE ENRICHED

Type of Wheat Flour 1 lb (0.45 kg)	Thiamin mg	Riboflavin mg	Niacin mg	Iron mg
Whole Wheat	2.5-2.7	0.54-0.80	19.7-27.2	14.4-15.0
White Unenriched	0.28	0.21	4.1	3.6
White Enriched (Can.)	2.0-2.5	1.2-1.5	16.0-20.0	13.0-16.5
White Enriched (U.S.A.)	2.9	1.8	24.0	40.0

Ways Whole Grain and Enriched Products Differ

Noting that present enrichment levels in the U.S.A. require more iron and vitamins B_1, B_2, and B_3 than are originally in the wheat, one might assume—as many have—that enriched products are as good or better than whole grain. In these four nutrients they may be. There are, however, many other essential nutrients for which wheat is a good source that are removed by milling and not returned in enrichment. If all of the benefit of whole grains are to be had, whole grains must be used. The chart on pages 92 and 93 will give some indication why.

The chart indicates that after wheat is milled to white flour there is only about one tenth of the vitamin B_1 left, one fourth of the B_2, one sixth of the B_3, one fourth of the iron, one half of the calcium, one fifth of the B_6, one fourth of the folacin, one tenth of the E, one fifth of the magnesium and phosphorus, one third of the zinc, one fifth of the manganese, half of the pantothenic acid, one fourth of the potassium, one tenth of the biotin, one fourth of the copper. While only about one tenth of the protein is removed, that includes about 30 percent of the lysine, the essential amino acid already the principal limiting factor of wheat protein.

Of all these, only four are required to be returned in enrichment programs in the U.S.A. and Canada. While they are included in generous amounts, especially in the U.S.A., there are eight known nutrients with RDAs established which are not replaced, each of which, except for calcium, is provided by wheat in significant amounts. In addition there are at least five others, whose need has been established, for which wheat is a good source, whose loss is not compensated by enrichment. Fiber, too, is proving a significant omission from the milled and enriched product.

(4) *Restored.* This term is applied to a milled product to which some of the nutrients have been returned, notably the four required in enrichment and sometimes lysine and other vitamins and minerals. There is no attempt to attack a specific nutritional disease, however, by adding more of a nutrient than was formerly present as occurs with enrichment.

(5) *Fortified.* This term is used when nutrients are added to a product that were not there originally or were there in short supply. Many of the new simulated foods must have nutrients added to them if they are to be of significant nutritional

NUTRIENTS IN WHEAT FLOUR, WHOLE GRAIN (____), WHITE (XXX), ENRICHED(---) U.S.A. 1974

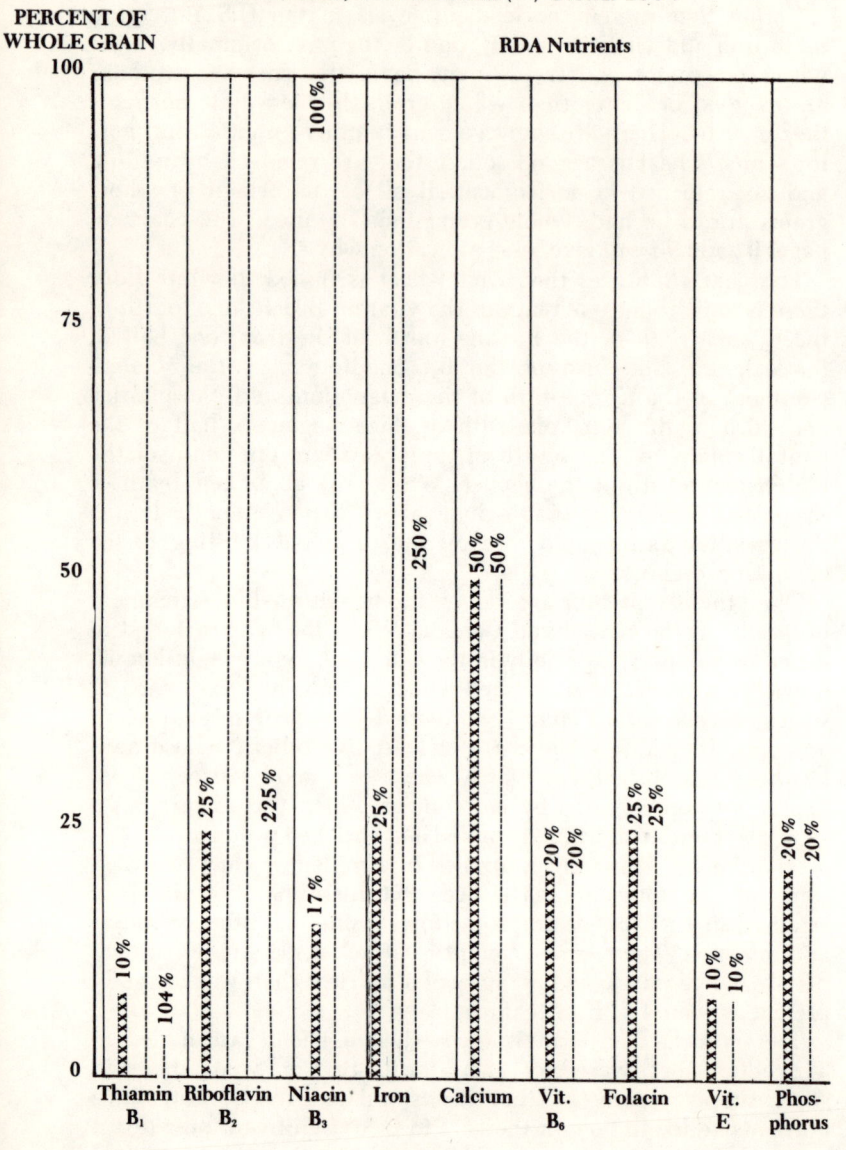

PERCENT OF WHOLE GRAIN

RDA Nutrients

Nutrient	Whole Grain	White	Enriched
Thiamin B$_1$	100%	10%	104%
Riboflavin B$_2$	100%	25%	225%
Niacin B$_3$	100%	17%	—
Iron	100%	25%	250%
Calcium	100%	50%	50%
Vit. B$_6$	100%	20%	20%
Folacin	100%	25%	25%
Vit. E	100%	10%	10%
Phosphorus	100%	20%	20%

ESSENTIAL NUTRIENTS NO RDA ESTABLISHED

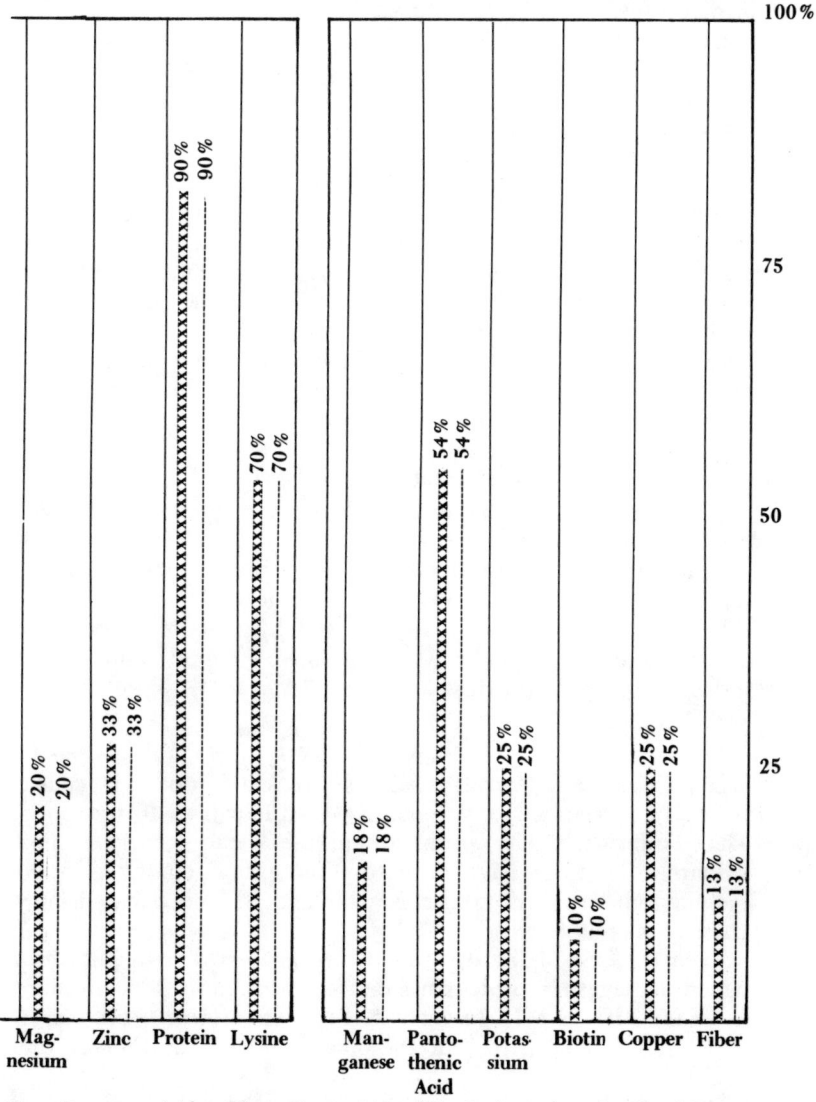

Nutrient	%
Magnesium	20%
Zinc	33%
Protein	90%
Lysine	70%
Manganese	18%
Pantothenic Acid	54%
Potassium	25%
Biotin	10%
Copper	25%
Fiber	13%

Note. Data are calculated from *Composition of Foods*, Agriculture handbook No. 8, *Home Economics Research Report* No. 36, and standard nutrition journals and texts.

value. Orange flavored crystals have no vitamin C until they are fortified with ascorbic acid. Pineapple and apple juice are vitamin C poor until fortified with the nutrient. Spun or extruded protein must be fortified with vitamins and minerals to provide nutrition approaching that of naturally occurring proteins. Margarine is fortified with vitamin A value to make it similar to butter. Milk has vitamin D added to help insure good utilization of its calcium. Salt is fortified with 0.01 percent potassium iodide to help prevent simple goiter.

(6) *Converted.* This is the term applied to cereal, especially rice, that is parboiled before the bran is removed. Moist heat distributes the B vitamins throughout the kernel and causes the scutellum and germ to adhere to the endosperm more tenaciously than normal so that more vitamins and minerals remain in the polished grain than when the grain is milled outright. It is superior to regular polished rice, inferior to whole grain rice in all nutrients, and unless enriched it has fewer of the four enrichment nutrients than enriched white rice.

Other Treatments for Cereals

In some areas of the world wheat is parboiled and dried before being marketed or stored. If the bran is removed—as it is traditionally—the resultant product (bulgur) is nutritionally inferior to the wheat from which it was made.

Wurled wheat has its bran removed by the use of lye in a process similar to that by which hominy is made from corn. It is depleted of many nutrients.

Ready-to-eat Cereals

Dry or instant cereals used as breakfast foods or snacks represent a tremendously expensive way in which to use grain. Those offering whole grains, bran, or wheat germ are most valuable. The rest have little to offer except energy and the included vitamins and minerals (which could be purchased more cheaply in other forms).

Even the best of the dry cereals are processed with high heat which damages the protein and destroys portions of such vitamins as folacin, B_1, and B_6. In enrichment or restorative processes, B_1 will likely be returned, but the others will not in Canada and may not in the U.S.A. (Read the label.)

Eating dry cereals as a snack is a particularly poor nutritional practice. Snack cereals generally get their flavor from large amounts of fat and sugar, empty calories of which we already have too many; and they are eaten without milk on which the processed cereal is dependent for protein value. Unfortunately, this is true of many of the "natural" grainolas (granolas) currently popular. A representative one has more sugar than any other ingredient but rolled oats and has 50 Calories of highly saturated coconut oil in every ounce (28 g) of the cereal. This ounce of grainola is concentrated in about one fourth cup (60 m.) yet offers 136 Calories—nearly as much as a whole cup (240 ml) of cooked wheat cereal or a cup and a third of plain wheat flakes.

FINALLY

Grains used in many forms make a tremendous contribution to the nutrition of the world's people in spite of our tampering with them. If we want everything of worth they have to offer, we must use the whole grain or all the fractions, and grains will best fill our needs in combination with milk and green leafy vegetables. The assertion of Dr. Henry C. Sherman of three decades ago is still valid:

> Recent research reinforces the time tested principle that the dietary should be built around bread and milk;...bread because as far as it goes it brings so much food value at so little cost; and milk because it so efficiently and economically supplements and balances the bread.... This principle does not exclude anything from the dietary.... When the dietary includes as much grain products as it well may for economy and as much milk as is desirable...the protein needs of good nutrition will have been very nearly if not fully met.... One moderate serving every day of meat or an alternative will be ample.[37]

In 1962 this principle was reiterated by nutrition specialists of the U.S. Department of Agriculture, Esther Phipard, Ph.D., chief of the Diet Appraisal Branch, Consumer and Food Economics Research Division, and her co-worker, Louise Page, Ph.D., when they suggested that a pound loaf of whole wheat bread, a quart of milk, and a cup of cooked kale would provide fully the protein, minerals, and vitamins recommended for an adult. A spread for the bread would add extra calories needed to meet energy requirements.[38] Of course this restricted diet is not recommended for anyone, but the statement indicates the high nutritive quality of the foods involved. It corroborates the word of the Lord that wheat was designed to be our staff of life, that the lands in which the Lord's people will live most happily will be "flowing with milk and honey," and that herbs were ordained for our use.

---

1. Frances Moore Lappé, *Diet for a Small Planet*, Ballantine Books, Inc., N.Y., N.Y., 1973, pp. 6-7, quoting *The World Food Problem*, a report of the President's Science Advisory Committee (U.S.A.) Vol. 2, May 1967, p. 338, and calculating from data in *National and State Livestock-Feed Relationships*, USDA Economic Research Service, Statistical Bulletin No. 446, Feb. 1970, p. 76.
2. *Ibid.*, pp. 8-9.
3. L. Jean Bogert, George M. Briggs, Doris Howes Calloway, *Nutrition and Physical Fitness*, Ninth Edition, W. B. Saunders and Co., Philadelphia and London, 1973, p. 89. Also Lappé, *op. cit.*, pp. 48-49.
4. Lappé, *op. cit.*, pp. 48-54.
5. National Academy of Sciences, *Recommended Dietary Allowances*, Eighth Edition, 1974, pp. 45-48.
6. *Nutrition Reviews*, Vol. 31, No. 8, Aug. 3, 1973, p. 238.
7. Denis P. Burkitt, M.D., F.R.S., F.R.C.S. (E), External Scientific Staff, Medical Research Council, London, England, quoted in "Western Civilization, Diet and Disease," *Drug Therapy*, January 1974, pp. 51-62.
8. *The Medical Letter on Drugs and Therapeutics*, Nov. 23, 1973, pp. 98-100. Also Denis P. Burkitt, and Neil S. Painter, "Diverticular Disease of the Colon: A Deficiency Disease of Western Civilization," *Br. Med. Journal*, Vol. 2, 1971, pp. 450-454.
9. Peter F. Plumley, and Brian Francis, "Dietary Management of Diverticular Disease," *Journal of the American Dietetics Association*, Vol. 63, Nov. 1973, pp. 527-529. Also N. S. Painter, and W. M. Stahl, "Questions and Answers," *Journal of the American Medical Association*, Vol. 221, Aug. 28, 1972, p. 1058, extracted in *Journal of the American Dietetics Association*, Vol. 61, Nov. 1972, p. 581.
10. Frank Goldstein, M.D. (Thomas Jefferson University, Philadelphia, Pa.), "Diet and Colonic Disease," *Journal of the American Dietetics Association*, Vol. 60, June 1972, pp. 499-502.
11. K. W. Heaton, "Are We Getting Too Much Out of Food," *Nutrition*, Vol. 27, Apr. 1973, p. 170, extracted in *Journal of the American Dietetics Association*, Vol. 63, Nov. 1973, p. 585.
12. FAO, "Wheat in Human Nutrition," pp. 32-33. Also Y. Pomeranz, Editor, American Association of Cereal Chemists Monograph, *Wheat Chemistry and Technology*, Second Edition, 1971, St. Paul, Minnesota, p. 71. Also F. L. Dunlap, Sc.D., *White vs Brown Flour*, Wallace and Teirman Co., Inc., Newark, New Jersey, 1945, pp. 149, 198.
13. Ruth Woods, "Vitamin Deficiency in Nervous and Mental Disease II. Clinical Studies," *Borden's Review of Nutrition Research*, Vol. 8, No. 1, Jan. 1947, pp. 2-4.
14. Belle Lowe, *Experimental Cookery*, Third Edition, John Wiley & Sons, Inc., London, 1943, pp. 456-457.
15. National Academy of Sciences, *Recommended Dietary Allowances*, Eighth Edition, 1974, p. 70. Also Bogert, *et. al.*, *op. cit.*, pp. 139-142.
16. William J. Darby, M.D., Ph.D., Kristen W. McNutt, Ph.D., and E. Neige Todhunter, Ph.D., "Niacin," *Nutrition Reviews*, Vol. 33, No. 10, Oct. 1975, pp. 289-297.
17. Bogert, *et al.*, *op. cit.*, p. 143, citing references. Also P. György, "Developments Leading to the Metabolic Role of Vitamin B_6," *American Journal of Clinical Nutrition*, Vol. 24, No. 10, Oct. 1971, p. 1250; Comprehensive Review, *Journal of the American Dietetics Association*, Vol. 60, No. 2, Feb., 1972, p. 143.
18. György, *ibid.*
19. R. J. Williams, *Nutrition Against Disease*, Pitman Pub. Corp., N.Y., Toronto, London, Tel Aviv, 1971, p. 76 (with documentation).
20. *Documenta Geigy, Vitamins*, reprinted from the *Geigy Scientific Tables*, Seventh edition, CIBA Geigy Ltd., Basel, Switzerland, 1970, pp. 473-476.
21. György, *op. cit.*, p. 1250.
22. *Documenta Geigy, Vitamins, op. cit.*, p. 476.
23. *Pantothenic Acid, Vitamin B_6 and Vitamin B_{12} in Foods*, Home Economics Research Report No. 36, Agricultural Research Service, USDA, by item.

24. Williams, *op. cit.*, pp. 59-60, citing numerous studies reported in the *Journal of Nutrition, Proceedings of the Society for Experimental Biology and Medicine*, and *Nutrition Reviews*, "Folic Acid and Pregnancy I," Vol. 25, 1967, p. 325, and "Folic Acid and Pregnancy II," Vol. 26, 1968, p. 5.
25. Susan Butterfield, and Doris Howes Calloway, Ph.D., U. of Calif., Berkeley, "Folacin in Wheat and Selected Foods," *Journal of the American Dietetics Association*, Vol. 60, Apr. 1972, p. 310.
26. National Academy of Sciences, *op. cit.*, pp. 56-59.
27. A. L. Tappel, Ph.D., "Vitamin E," *Nutrition Today*, July/Aug., 1973, pp. 4-12.
28. National Academy of Sciences, *op. cit.*
29. Tappel, *op. cit.*
30. *Ibid*. Also Wilfrid E. Shute, M.D., *Vitamin E for Ailing Hearts*, Pyramid Books, N.Y., 1972.
31. Pomeranz, *op. cit.*, p. 565.
32. H. T. Slover, Joanna Lehmann, and Valis, "Nutrient Composition of Selected Wheats and Wheat Products III. Tocopherols," *Cereal Chemistry*, Vol. 46, No. 6, Nov. 1969, pp. 635-641.
33. H. T. Slover, and Joanna Lehmann, "Effects of Fumigation on Wheat in Storage. IV. Tocopherols," Human Nutrition Research Division, USDA, Beltsville, Maryland 20705, *Cereal Chemistry*, Vol. 49, 1972, pp. 412-415. (Also personal communication from Martha Louise Orr, Nutrition Analyst, USDA Agricultural Research Service.)
34. V. H. Booth, and M. P. Bradford, "Tocopherol Contents of Vegetables and Fruits," Dunn Nutritional Laboratory, University of Cambridge and Medical Research Council, *British Journal of Nutrition*, Vol. 17, 1963, pp. 575-581. (Also private communication from Vernon Booth and others of his papers on tocopherols in foods.)
35. D. S. Fischer, R. Parkman, and S. C. Finch, "Acute Iron Poisoning in Children, the Problem of Appropriate Therapy," *Journal of the American Medical Association*, Vol. 218, Nov. 15, 1971, p. 1179, extracted in the *Journal of the American Dietetics Association*, Vol. 60, Feb. 1972, p. 154.
36. Maxwell M. Wintrobe, "The Proposed Increase in the Iron Fortification of Wheat Products," *Nutrition Today*, Nov./Dec., 1973, pp. 18-20.
37. Henry C. Sherman, *Principles of Nutrition and Nutritive Values of Food*, USDA Misc. Pub. No. 546, pp. 31-33.
38. Esther F. Phipard, Ph.D., and Louise Page, Ph.D., "Meeting Nutritional Needs Through Food," *Borden's Review of Nutrition Research*, Vol. 23, No. 3, July-Sept., 1962, p. 33.

CHAPTER 5

Meats to Be Shared

Yea, flesh also, of beasts and of the fowls of the air I, the Lord, hath ordained for the use of man.—Doctrine and Covenants 86:2b.

The need for high quality protein in human diet is well established. Because meats are high quality protein and have traditionally formed the basis of menu planning in affluent countries, many believe that generous and constant use of meats is necessary to good health. The prophet's statement of the way they are to be used is at variance with this general conception. Once again, the testimony of the science of nutrition is that the prophet was more than a century ahead of his time.

God's Instructions on the Use of Meats

God tells us he has ordained the flesh of beasts and fowl for our use "with thanksgiving. Nevertheless, they are to be used sparingly; and it is pleasing unto me that they should not be used only in times of winter, or of cold, or famine. All grain is...to be the staff of life, not only for man, but for the beasts of the field, and the fowls of heaven, and all wild animals that run or creep on the earth; and these hath God made for the use of man only in times of famine and excess of hunger."[1]

The Lord has made meats available for our food. There is no hint of mandatory vegetarianism in this or related scriptures. Writing to Timothy, Paul prophesied:

> Now the Spirit speaketh expressly, that in the latter times some shall depart from the faith, giving heed to seducing spirits, and doctrines of devils; speaking lies in hypocrisy; having their conscience seared as with a hot iron; forbidding to marry, and commanding to abstain from meats, which God hath created to be received with thanksgiving of them *which believe and know the truth* [italics mine]. For every creature of God is good, and nothing to be refused, if it be received with thanksgiving; for it is sanctified by the word of God and prayer.[2]

Centuries later Joseph Smith encountered this problem. Some who wanted to be a part of the Restoration movement had previously believed they should eat no meat and felt that such abstinence should be the practice of the Restoration. In response to his inquiry of the Lord, the young prophet received instruction that anyone who taught that the Saints must not eat meat was "not ordained of God; for, behold, the beasts of the field, and the fowls of the air, and that which cometh of the earth, is ordained for the use of man, for food, and for raiment, and that he might have in abundance, but it is not given that one man should possess that which is above another; wherefore the world lieth in sin; and woe be unto man that sheddeth blood or that wasteth flesh and hath no need."[3]

While meat is designed to be used by man, the Lord has set some restrictions. It is to be used by those who believe and know the truth, *with thanksgiving, sparingly*, and *at stated periods of time*. Any excessive use of it by one segment of the population, while in another part of the world there is not only little if any meat but not enough food of any sort, is condemned by the Lord in no uncertain terms.

The principle is reinforced in the Word of Wisdom itself. Flesh of beasts and of fowls is to be used sparingly, and it is "pleasing" to the Lord if they are not used "only in times of winter, or of cold, or famine... and excess of hunger."[4]

The wording of this portion of the instruction has caused much discussion in the church. Some have felt that it says that meats are to be used at all times. Knowledge of the language Joseph Smith was accustomed to using, however, makes it abundantly clear that this is not the case.

In the first verse of the Word of Wisdom, identical terminology is used, but it is obscured by the construction of the sentence. In paragraph one of this instruction, we are told that to drink wine or strong drink is "not good, neither meet in the sight of your Father, only in assembling yourselves together to offer up your sacraments before him."[5] For nearly a century and a half church members have understood this sentence to mean that it is not acceptable to take wine or strong drink *except* in the Communion service.

This understanding is consistent with the direction of the Lord given some three years earlier that no wine or strong drink should be used for this service except it had been made new by the Saints.[6] Canning was just being introduced. Nicholas

Appert had invented the process in France in 1807, and it was not widely known or practiced in the U.S.A. until much later. Grape juice pressed in the fall was fermented before long. If it was to be used in the sacrament until the grape season of the following year, there was no choice but to use it fermented. Even this homemade wine was not to be used, according to the prophet, *except* in the service of Communion.

The same terminology appearing in the second verse of this document undoubtedly has the same meaning. It is pleasing to our heavenly Father if we do not use the flesh of beasts or of fowls *except* in times of winter, cold, famine, and excess of hunger. If we say that the Word of Wisdom instructs us to eat meat at all times, to be consistent we have to say that the Lord also instructs us to use wine and strong drink at all times; for he says that to eat certain meats is not good *only* at certain times and that to drink wine and strong drink is not good *only* in offering up our sacraments.

That the word *only* was commonly used to mean *except* in Joseph's day is evident from other revelations. Doctrine and Covenants 59:3a instructs us that on the Lord's day, we are to "do none other thing, only [except] let thy food be prepared with singleness of heart...." According to 98:5 salt that has lost its savor is "good for nothing, only [except] to be cast out...." And there are numerous other examples in the Scriptures, including these from the King James version of the Bible, which was Joseph's chief source of literary instruction during his youth: Genesis 19:8 and 24:8; Exodus 21:19; Numbers 18:3; Deuteronomy 12:15-16.

God's Instruction and the World Food Situation

Whether or not there are nutritional reasons for our eating meats only in winter, cold, famine, or excess of hunger, in terms of the needs of the peoples of the world this is perhaps the most profoundly prophetic declaration of the Word of Wisdom. A loving heavenly Father looks at all his creation. He knows that, rightly used, there is enough food for all who inhabit the earth. He also knows that circumstances distribute that food inequitably over the earth. For food to be distributed so all may live healthfully, he will have to have a people sufficiently concerned about the needs of others to find a way to bring about the necessary distribution.

God knows, too, that the inordinate use of primary foods in the production of meats will be one of the greatest sources of waste of food resources and of discontent among the underprivileged people of the earth when they realize that they hunger while others eat extravagantly of the foods that would bring life and health to them. Although the problem was remote in 1833 it has been very apparent to those concerned with feeding the world. Nearly three decades ago an editorial titled "Wheat and World Hunger" reprinted from the *Journal of the American Medical Association* stated:

> There is no escape from the fact that cereal grains used directly and indirectly as food are the bulwark of sustenance for most of the world's human population. The excessive production of animal converted foods—especially top quality meats which require extra grain for fattening—is a waste of food calories during a world food crisis.... Shortage of feed grains... should tend to be balanced by appropriate reduction in livestock.[7]

Until the sudden realization that there is a world shortage of food alerted the general population recently, those who spoke of the wastage of food resources inherent in the heavy use of meat went largely unheard. Now, however, national magazines of many descriptions have taken up the theme. Prelates of many churches urge their followers to reduce their meat consumption in deference to the needs of their fellowmen. Representatives of many nations gather to discuss food problems and to urge that grains be spared for human consumption by reduced usage for finishing livestock and even by the reduction of the alcohol consumed in the form of beer, whiskey, and other distilled liquors.

Again the American Medical Association pointed out the problem in *Today's Health*. Quoting the biblical proverb "When [sic] there is no vision, the people perish" (Proverbs 29:18), Daniel Grotta-Kurska points out:

> There is now approximately one acre of arable land for every person in the world [according to WHO figures]. The meat eaters need 1.63 acres to feed themselves for one year; vegetable eaters need only 0.5 to 0.6 acres.... Those who eat beef or other flesh foods are using more than their fair share of the land.[8]

The world Food and Agriculture Organization of the United Nations estimates that two thirds of the world's people live in countries in which diets on the national average are inadequate. That means that if every person got a fair share there would not be enough to feed everyone adequately. Since some do get more than their fair share they live healthfully while others suffer severely, and some do not survive. FAO says there are no reliable statistics on those who starve. Much of the world's hunger is beyond the reach of statisticians.

We do know, however, that the portion of the world in which food supplies are grossly inadequate includes large portions of Asia, most of Africa, part of South America, almost all of Central America, and the islands of the Caribbean. That portion in which there is generally enough food if it is properly distributed includes the U.S.A., Canada, Brazil, Argentina, Chile, the tip of South Africa, Oceania (Australia, New Zealand, Polynesia), Japan, the U.S.S.R., and the countries of Europe.[9]

Although the primary need of the deprived areas is for calories, the greatest disparity between the foods available in the "have" nations and the "have-nots" is their supply of protein—especially animal protein. This is apparent from the following chart which shows how different the supplies of Canada and the U.S.A. are from those available in the poorest of the nations, and also how these supplies differ from the accepted needs of the people:

SOME PROTEIN NEEDS AND SUPPLIES BY WORLD AREAS[10] (1969)

Area	Grams Protein/Person/Day Animal	Total	Reference Adult RDA Males	Females
FAO Desirable Goal	10.0	60		
Communist Asia	3.2*	48		
West Central Africa	3.2	48		
Canada	64.0**	96	46-55	35-43***
U.S.A.	64.0	95	54-56	46-48

*3.2 grams animal protein is equivalent to ½ egg, or ⅓ glass milk, or ½-⅔ ounce (14-16 grams) fish or meat.
**64.0 grams animal protein is equivalent to two large servings meat plus a pint (480 ml) milk plus an egg.
***Pregnant females RDA adds 10 grams protein, lactating 10-20, in Canada. Pregnant females RDA adds 30 grams protein, lactating 20, in U.S.A.

It is apparent that the U.S.A. and Canada have many times the animal protein that the FAO even hopes other nations may have someday—in fact, *must* have if all are to live healthfully. According to the FAO World Food Survey of 1963, in those areas in which animal proteins constitute less than 1/5 of the protein of the diet, there is increased evidence of retarded growth in children, poor physical health of adults, low resistance to disease, especially among those five years of age or younger, high mortality rates among infants and young children, and a low life expectancy.[11]

The disparity between the "have" and the "have-not" countries is obvious when meat supplies are considered. In 1973 Americans ate an average of 176 pounds (79.9 kg) meats per person. The people of India had less than 3 pounds (1.35 kg) each. Americans ate an average of 116 pounds (52.2 kg) of beef—the animal requiring the greatest amount of primary food for its production—in 1972. The English consumed 50 pounds per person (22.5 kg) that year. The people of Japan, also among the nutritionally favored nations, ate only 6 pounds (2.7 kg) apiece. As is evident from the preceding chart, communist Asia and West Central Africa scarcely had enough to measure. For at least a third of a century concerned persons have been speaking of this disparity in terms of political unrest, revolution, and war. Certainly it is a situation that cannot continue among people who develop a sense of social justice.

Hunger is not new. Nanking University figures show 1,828 famines between 108 B.C. and A.D. 1911. The British Isles recorded 201 famines between A.D. 10 and 1846, an average of one almost every nine years.[12] Willard W. Cochrane suggests that three hundred years ago most of the people were hungry most of the time.[13]

What is new is our awareness of hunger and our intention to help alleviate it, an awareness and an intention to which the Lord called his people more than a century and a third ago. New methods of agriculture, new sources of food, decreasing birthrate as countries become more developed economically and socially and the people are assured of the survival of the majority of their children, increased educational opportunities, increased concern of people who have food resources to share lead us to hope that someday all may be adequately fed.

If the situation does improve, G. I. Burch reminds us that there is the possibility of intensified political unrest until the inequities are solved. A starving man does not fight. He lies down and dies. But a man who has enough food to survive and enough knowledge of the rest of the world to be aware of the fact that he and his are being left out will fight for what he feels is rightfully his. In developing countries now, Burch reports, men are not comparing their food supply with that of their fathers but with that of their neighbors and the new standards they seek. If we really want peace, we must demonstrate our intention to make certain that one man does not have more, or more desirable, food available than another anywhere in the world.[14]

Where regular meat supplies are available, they testify to the abundance of food that God has supplied to that nation in which it is possible to use food to feed meat-producing animals. Those privileged to live in such abundance should be aware of that blessing and eat with thanksgiving!

Those who are truly thankful desire that others may share their rich blessings. Thanksgiving turns into action—in this case:

(1) using meats sparingly that there be no damage to health and no waste, even that occasioned by eating more than is needed;

(2) fasting from the use of the flesh of beasts and of fowls during a portion of each year as a reminder of the needs of others and strengthening resolves to do something about those needs.

The Lord spoke strongly of his expectations in the matter when he said, "It is not given that one man should possess that which is above another; wherefore the world lieth in sin; and woe be unto man that sheddeth blood or that wasteth flesh and hath no need."[15]

Fish and Milk as Protein for World Feeding

Because they use the least of the world's primary foodstuffs in their production and are so widely available, milk and fish have long been advocated by the World FAO to provide the animal protein so desperately needed in developing countries. In the Lord's instruction concerning those flesh foods from which there should be an annual fast, fish was not mentioned.

That the Lord is aware of the difference in the flesh of fish and that of others of his creation is evident, not only from the fact that he is the creator but also from Paul's assertion that, "All flesh is not the same flesh; but there is one kind of flesh of men, another flesh of beasts, another of fishes, and another of birds."[16] That Christ considered fish desirable food is also evident from the records of Matthew, Mark, and Luke. Each of these early writers testifies that he fed a multitude of people with five loaves and two fish. Luke tells of the resurrected Lord eating a piece of broiled fish and a honeycomb.[17] John records that the Master gave fish and bread that had been prepared in a fire of coals to Peter and the other disciples who had gone fishing after his death and surrection.[18]

Since God knows the flesh of fish to be a common food eaten and served by his Son and did not advise its limited use as a flesh food, it is apparent that no such limitation was necessary either to bring his followers good health or to please him by showing their intent to feed all mankind adequately. There is always the imperative that all food be used with prudence so that a disproportionate amount of no one kind will be consumed; this limits the use of fish, as of all foods, to a reasonable place in the dietary.

Fish flesh *is* different from that of land animals. Its protein rates 80 on the World Health Organization utilization scale that places the average for meats at 67 out of 100.[19] The fattest of fish (among them some herring, chinook salmon, and lake trout) have only enough fat to compare with the lean that can be separated from the fat of beef and pork.[20]

Fish fat is much less saturated than the fat of other animals and even of vegetable oils. The vegetables that provide polyunsaturated fatty acids usually have two double bonds per molecule with which to react with other nutrients in the body. Many of the polyunsaturates of fish have five or six such bonds. In addition, fish have supplies of vitamin B_6, needed for metabolizing both protein and cholesterol, generally more generous than those of land animals, and require less cooking time so less of the B_6 is destroyed.[21]

All fish have about 0.5 percent of their fat in the form of phospholipids. These are substances, including lecithin, that emulsify fats and so assist in their transportation to and absorption into cells where they are needed instead of allowing them to be deposited on vessel walls where they do damage.

Fish is the only food known to contain sizable amounts of the highly unsaturated fatty acid, docosahexaenoic acid, which recent research has indicated may be needed to prevent multiple sclerosis. Most people make the amounts needed in nervous system tissues from other dietary fats, but some lack the necessary enzyme to produce it and must have it preformed in their diets.[22]

Fish store much of their fat in their livers. For example the liver of cod is approximately 10 percent of the wight of the fish and 50 to 80 percent oil. The liver oil is largely triglycerides, not PUFA, and is generally rich in vitamins A and D.

The tail part of the fish may be only 30 to 60 percent as fat as that approaching the head. Dark colored flesh is generally fatter than light, stronger flavored and may become rancid more quickly in frozen storage so has a limited storage period.[23]

As for feeding the world, fish are very different from land animals and fowls. In their natural habitat in oceans, lakes, and streams, fish do not use primary foods. Fish culture as promoted by the FAO/WHO of the United Nations requires only sunlight and some inorganic fertilizer to encourage the growth of plankton and algae to produce food for the fish.

Although supplies of fish are not unlimited and require skillful management to maintain, since fish eat foods that man does not ordinarily use, to refrain from eating them does not release primary foods to benefit the hungry. On the other hand, an increase in the use of fish could assist greatly in alleviating hunger by providing needed protein, both for those who are now without adequate food supplies and for those who choose to share the primary foods available to them with people instead of animals.

An increased harvest of the sea is considered possible as well as desirable. With present technology and proper management, we could harvest up to two billion tons of sea plants and animals without depleting the source of supply. Our 1969 harvest totaled about 63.1 million tons.[24]

Knowing all of this, the Lord called us to be concerned about the needs of the world's people before they became crucial. He asked us to express this concern by sparing use of those foods that take a disproportionate share of the world's resources in production and by fasting from their use a part of every year, not only to conserve food but to remind us and our children of the necessity of finding a way to feed all of mankind and of our calling to be the genesis of that way. Fish may well help provide necessary protein and needed variety to our diets as we follow the counsel and will of our Father.

Word of Wisdom Provision for Special Needs

There is a specific provision for our use of meats in time of excess of hunger. Some have thought this means that when a man works hard or an athlete has a race to run or a game to play, he should have lots of meats. Such is not the case. Protein needs are linked with the size of the body and the demands made on it for growth and repair.[25] For work, one needs calories coupled with the nutrients needed to use them—especially some of the B vitamins. Recent research indicates that carbohydrates—not proteins—are linked with endurance.[26]

Some people are hungriest, however, when they have little desire to eat. This is the situation in some anemias when there is little or no appetite for food although it is urgently needed. Liver holds the richest known food supply of nutrients needed for the restoration of health. When meat carries the nutrients needed in the form most acceptable to such an individual with an excess of hunger, the Lord has provided for its use.

The same is true when other foods are not available from any of a number of circumstances. If it is a famine that precipitates the situation, it is wisdom, as Professor Frank Pearson, Cornell U., Ithaca, N.Y., has indicated,[27] to eat the livestock before they become decimated with hunger and then to eat the foods they would have eaten had they lived.

Because we largely failed in our mission to find a way to feed the world, God has called on others, including the FAO, to bring about the solution to world hunger. Even many of the new youth culture see the need and dramatize it in ways, some of which are injurious to themselves and to their children.[28]

Validity of Word of Wisdom Instructions

Following the Lord's instructions is injurious to no one. To use the flesh of fowls and beasts sparingly is sound nutritional advice.

To fast from them part of every year is in no way harmful if use is made of other good protein foods. Here are some of the reasons:

(1) Flesh foods are good protein but are not the best. Eggs hold that favored position with milk second, fish third, and meats fourth at best. (See WHO chart in Cereals chapter.) The relative values of these and other proteins were discovered during World War II in the search for a protein food that could be included in lifeboat rations of allied air- and seaman who were likely to be stranded on the ocean for long periods of time without adequate water.

Meat in any diet requires water to flush away the products of protein metabolism, and fresh water supplies were limited on lifeboats. Protein wastes cannot be handled by the kidneys unless properly diluted. Neither can salt, and sea water is too salty for the kidneys (drinking it just increases the need for additional water). Consequently meat protein could not be used on lifeboat rations.

Protein metabolism is always going on in the body, however. If one is fasting, the body first uses reserves in muscle and blood then tears down its own tissue for use, and some wastes from the process must be excreted even if no food is eaten. Investigators fasted rats to determine the level of excretion without dietary protein. Then they added rations with different proteins included. As was expected, when meats were added, the protein wastes in the urine increased. When they tried eggs, however, they were delighted to find that the wastes dropped far below the amount discarded when the animals were fasting.

When it was demonstrated that human subjects reacted in the same way, eggs were added to survival rations, bringing greater satisfaction and health to unfortunate servicemen while reducing their need for water. Eggs became the standard by which we measure the efficiency with which proteins are used in the body. Soon we learned the value of milk, fish, and plant protein and the principle of supplementation (discussed in the chapter on cereals) which is the key to feeding the world.

(2) To use more protein than is needed is wasteful of our most expensive food and imposes a needless metabolic burden on our bodies. After our current need for amino acids is supplied, the rest of the protein is broken down. Most of the carbon,

hydrogen, and oxygen is remade into carbohydrates or fats to be used for energy or stored in the tissues as glycogen or fat. The nitrogen fractions of the molecule must be excreted. One form of such excretion is urea. Under some circumstances, and especially if the person is not drinking enough water, uric acid crystals are formed that may lodge in the tissues and cause problems. Gout and kidney damage are two forms these problems may take.

Generous quantities of protein are needed for safety, but excesses are at best wasteful and at worst dangerous. In recognition of this fact, the 1973 RDA* for the American reference adult male was reduced from 65 g to 56 g, and that for the adult reference female from 55 g to 46 g. The U.S.A. RDAs still provide for generous amounts of protein intended to cover variations in need and in the quality of food eaten. WHO recommendations are lower.

Using excessive amounts of protein also wastes calcium and vitamin B_6 it requires. Recent studies revealed persons with 47 grams protein in their diets retaining calcium in their bodies well. When the protein was raised to 95 grams, however, with the same amount of calcium present, hardly any of the calcium was retained at all. When the diet contained 142 grams protein the subjects were actually losing calcium even though they were still consuming the same amount as before.[29]

(3) Eating meats sparingly will leave a place in the diet for other needed foods that will not be obtained if the appetite is satisfied with meat. Recent dietary studies in the U.S.A. indicate that of adults between the ages of 20 and 34, men got five times as much high protein foods, except milk, as the daily food plan recommends but only one seventh of the green and yellow foods and one third of the vitamin C foods recommended. Women got three and one fourth times the recommended high protein foods, other than milk, that the food plan suggests, with as little of the vitamin C foods and the green and yellow ones as the men. The men did get the milk called for in the plan with a little to spare, but women failed to get enough to fill the recommendation.[30]

---

*Protein requirements are based on ideal body weight—0.8 grams/kilogram ideal weight. Pregnancy, lactation, and illness increase the need.

Unfortunately, the foods that get crowded out of these high meat diets are those most likely to contribute nutrients that would enrich health and increase the prime of life—calcium, vitamins A and C, folacin, and riboflavin, to name a few. No meat supplies calcium in appreciable amounts unless one uses the bones. Only liver offers vitamins A and C. No meat other than liver can support its own calories with vitamins B_1 and B_2. Folacin appears in meats in small amounts, but much of it is destroyed by cooking processes. Meat offers no fiber for the digestive tract. And the cost of meats is so high that there is just not enough money left for the purchase of needed fruits, vegetables, and milk. It is readily understandable that those who conduct nutrition studies in the U.S.A. consider that one reason for deficiencies noted is the great emphasis that has been placed on eating meat.[31]

(4) Eating meat sparingly reduces the amount of hard (saturated) fats in the diet. These fatty acids are thought to be harmful in large quantity, especially if the proportion of essential fatty acids is low.

Fats are needed in every diet—not only to provide energy, satiety, and flavor and to support and protect organs, prevent heat loss, and provide reserve energy, and flavor—important as these are—but for life itself. Without the essential fatty acids (once called vitamin F) and other lipids (fats and fat-like substances) with which they work, there can be no growth, reproduction, or healthy living tissue. Skin becomes rough and eczematous when they are in short supply, and kidneys often fail. Fats are necessary for many enzyme systems, in cell membranes, for the preparation and regulation of hormones, in maintaining blood vessel structure, in the production and use of energy, digestion, brain development, transmission of nerve impulses, and memory storage. Without compounds created from these fatty acids, the stomach does not secrete the proper digestive juices, the pancreas cannot function properly, pituitary hormones are not released as needed, and the smooth muscles cannot metabolize food available to them. Fat soluble vitamins are brought to the body, transported, stored, and used with fats. Fats are not to be eliminated from any diet.

On the other hand, excessive amounts of fats are apt to be

harmful. They slow digestion. In moderation this helps allay hunger, but extended delay can cause distress. They contribute to obesity because they are concentrated energy. One gram of fat provides nine Calories. By contrast, a gram of protein or carbohydrate provides only four. Fats can cause the intake of essential nutrients to be low by satisfying hunger quickly, especially since they rarely carry vitamins other than A, D, E, and K, and are free of minerals and fiber. They may lead to the accumulation of cholesterol and triglycerides in the bloodstream, especially if they are saturated fats. Although all of the data are not in, fats have been suspected of being a factor in the production of heart and circulatory disease[32] and colon-rectal cancer.[33]

The North American dietary is, for most people, very rich in fats. A reasonable proportion of fats for healthy hearts and optimum weight is thought to be close to 25 percent of the calories in the diet. Canadians and citizens of the U.S.A., Holland, Denmark, and New Zealand average 40 to 45 percent of their calories from fats. Many get more, for those included in the "average" who restrict their meat eating get far less. The Asian countries average only 10 percent of their calories from fat, and most Europeans get 10 to 25 percent of theirs from this source.[34]

Essential Fatty Acids

The essential fatty acids needed by adults can be synthesized by normally healthy people from one of the polyunsaturated fatty acids, linoleic. This acid is abundant in most, but not all, vegetable fats but scarce in animal products. Animal fat does provide arachidonic acid, which the body must have; this can also be made from the linoleic. Adults need from 1 to 2 percent of their calories from essential fatty acids. Infants need a minimum of 3 percent. Premature infants may need up to 4.5 percent.

For those living in affluent countries it is easy to obtain needed essential fatty acids. One tablespoon corn, cottonseed, or soybean oil provides about seven grams of the substance, offering 63 Calories—enough to supply the maximum need of a man using 3,000 Calories a day. Half a tablespoonful will supply his minimum need and is in the range of the need of most women. This is easily obtained in margarine, bakery products, or salad dressings, made with oils high in linoleic acid, and from nuts, fruits, and vegetables.

Some vegetable oils are not high in linoleic acid. Coconut oil, although frequently used to substitute for dairy products, is more saturated than the milk fat it replaces, and has only traces of the essential acid. Olive oil, frequently used in Southern European cuisine, is not highly saturated but has few polyunsaturates. Rapeseed oil, used for cooking and in the making of margarine in Canada and the Orient, is very low in both polyunsaturates and saturated fatty acids and is composed largely of long chain fatty acids whose effect on the body is not adequately understood.*

All animal fats carry arachidonic acid which can partially spare the linoleic. In animals, significant supplies of linoleic acid, however, are limited to pork and poultry. Beef has only traces of this essential nutrient. To get needed amounts of essential fatty acids from meats would require one to eat the skin of poultry and the visible fat of other meats. This is not generally the practice nor recommended for a people already eating an excess of fat. For those on marginal diets, however, in which the fat is needed for calories, there is a significant contribution of these essential fatty acids from animal fats.

Note this contrast between broiled bacon and vegetable oils high in PUFA as sources of linoleic acid needed by one consuming 2400 Calories daily:[35]

Source of Five Grams (45 Calories) Linoleic Acid

Food	Amount Required	Calories	Saturated Fatty Acids
Bacon, broiled	100 g (3½ oz.)	Over 600	17 g—153 Calories
Oils, Corn, soybean, cottonseed	10 g (⅓ oz.)**	Under 90	1-2.5 g—9-23 Calories

*One of the fatty acids in rape, erucic acid, was thought to be responsible for interfering with enzyme systems in rats causing fatty acid deposits and muscle damage to their hearts. New varieties with reduced erucic acid were introduced, and the term "canbra" applied to them. Unfortunately, laboratory animals fed the canbra (rape) oil also develop heart damage. In the American Medical Association's *Today's Health* for May 1971 concern was expressed for the continued use of these oils in foods. Since Canadian law does not require the listing of oils used in margarine, except to designate if vegetable, animal, or marine oils are used, to learn what oil is used in margarine there, it is necessary to write to the manufacturer.

**This amount equals ¾ of 1 tablespoonful.

In general, it is easier to get needed linoleic acid from seed oils than from animal sources. The following chart indicates the amount of fat that one purchases with some common foods, the proportion of that fat which is saturated (hard fat), and the proportion of the total fat that is the essential linoleic:[36]

Fats and Fatty Acids Found in Some Common Foods

Food	Percent Fat as Purchased by Weight	Proportion Saturated	Fatty Acids Ratio Linoleic to Total Fat
Coconut	35.3	85%	Traces
Beef, very lean*	10-12	1/2	Traces
Beef, regular	20-38	1/2	Traces
Pork, lean only	7.5-10.5	1/3	1 gram in 12
Pork, regular	25-33	1/3	1 gram in 12
Turkey and mature chicken	15-25	1/3	1 gram in 5-6
Chicken, young	5.0	2/5	1 gram in 5
Tuna, in vegetable oil	20.5	1/4	1 gram in 2.5
Tuna, in water	3-4	1/4-1/3	1 gram in 5
Soybeans, mature	17.7	1/6	1 gram in 2
Wheat, germ	10.9	1/5.5	1 gram in 2
Milk, whole	3.7	1/2	Traces

Fats Combined with Protein in Nature

Whatever protein one eats, it is almost certain that there will be fat included if the protein is from nature. Some animal proteins have an especially large amount of fat attached. From others it can be separated quite successfully. The accompanying chart indicates the amount of fat that accompanies one gram of protein in a number of foods and the number of fat Calories that come with 100 protein Calories in those foods:[37]

---

*Beef and milk have been produced experimentally with fewer saturated and more unsaturated fatty acids by feeding PUFA protected from the bacteria of the rumen by formaldehyde.

Protein-Fat Ratios in Common Foods

Food	Grams Fat per Gram Protein	Calories Fat per 100 Calories Protein
Bacon, lean, broiled crisp	2.5	560
Bologna	2.4	525
Weiners	2.2	495
Poultry, skin	1.0	225
Poultry, dark meat, skinned, roasted	0.23	52
Poultry, light meat,	0.11	25
Hamburger, regular, in casserole	1.2	270
Hamburger, regular, broiled	0.8	180
Hamburger, lean, broiled	0.5	113
Beef Roasts, no visible fat	0.5	113
Beef steak, broiled, no visible fat	0.2	45
Beef, lean pot roasts, no visible fat	0.2	45
Pork, roast, no visible fat	0.4	75
Ham, broiled, no visible fat	0.4	75
Milk, whole	1.0	225
Milk, skim	0.028	6.3
Eggs	0.8	180
Tuna, canned in oil - total	0.85	190
Tuna, canned in oil - drained	0.3	65
Tuna, canned in water	0.03	6.5
Salmon, king, canned (also mackerel)	0.7	159
Salmon, red, canned	0.46	104
Salmon, pink, canned	0.3	65
Salmon, king, baked or broiled	0.3	65
Mackerel, baked or broiled	0.3	65
Soybeans	0.5	113
Wheat, Hard	0.15	34
Wheat, Soft	0.2	45

Of the foods chosen for the chart, skimmed milk and tuna canned in water provide the lowest possible amount of fat for each unit of protein. Skinned light meat of roasted or broiled poultry ranks next with wheat followed by very lean pot roasts or broiled steaks with all visible fat removed next in line. While some fish and soybeans may have a little more fat for each unit of protein than these very lean meats, their fats, like those of the wheat, are far less saturated than those of the meats. Still other fish, like cod, are extremely low in fat.

Pork is generally thought of as being fatter than beef. Trimmed closely and baked or broiled as much pork is, however, it compares favorably with many forms of beef. Pork fat, like that of poultry, is far less saturated than beef fat and contains a higher proportion of the essential fatty acids.

Bacon and sausages of any derivation are extremely high in fat. Incidentally, both bologna and frankfurters made with cereal or cereal and milk solids have a little higher percentage of protein that those made with all meat. These "fillers" replace some of the fat. In purchasing, one needs to be aware that "all meat" does not mean "all *lean* meat." Fat is also meat.

Much poultry fat can easily be removed with the skin. This practice does, however, constitute a waste since the skin is also a good protein food ranking with broiled regular hamburger in fat-to-protein ratio. Using only white meat of the poultry also reduces the fat eaten. At the same time, one should be aware that the dark meat is nearly twice as rich in iron as the light and carries more vitamins B_1 and B_2. Light meat does have more niacin.

Cereal proteins in general have low fat ratios. Whole wheat has only one gram of fat for every five to seven grams protein. Of the fats present, over half are unsaturated, and over half of these are linoleic. The oil of wheat is also the richest known food source of vitamin E needed to support the polyunsaturated fatty acids in the diet.

Of the legumes, soybeans are perhaps the highest in fat with about equal calories of fat and protein in the intact bean. These fats are almost entirely unsaturated with three fourths of the unsaturated fats linoleic, however; and the protein content and quality is so high that soybeans have long been dubbed the "meat without bones" of the Orient. Many of the new textured soy products have nearly all of the oil removed.

Saturated Fatty Acids and Disease

Just how significant the saturated fatty acids are in the development of disease is not yet absolutely certain. For a long time they have been suspect in the development of heart and circulatory disease. Now they are being suspected, along with the absence of sufficient fiber in the diet, in the development of disease of the colon-rectum, including cancer, as was revealed in the chapter on cereals.

Diet began to be suspected in the development of colon-rectal cancer when it was noted that the disease was concentrated in areas in which large amounts of meats, especially beef, were eaten—Canada, the U.S.A., New Zealand—and rarely occurred in areas in which meat was scarce—Japan, Chile, several Latin American and African countries. Recently the suspicion seemed to be substantiated when it was found that Japanese who migrated to Hawaii some forty to fifty years ago and revised their diet to include more beef and fewer fish and vegetables had a colon-rectal cancer rate much higher than their relatives who remained in Japan. American Negroes, who once had rates for the disease far below that of their white neighbors, are contracting the disease at an increasing rate that has brought them nearly up to the rate of the whites as they have become more affluent and have adopted the eating practices of the affluent. Studies in Scotland, England, Denmark, Argentina, Uruguay, and New Zealand all support the thesis that associates the disease with heavy beef eating.

These studies have led Dr. John Berg of the National Cancer Institute (U.S.A.) to state, "There is now substantial evidence that beef consumption is a key factor in determining bowel cancer incidence."[38]

Dr. Ernest Wynder, president of the American Health Foundation, believes that it is the large amount of hard fats consumed in beef that causes the problem.[39] The products of such fat metabolism result in an intestinal bacterial flora that produces chemicals known to be carcinogenic (cancer producing). When these substances are in contact with the tissues for long periods of time, damage may occur. Whether it is the absence of fiber, the presence of hard fats, or a combination of the two that is associated with the problem, certainly increasing incidence of the disease in many areas of high meat (especially beef) consumption along with a highly refined diet indicates a need for a change of dietary patterns in these areas.

One of the changes that has already occurred is the trend toward the adoption of the view that polyunsaturated fatty acids should replace saturated ones in the diet if there are to be healthy hearts. Diets high in saturated fatty acids are frequently associated with high levels of cholesterol and triglycerides in the bloodstream, and these characteristics seem related to the development of heart and circulatory problems. It will be some time, however, before there are complete answers to all of the problems involved in settling on the diet most likely to aid in the control or prevention of heart disease.

Cholesterol

Although cholesterol has gained a bad reputation because of all of the emphasis that has been put on it with respect to heart disease and atherosclerosis, cholesterol is not bad. In fact, it is so essential a part of life processes that if it is not provided in the diet the liver, skin and/or other tissues have to produce it for our bodies to use. It is a necessary part of our digestive juices—especially the bile that helps digest fats. It is essential in the formation and functioning of nerve tissue, including our brains. It is the substance from which our bodies make vitamin D. It is a part of our bone marrow, liver, muscles, connective tissue, and sex hormones. Normal adults metabolize approximately 2 grams (2,000 mg) of the substance daily.[40]

Since the body synthesizes cholesterol, the cholesterol that is eaten is not solely responsible for the cholesterol that appears in the blood. And the body can make cholesterol from any fat, including the polyunsaturates, whether it comes from food or is prepared in the body from an excess of calories. In fact, the triglycerides formed from excess calories and being prepared for storage in the body may be as important as cholesterol to the health of heart and blood vessels.

There is no single cause for high cholesterol levels in the blood, and there has been no demonstration that high cholesterol levels actually cause either heart disease or atherosclerosis. They do seem to indicate the presence of a problem, however. It is generally thought—and recommended by the American Medical Association—that each person should learn his distinctive cholesterol level early in life and make necessary adjustments in life-style, diet, and activity if needed from time to time to keep it within range as he grows older.[41]

Many factors influence the way our bodies handle cholesterol. Heredity is an important one. Breast-fed children seem to have a better mechanism for utilizing it efficiently than those who are artificially fed. Obesity is associated with high blood levels of triglycerides and cholesterol. Caffeine elevates the blood level. Smoking, tension, disease factors, and exercise or lack of it all play a part.

Vitamin B_6, whether from food or bacterial synthesis in the intestines, plays a significant role in the metabolism of cholesterol in the tissues that require it instead of allowing it to circulate in the bloodstream where it can do damage.[42] Incidentally, the presence of large amounts of PUFA in the diet suppresses the intestinal synthesis of the vitamin.

Emulsifiers—the phospholipids which include lecithin—help transport the fat to tissues where it is needed. Some fatty foods such as eggs, soybeans, and liver provide lecithin, and the body synthesizes that which it needs in addition to dietary lecithin if the diet provides necessary raw materials—choline (one of the B vitamins found in cereals and meats), methionine (an amino acid especially abundant in eggs), inositol (a part of the phytate molecule released during the preparation of whole grain or by metabolism when there is vitamin B_6 present, or itself synthesized in the body). With the necessary dietary ingredients and normal body functioning, the body is equipped to keep the cholesterol and phospholipid content of the blood in balance.

Vitamin C is necessary for the conversion of cholesterol to bile acids needed for the digestion of fats, and is essential to the integrity of heart tissues and blood vessels (see vitamin C foods). Dietary fiber needs to be present to expedite the removal of the bile salts when they have finished their work. Pectin of fruits, some vegetables such as carrots, and guar gum from seaweed help to keep the cholesterol level under control. So also do green vegetables and onions. Sugar (sucrose) in the diet, for some reason still unknown, increases the cholesterol level of blood, while starches, as those in bread and potatoes, lower that level.

The amount of cholesterol eaten does affect the level of the substance in the blood, but to try to control that level simply by eliminating cholesterol from food is, as the American Medical Association cautioned a decade ago, foolish and futile and carries the risk that many good foods needed for health may be eliminated. The use of milk, for example, has decreased alarmingly during the past few years, at least partially due to an effort to avoid cholesterol. Actually, if the two cups of milk each day recommended for adults in the U.S.A. are taken as whole milk, only about 50 mg of cholesterol would be obtained from the milk. If the milk is skimmed, there is practically no cholesterol present.

Egg consumption has likewise fallen for the same reason. A large egg does provide from 250 to 300 mg cholesterol, but it also provides the best protein available, a number of essential vitamins and minerals in generous quantity, is one of the best sources of lecithin known, and is the best known source of methionine needed for the body to produce more lecithin. Dr. Roger Williams points out that in actual tests, giving a man the equivalent of 10½ eggs a day increased the amount of cholesterol circulating in the blood but did not increase the amount deposited in blood vessels where it could do damage. With rats, Dr. Williams notes, those given 10 percent of their diet in eggs (the equivalent of 2½ to 3 eggs a day for one needing from 1,800 to 2,400 Calories) lived longer than controls given what appeared to be an equally adequate diet.[43] This does not necessarily mean that one should eat three or four eggs a day. Even cholesterol restricted diets, however, usually recommend the use of some eggs, and the "prudent" diet designed to promote healthy hearts recommends seven eggs a week for children.[44]

Many who study the problems of diet and heart disease find the theory that dietary cholesterol causes heart disease is not borne out in population studies. Persons in northern India have a diet containing ten times as much fat, most of it animal fat, as those in southern India; yet southern India has a heart disease rate 15 times as high as northern India. The Masai tribe of Tanganyika have a diet heavy with milk, milk products, and meat, but the people have low blood cholesterol and little if any evidence of atherosclerotic disease. Eskimos, whose high animal fat diet has long been documented, began to experience problems with heart disease only after they adopted refined flour and sugar as staples of their diets. And prisoners of war have widespread fatty deposits in their arteries with little fat of any kind in their diets.

A June 1973 review of the evidence concerning diet and heart disease points out that no one really knows what normal or safe levels of either cholesterol or triglycerides are. In addition to reference to the situation among the Masai, the review refers to a "Farmington" study of 1,000 dietaries showing no correlation between consumption of animal fat or cholesterol and the presence of high cholesterol levels in blood or incidence of atherosclerosis. They do point out that 80 percent of those who suffer death or disability from these diseases demonstrate one or more of the risk factors—hyperlipidemia (high level of fats in the blood), high blood pressure, or cigarette smoking. They also find other factors of importance including personality type, occupation, obesity, heredity, and diabetes mellitus.[45]

At the USDA Agriculture Research Center, Beltsville, Maryland, rats of varying heredity were fed 25 percent of their diet as egg (high cholesterol). When the egg was combined with starch or glucose (a simple sugar that occurs naturally in fruits, also called dextrose) there was little change in blood cholesterol levels from that produced by the stock diet. When sugar (sucrose) was used with the egg, however, there was a marked rise in the cholesterol level. The rise was much greater in one strain of rats than in another, and the researchers concluded that the amount and kind of fat in the diet may not be as important in determining blood cholesterol levels as the kind of carbohydrate combined with it and the inheritance of the individual.[46]

Dr. John Judkin, Professor of Nutrition, University of London, England, has also found sugar consumption related to high cholesterol levels and heart disease. He has found those eating 110 g (about 4 ounces) sugar daily to be five times more likely to develop myocardial infarction (one type of heart disease) than those using 60 g (2-1/7 oz.). If the blood fat is already high, he finds the effect of sugar multiplied. Dr. Judkin points out that at the turn of the nineteenth century the average sugar consumption in England was in the order of 10 grams (about ⅓ oz.) daily. It gradually increased until 1900. Since then it has doubled until daily consumption now approximates 125 grams (about 4½ oz.) in the U.S.A. and more in Britain, with a third or more of the U.S.A. population eating in excess of 150 grams (5⅓ oz.) daily.[47]

Dr. Wilfrid Shute of the Shute Institute for Medical Research, London, Ontario, reminds us that the rise in the incidence of heart and circulatory ills in the U.S.A. and Canada has coincided with the depletion of many breads and cereals of the vitamin E that occurs in the whole grain. Dr. Roger Williams recognizes the possible involvement of a vitamin E deficiency, saying, "Vitamin E is an essential nutrient for our bodies, and there is no reason to doubt that its lack can be a basic cause of atherosclerosis and heart disease."[48] Others—many of whom have not tried the vitamin E therapy that Dr. Shute finds effective or have tried it with limited dosage—declare that vitamin E is not implicated in the problem.

Whether the dietary problems related to heart disease are with saturated fats, cholesterol, triglycerides, vitamin E, vitamin B_6, sugar, or whatever, eating the flesh of beasts and of fowls sparingly and heeding the scriptural injunction that it is not wise to eat much honey (sweet)[49] helps to put one in the position of eating what has been known as the "prudent" diet that has been demonstrated, at least with monkeys, to result in fewer damaged hearts. The "prudent" diet,[50] originated by the late Dr. Norman Jolliffe of New York's City Health Department, reduces hard fats in the diet, eliminates the "empty calories" (made empty by refinement of grains, sugar, and fats), and replaces the less nutritious foods with fish, skim milk, lean meats, whole grains, vegetables, and fruits. It restricts quantities to maintain normal weight and provides for exercise. It is, in short, similar to the U.S.A. Daily Food Plan interpreted by the Word of Wisdom.

Other Nutrients in Protein Foods

There are a number of nutrients other than proteins and fats for which the protein food group is included in the food plans of all nations. With the exception of vitamin B_{12} these nutrients, like protein, do not appear exclusively in animal foods nor is each of the protein foods an equally good source of each nutrient. To be sure that nothing is missing or in short supply, we should eat a variety of foods, including some from every food group designated by governments and the Lord.

Iron

We generally think of meats as containing rich supplies of iron. The content may vary, however, from 1 mg in 100 g (3½ oz.) of light meat of turkey to 2 mg for the same size serving of dark meat of turkey, to 2.7 mg for that much hamburger or ham, up to 6.5 mg for a similar serving of beef liver or 19.2 mg for that much pork liver. Whole wheat bread has nearly three times as much iron as the same weight of light turkey meat but does not approach the iron content of pork liver. Fish is generally low in iron, but mackerel ranks with eggs and dark meat of turkey in the mineral—just a little below hamburger and ham.

Iodine

On the other hand, seafoods are the only ones of the protein group likely to contain much iodine. Even fresh water fish are not a reliable source of this nutrient. Iodine is required by the thyroid gland for the production of thyroxine, the hormone which regulates many body functions, including the rate at which energy is used. Without sufficient thyroxine, the basal metabolism is slowed and the body tends to store fat. Goiters develop as the gland struggles to produce the required amount of the hormone.

A malfunctioning thyroid, whether from lack of iodine or some other cause, always affects mental, emotional, and physical health. The nerves, rate of heartbeat, and appetite are affected. In infants, cretinism—a serious defect in mental and physical development—occurs most often when the mother's diet lacks needed iodine. The child is squat and potbellied, its skin rough and dry, its face bloated (usually with flaring nostrils and thick lips). Cretins are usually passive and good-natured—but foolish Many never learn to walk or talk clearly and often have defective hearing. Fortunately, if the defect is noticed early enough in life, the administration of thyroxine can prevent permanent disability. Treatment must usually continue a lifetime.

In adults, especially women, myxedema may result from a malfunctioning thyroid. The disease is characterized by a special type of puffiness, especially of the face. They become very sensitive to cold. Their skin becomes dry, rough, and yellowish. They lose energy and sometimes their hair. Other symptoms can be detected by a doctor. If not treated, they become lethargic and mentally retarded. Once the disease develops, as with cretinism, treatment must usually continue for a lifetime.

While seafoods would help provide for the iodine need of

persons all over the world, they are not always available or regularly selected in dietaries. An alternate source of the mineral has been provided in many areas. Salt is iodized at a rate of 0.01 percent potassium iodide and offered as a cheap, generally well accepted source of the nutrient. Canada requires by law that all table salt be so fortified to protect Canadians from iodine deficiencies. The U.S.A. gives a choice of iodized or plain salt, and about half the people choose the plain, probably because they do not understand their need for the nutrient, especially in areas in which iodine is in short supply in the soils.

Although iodine deficiency diseases that were once rampant in the goiter belts of the U.S.A. and Canada have been reduced dramatically by the use of iodized salt, goiter is still one of the most prevalent nutritional deficiency diseases known in Austria, Northern India, South and Central America, Yugoslavia, and some areas of Africa, according to the World Health Organization. In one area of what was the African Congo, 54 percent of the people are reported to be goitrous, and according to FAO estimates there are 200,000,000 cases of simple goiter in the world.

Recommended Dietary Allowances for iodine were first set in 1968. For men the RDA is 140 micrograms a day, and for women up to 125 micrograms (with pregnant women requiring the largest amount). This quantity is obtained in a little over one third of a teaspoon of salt fortified at the level at which Canada and the U.S.A. fortify their salt.

There are a few cases in which iodized salt should not be used. Some skin disorders clear more readily without it, and some types of goiter not related to iodine deficiency respond to treatment better without it. Plain salt may make more crisp sauerkraut or pickles and may help canned green beans to retain their color. In other cases, however, unless seafoods are being eaten regularly or it is certain that the soil in which fruits and vegetables being consumed were grown is rich in the nutrient, iodized salt is a wise choice. Sea salt available from some markets is an uncertain source of the nutrient. Iodized salt is effective, reliable, and cheap.

B Vitamins

Meats are often thought of as especially rich in B vitamins. Liver is, and other meats have significant amounts of some of the B vitamins. Meats supply niacin (B_3) generously. A 100 g (3½ oz.) serving of hamburger offers as much niacin as 1½ tablespoons peanut butter or five ounces (140 g) whole wheat bread. Pork is rich in thiamin (B_1), but a 3½ oz. (100 g) serving of beef, chicken, or fish will give B_1 about equal to that present in a 1 oz. (28 g) slice of whole wheat bread, one large egg, one small tomato, or half an orange. Rich as pork is in thiamin, one cup of cooked green peas will about equal a 3½ oz. (100 g) serving of cured ham in the nutrient. Fresh cooked pork carries twice the B_1 as the cured, however. Other B vitamins occur in varying amounts in meats but rarely in sufficient amounts to care for body needs without supplementation—with the exception of vitamin B_{12}.

Vitamin B_{12}, as far as we know, is found only in animal foods. It is not synthesized by plants, man, or higher animals, yet it is found in milk, eggs, seafoods, and meats. Apparently it is produced by the bacteria and fungi that live by the millions in the soil and in the rumen and intestines of animals. From the rumen of some animals and/or intestines of others the vitamin enters the animal products. We have no other known food source of the vitamin except that some may adhere to vegetables grown in soil with high bacterial count if the plant is not thoroughly washed.

We need extremely small amounts of vitamin B_{12}. The RDA for all adults since 1973 has been only 3 micrograms (0.000003 g) with the exception of pregnant women, whose RDA has been set at 4 micrograms. The 1968 RDAs, the first that listed vitamin B_{12}, provided for twice the present adult RDA for all adults past 55 years of age. Either amount is so small that it cannot be seen without a powerful microscope, yet it is so important that without it there can be neither health of body or of mind.

Vitamin B_{12} is best known as the "extrinsic factor" needed to prevent irreparable degeneration of the nervous tissue of victims of pernicious anemia. It plays a significant role in the formation of all nucleic acid and is therefore needed in the formation of all cells. As with other nutrients, it never works alone. One of its most vital partners is folacin, found chiefly in plants.

Vitamin B_{12} was first discovered in 1948 in liver, which had been used for nearly a quarter of a century to save the lives of those with pernicious anemia. In this disease it is frequently not the lack of the vitamin in the diet but the absence of a substance (intrinsic factor) in the intestines of the victim that prevents the absorption of the vitamin into the bloodstream. For this reason, victims of the disease must frequently be treated by injection rather than by diet.

With pernicious anemia, mental problems may be the first sign of disease. These may vary from mild difficulty in remembering or concentrating to severe depression, agitation, hallucinations, manic or paranoid behavior. Persons affected may appear very like schizophrenics. Prompt treatment brings relief. Neglect can result in irreversible brain damage. Routine testing for B_{12} in the blood of all mental patients has been recommended to determine whether the problem may really be need for vitamin B_{12}.[51]

Vegetarians need to be particularly mindful of their need for B_{12}. Children are especially vulnerable. Their tongues get sore; they become weak, apathetic (uninterested in their surroundings); their skin becomes highly colored; nervous abnormalities and anemia may develop. Nerve tissues deteriorate in all age groups; and as has been noted in duscussing folacin, irreparable damage may occur before it is detected if the folacin supply is extremely high.

Dietary needs for vitamin B_{12} are easily filled by one who eats an omnivotous (mixed plant and animal) diet or an ova-vegetarian one (emphasis on plant food but including milk and eggs). Shellfish and organ meats, especially liver, are very rich in the substance. Milk and eggs used regularly contribute the vitamin generously. Muscle meats are less effective in filling the need, but contribute significantly. The amounts supplied by some typical foods are noted in the chart on page 126.

It is well to note that if textured proteins are used instead of animal proteins, they must be fortified with B_{12} or it will not be present.

Unlike other B vitamins, vitamin B_{12} is stored in the tissues for two or three years or more. It is not, then, necessary to have it daily; and deficiency disease from lack of it may be a long time in becoming manifest. New vegetarians should be aware of this lag in the development of disease from the absence of the nutrient in their diets.

While animal products are needed, as far as we know, to

Comparison of Food Sources of Vitamin B_{12} for Adult[52]

One Serving Food*	Micrograms B_{12}	Approximate Day's Need Filled
Beef liver	80.0 (allow 30% cooking loss)	10
Pork liver	32.0 (allow 30% cooking loss)	7
Beef muscle	1.4 (allow 30% cooking loss)	1/3
Pork muscle	.55 (allow 30% cooking loss)	1/8
Chicken muscle	.40 (allow 30% cooking loss)	1/11
Eggs	2.8 (allow 30% cooking loss)	1/2
Oysters	18.0 (allow 30% cooking loss)	4
Clams	98.0 (allow 30% cooking loss)	20
Trout	5.0 (allow 30% cooking loss)	1⅓
Mackerel (canned)	7.7	2½
Salmon (canned)	6.9	2
Tuna (canned)	2.2	3/4
Milk, pasteurized	.96	1/3
Milk, dry reconstituted	.96	1/3
Milk, evaporated diluted	.19	1/15
Yogurt	.26	1/12

provide vitamin B_{12}, it does not have to be from the flesh of beasts or of the fowls of the air. These can augment the supply when they are available during the times the Lord has specified for their use.

Beneficence of the Lord's Instruction for the Use of Animal Flesh

It is interesting that the Lord made provision for the use of the flesh of beasts, fowls, and wild land animals both in times

---

*One serving meat or fish is 3½ oz. (100 g).
 One serving egg equals two large eggs.
 One serving milk or yogurt equals 1 cup (240 ml).

of winter and of cold. Some have thought this a needless repetition. It is, however, a thoughtful provision of a loving Father who finds joy in the joy of his creation. Had the eating of these meats been limited to the time of cold, there would have been many in the world completely forbidden the pleasure of eating them. There is a season called winter, however, in every part of the world. It may never get cold, but it is a time the Lord has designated in which the fast may be broken.

This action on the part of the Lord is consistent with his revelation of his way with men:

> Inasmuch as ye do this the fullness of the earth is yours: the beasts of the fields, and the fowls of the air, and that which climbeth upon the trees, and walketh upon the earth; yea, and the herb, and the good things which come of the earth, whether for food or for raiment, or for houses or for barns, or for orchards, or for gardens, or for vineyards; yea, all things which come of the earth, in the season thereof, are made for the benefit and the use of man, both to please the eye, and to gladden the heart; yea, for food, and for raiment, for taste and for smell, to strengthen the body, and to enliven the soul.
>
> And it pleaseth God that he hath given all these things unto man; for unto this end were they made, to be used with judgment, not to excess, neither by extortion: and in nothing doth man offend God, or against none is his wrath kindled, save those who confess not his hand in all things, and obey not his commandments.[53]

There is no disposition on the part of the Lord to discipline or deprive us of any of the things that he made for us to enjoy. There is only concern that we use them in such a manner that they prove a blessing to all his creation.

---

1. Doctrine and Covenants 86:2b-c.
2. I Timothy 4:1-5.
3. Doctrine and Covenants 49:3d-f.
4. *Ibid.*, 86:2b-c.
5. *Ibid.*, 86:1b.
6. *Ibid.*, 26:1d.
7. Editorial, "Wheat and World Hunger," *Journal of the American Medical Association*, Vol. 136, Jan. 31, 1948, p. 330.
8. Daniel Grotta-Kurska, "Before You Say 'Baloney'...Here's What You Should Know About Vegetarianism," *Today's Health*, Oct. 1974, pp. 18-21, 73.
9. Willard W. Cochrane, *The World Food Problem—A Guarded Optimistic View*, T. Y. Crowell, 1969, pp. 36-37. Also Herbert L. Marx (Ed.), *World Food Crisis*, H. W. Wilson Co., N.Y., 1975, pp. 24, 45.
10. *Ibid.*, p. 44.
11. *Ibid.*, pp. 48-49.
12. G. I. Burch, "Population Reference Bulletin" contained in symposium edited by Clifford M. Hardin, *Overcoming World Hunger*, Prentice Hall, 1969, p. 50.
13. Cochrane, *op. cit.*, p. 63.
14. Burch, *op. cit.*, p. 46.
15. Doctrine and Covenants 49:3e-f.
16. I Cor. 15:39.
17. Luke 24:40-42.

18. John 21:1-13.
19. See chart of protein utilization in chapter on Cereals.
20. USDA, *Composition of Foods*, Agri. Handbook No. 8, by items.
21. USDA, *Pantothenic Acid, Vitamin B_6 and Vitamin B_{12} in Foods*, Home Economics Research Report No. 36, by item.
22. Maurice E. Stansby, U.S. Dept. of Commerce, Seattle, Washington, "Polyunsaturated Fatty Acids and Fat in Fish Flesh," *Journal of the American Dietetics Association*, Vol. 63, Dec. 1973, pp. 629-630.
23. *Ibid.*
24. E. R. Pariser, "The Potential, the Problems and the Status of Using Proteins of Aquatic Origin as Human Food," *Food Technology*, Vol. 25, Nov. 1971, p. 89. Extracted in *Journal of the American Dietetics Association*, Vol. 60, No. 2, Feb. 1972, p. 149.
25. National Academy of Sciences, *Recommended Dietary Allowances*, 8th Ed., 1974, p. 43.
26. Paul Slovic, Ph.D., "What Helps the Long Distance Runner Run?" *Nutrition Today*, Vol. 10, No. 3, 1975, pp. 18-21.
Also Harold Elrick, M.D., James Crakes, M.D., William Phillips, Ph.D., Alexander Leaf, M.D., Robert Vinton, M.D., "Indians Who Run 100 Miles on 1,500 Calories a Day," *The Physician and Sports Medicine*, Feb. 1976, pp. 38-42 (includes documentation).
27. Clifford M. Hardin, *Overcoming World Hunger*, Prentice Hall, 1969, p. 42.
28. Darla Erhard, R.D., M.P.H., "The New Vegetarians" and "A Starved Child of the New Vegetarians," *Nutrition Today*, Vol. 8, No. 6, Nov./Dec., 1973, pp. 4-12. Also "The New Vegetarians, Part II," *Nutrition Today*, Jan./Feb. 1974, pp. 20-27.
29. R. M. Walker, H. M. Linswiler, "Calcium Retention in Adult Human Males as Affected by Protein Intake," *J. of Nutrition*, Vol. 2, Sept. 1972, p. 1297. Abstract in *Journal of the American Dietetics Association*, Vol. 62, No. 2, Feb. 1973, p. 204.
30. Ronald M. Deutsch, *The Family Guide to Better Food and Better Health*, Creative Home Library in association with Better Homes and Gardens, Meredith Corporation, Des Moines, Ia., 1971, p. 12.
31. "Highlights from the Ten State Nutrition Survey," *Nutrition Today*, July/Aug. 1972, pp. 7-8.
32. L. Jean Bogert, and others, *Nutrition and Physical Fitness*, 9th Ed., W. B. Saunders Co., Phil. and London, 1973, p. 70.
33. "Diet, Intestinal Flora and Colon Cancer." *Nutrition Reviews*, Vol. 33, No. 5, May 1975, p. 136.
34. Bogert, *et. al.*, pp. 69-70.
35. "Selected Fatty Acids in Foods," USDA *Composition of Foods*, Agri. Handbook No. 8, pp. 122-145, by item.
36. *Ibid.*
37. USDA, *Composition of Foods*, Agri. Handbook No. 8, by item.
38. Jerry E. Bishop, "Cancer vs. What you Eat," *Science Digest*, Mar. 1974, pp. 10-14. Also Nicholas Gonzalez, "Preventing Cancer," *Family Health/Today's Health*, May 1976, p. 33.
39. *Ibid.*
40. Bogert, *et. al.*, p. 69.
41. "Recommendations on Diet and Coronary Heart Disease" (from a joint statement of the Food and Nutrition Board NAS/NRC, and the AMA Council on Foods and Nutrition), *Nutrition Today*, July/Aug., 1972, p. 21.
42. Roger J. Williams, *Nutrition Against Disease*, Pitman Pub. Corp., N.Y., Toronto, London, Tel Aviv, 1971, pp. 79 and 249-250.
43. Williams, *ibid.*, pp. 68-69.
44. Kurt A. Oster, M.D., "In Answer to Your Letters," *Medical Counterpoint*, Nov. 1974, p. 42.
45. Robert E. Shank, M.D., "Status of Nutrition in Cardiovascular Disease," *Journal of the American Dietetics Association*, Vol. 62, June 1973, pp. 611-616.
46. USDA Agricultural Research Center Publication No. 341, *Toward the New*, Apr. 1970, pp. 12-14.
47. John Judkin, M.D., "Sucrose and Heart Disease," *Nutrition Today*, Spring 1969, pp. 16-20. Also "More About Sucrose and Atherosclerosis" (Dr. Judkin's reply to criticisms), *Nutrition Today*, Autumn 1970, p. 15. Also Williams, *op. cit.*, p. 85, with documentation of three Judkin papers on page 264.
48. Williams, *op. cit.*, p. 75 (with references to literature, pp. 242-244).
49. Proverbs 25:27.
50. Williams, *op. cit.*, pp. 261-262 (with references).
51. R. J. Hart, Jr., P. R. McCurdy, "Psychosis in Vitamin B_{12} Deficiency," *Archives of Internal Medicine*, Vol. 128, Oct. 1971, p. 596, abstract, *Journal of the American Dietetics Association*, Vol. 60, Jan. 1972, p. 57.
52. USDA, *Pantothenic Acid, Vitamin B_6 and Vitamin B_{12} in Foods*, Home Economics Research Report No. 36, by item.
53. Doctrine and Covenants 59:4b-5b.

CHAPTER 6

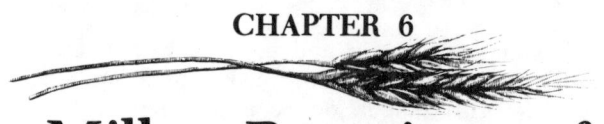

Milk, a Repository of Nutrients

And I hold forth and deign to give unto you greater riches, even a land of promise; a land flowing with milk and honey, upon which there shall be no curse when the Lord cometh....—Doctrine and Covenants 38:4d-e.

Although it was not mentioned in the Word of Wisdom, milk was obviously intended for the use of man. Though not an essential food in the sense that man cannot live without it, it is one of nature's marvels in providing essential nutrients economically. For this reason it has been set apart as a separate food group by Canada, the U.S.A., and a number of other nations, and its daily use is recommended for most people.

Of the vast number of nutrients available in milk, at least four are particularly significant:

(1) Vitamin B_{12} has already been discussed. Mention need only be made here that each cupful of milk which has not received severe heat treatment provides about one-third the RDA of the vitamin for most people. Evaporated milk and that made into yogurt have each lost much of their potency in the vitamin. Pasteurizing or drying milk does not affect it significantly.

(2) Protein of milk, as previously noted, is complete, of high biological value, and may be obtained almost completely free of fat when that seems desirable. One U.S.A. quart (0.95 liter) provides 36 grams of protein—more than the minimum daily requirement of adult males weighing 70 kg (154 pounds), and more than two thirds of the most generous RDA for the highest demand groups of reference size, except pregnant and lactating mothers (and even these can get more than half their RDA from this quantity of milk alone).[1] It has the additional value of complementing plant protein in the diet, making the total protein of high biological value.

Both as a complete protein and as a complement for plant protein, milk is one of our most economical protein foods. At present prices in Canada one can purchase this excellent protein in the form of whole, pasteurized milk at slightly over half the cost of an equal quantity of protein as regular hamburger. As nonfat dry milk, the protein may be had for less than one-fourth the cost of hamburger protein.

(3) Riboflavin, vitamin B_2, is necessary if children are to develop normally before or after birth, and if persons of any age are to see, have healthy skin, and metabolize food properly. When there is not enough of it available, one of the first symptoms noticed may be an extreme sensitivity to light. Dark glasses may become a necessity, and the eyes become bloodshot, itch, burn, and feel sandy. (The bloodshot eyes of an alcoholic are at least partially attributable to a riboflavin deficiency created by the consumption of many calories of alcohol without the necessary B vitamins, including riboflavin, to metabolize them.) Scaly, greasy cracks form at the angles of the mouth and at the edge of the nostrils as the deficiency persists, wounds will not heal, stamina and resistance to disease are lowered, nervous disorders similar to those associated with other B vitamin deficiencies appear.

In experimental animals, if riboflavin is removed during the time the fetus is forming, the young are often born with deformities that include cleft palate, club feet, receding lower jaws, misplaced or incomplete organs and open abdominal cavities. Just how much riboflavin deficiency affects human pregnancies can only be conjectured, but we do know that congenital malformations occur much more frequently in children born to mothers whose diets are inadequate or in whom there is interference with the utilization of the nutrients by the intervention of drugs or other environmental factors (see chapter on Well Born Children).[2]

It is recommended that we have 0.6 mg riboflavin for every 1,000 Calories we consume. One liter (1.06 U.S.A. quarts) of milk will fill the need of those eating up to 3,000 Calories. So, also, will a small serving (56g—2oz.) of liver; but to get that amount from muscle meats would require about eight servings, 3½ oz. (100g) each. From broccoli or kale, two of the green vegetables richest in the substance, it would likewise require eight similar servings. From other vegetables, it would require twice that much or more. Currently milk provides approximately 45 percent of the riboflavin of the American dietary. For those who use no milk, there should be added portions of liver, legumes, eggs, green vegetables, enriched or fortified cereals or supplements to fill the need.[3]

As with all water soluble nutrients, vitamin B_2 must be carefully preserved in food preparation. The iridescent substance will be found in cooking liquids, whey from cheese making, and in the drippings of meats. Cooking temperatures have little effect on it, but the addition of soda is destructive. It is particularly sensitive to light. Milk delivered in clear bottles and allowed to stand on the doorstep in sunlight for one hour will lose up to one half its B_2. In two hours, it will have lost up to three fourths its supply. Even in lighted display cases, milk needs the protection of opaque containers or those treated to turn back light rays. Delivered at home, milk needs a dark, insulated container until it can be refrigerated. Served on a sunlit table, it needs protection from the light.[4]

Because whey is discarded in cheese making, cheese is a variable source of riboflavin. Cottage cheese retains about half its vitamin B_2. Cheddar cheese retains some more. Fortunately, the whey is now being utilized in a number of food products, including a nutritious soft drink now becoming popular in some areas of the world. Its use represents good ecological stewardship as it prevents wastage of essential nutrients while relieving the basic hungers of the world.

(4) Calcium accounts for a larger portion of the body weight than any other mineral except water, which is rarely thought of as a mineral but which fits the chemical definition. Most of the weight is in the teeth and bones, but very essential amounts of the mineral are dissolved in body fluids where its presence is necessary to life itself. It works on a team that includes phosphorus, with which it must always be in balance for good health, vitamins D and C, magnesium, flourine, protein, and others.

Without calcium, there can be no reproduction or growth. Cell membranes must have the proper calcium balance to allow nutrients and wastes to pass through them. Without this process of feeding tissues and eliminating wastes, there can be no life.

Nerve impulses do not pass through the body without calcium.

Muscles cannot contract and extend properly without it, and deficiencies are manifest in calcium tetany—cramps in legs, toes, and other muscles. The most important muscle of the body requires it, for the rhythm of the heartbeat depends on the presence of adequate amounts of calcium. Blood will not clot without it.[5]

Tooth and bone development and maintenance require calcium. This fact is well understood with respect to children, but few realize how significant it is for adults. This lack of understanding has led to an unjustifiable reduction of milk and other high calcium foods in the diets of older youth and adults.

Children who have inadequate supplies of calcium and/or its teammates frequently develop rickets. Legs become bowed, backs hunched, ribs have knobs down the chest characterized as rachitic rosary, teeth are underdeveloped, malformed, and decay easily.

Rickets does not occur in adults for the bones and teeth are no longer growing, but the tissues are not static. They form the storehouse for calcium from which the body draws calcium for use in blood, nerves, and muscles daily. If there is not sufficient calcium to replace that withdrawn, disease results.[6]

Osteoporosis, a condition in which the bones lose their mass or density, occurs in many adults, especially women.[7] As the bone deteriorates, losing strength and elasticity, there is pain in the lower back and ribs, bones break easily, and for many there is collapse of bony structures that leaves them stooped—often with loss of inches in height. After the age of forty, there is loss of bone material that averages 3 percent per decade for men but a more critical 8 percent per decade for women unless special care is taken to prevent it. The incidence of hip fractures in women doubles with each five years of life over fifty unless this team of nutrients is supplied generously. It is women who most frequently bend with age when 30 to 50 percent of the calcium is gone from their bones.[8] Studies at Iowa State University years ago showed that women past fifty still need calcium equivalent to that contained in three cupfuls (720 ml) milk daily to keep in calcium balance, assuming they have a moderate intake of protein and other favorable dietary factors. Those who want to remain healthy and delay or obviate this disease of aging will find milk consumption one of the easiest ways to provide the nutrients needed to do it.

Osteomalacia is also prevalent in many areas of the world, especially in areas of low calcium intake in which conditions of weather, living habits, or dress shield bodies from the sun. In this disease, bones soften with accompanying pain, tenderness, muscle weakness, loss of appetite, and loss of weight.[9]

In every age, there is tooth and gum disease that accompanies poor calcium nutrition. Problems with the formation of the dentin and the enamel of the teeth begin before birth and extend into childhood for the calcium-poor infant. The problems are increased for the premature, who are born with less than half the calcium of the full-term children and suffer more malformations as a result unless this need is properly filled. Decay and gum disease continue to plague the calcium deprived through childhood and adult life.[10]

Other Needs for Good Calcium Nutrition

Manifestations of poor calcium nutrition do not always denote a simple lack of calcium. There may be plenty present, but it may be unavailable because there are insufficient amounts or excesses of other members of the calcium nutrition team.

To assure sufficient vitamin D for good calcium nutrition, much milk—fresh, dry, and evaporated—is fortified with the nutrient. If fortified milk is not used and the body is not regularly exposed to the sun for the formation of vitamin D by the skin, some other source of the vitamin is imperative. With present practices of fortifying many foods with vitamin D, wearing skimpy clothing, and using supplements freely, however, it is necessary to warn against having too much of the nutrient in the body.[11] Left on its own, the body can regulate the amount it makes by darkening the skin, but it cannot adjust to excessive amounts in dietary or supplemental form without damage. It reacts by drawing calcium and phosphorus from the bones, circulating them in the blood, and excreting valuable supplies of these minerals in the urine. Some of the circulating mineral is taken up in soft tissues, including kidneys and blood vessels. In children the skin becomes loose and dry, the legs tremble, there is loss of muscle tone, and eventually the heart and kidneys become affected. Adults lose their appetites, develop gastrointestinal disturbances, pain in the head and joints, and muscular weakness. Death sometimes occurs from kidney failure. Special care must be taken by pregnant mothers whose own accumulated dose may not be critical for their tissues but may be too much for their developing infant.[12]

The Recommended Dietary Allowance of vitamin D for all ages is 400 IU. Children in England now easily get 1,200 IU per day from food alone. Their Canadian and U.S.A. counterparts may easily get 2,000 IU per day. When overanxious parents add supplements to these foods, intake could become critical.

Phosphorus must also be kept in balance with the calcium. One prevalent problem is that the consumption of large amounts of meat teamed with soft drinks high in phosphoric acid, as cola beverages are, with low calcium intake results in an excess of phosphorus. With this imbalance, calcium cannot be retained in the tissues and much is excreted in the urine, producing calcium deficiencies with all the problems that accompany such a state. On the other hand, large supplements of calcium without attention to balancing them with team minerals can result in serious deficiencies of phosphorus and magnesium and other minerals. Milk provides phosphorus at a rate of about 80 mg to every 100 mg calcium. In a well balanced diet of milk, whole grains, and meats additional phosphorus is easily supplied to provide about equal amounts of the two minerals, as the RDAs suggest.

Protein, too, must be kept in moderate supply in the dietary of one who hopes to maintain good calcium nutrition. Excesses prevent retention and utilization of the nutrient (see preceding chapter, reference 29).

Other Sources of Dietary Calcium

Milk does not have to be drunk. It can be used in cream soups, milk puddings and custards, ice cream, ice milk, yogurt, or cheese. One does need to be aware that they are not all equally valuable, however.

Some cheeses, for example, lose a lot of calcium along with the riboflavin in the whey. One hundred Calories worth of skim milk will provide 340 mg calcium, while 100 Calories worth of cottage cheese made from skim milk has only 100 mg of the calcium left. A teen-ager wanting to fill his calcium need from cottage cheese would have to eat eight cupfuls (1,920 ml)— almost 3½ pounds (1,600 g) a day. That would drastically reduce the variety of foods available for the day and be extremely wasteful of protein.[13]

Cheddar cheese retains more of its calcium than cottage cheese does, so that for every 100 Calories worth of cheddar there are approximately 190 mg of calcium. Processed cheeses generally have less calcium than cheddar. Processed cheese foods may have much less. The percentage of water listed on their label may help give some hint as to the amount of cheese actually present.

If milk or milk products are not chosen or are not available, bones may provide dietary calcium. In some cultures they are prepared by softening in food acids, such as vinegar, and added to other foods. Some use bone-meal as a supplement. Fish bones are particularly likely to be used in developing countries as whole fish is processed into fish meal used to fortify local foodstuffs. Fish bones are even available in the U.S.A. and Canada in canned fish, in the processing of which the bones are softened so their presence is hardly noticeable. For best nutrition they should not be removed from the canned fish before serving.

Dark, green leafy vegetables, when included in a well balanced diet, contribute to good calcium nutrition. Used alone, however, they are hardly adequate. It would take a pound and a half (0.68 kg) or more of the richest ones we know to provide calcium equivalent to that contained in one liter of milk.

In addition to the major contribution that milk makes to the diet in protein, riboflavin, calcium, and vitamin B_{12}, it makes significant offerings of a number of other RDA nutrients—vitamin B_6, folacin, and vitamin A to name a few. Of the 2.0 mg vitamin B_6 recommended for daily use by most adults, each cupful (240 ml) of fresh pasteurized or reconstituted dry milk provides about one eighth (0.24 mg). Evaporated milk has the B_6 content reduced by about one third. Of the 400 micrograms folacin required by nonpregnant, nonlactating adults, one cupful of milk provides nearly a tenth. Similarly, a cupful of whole milk provides about one ninth of the RDA of vitamin A for most adult women—but only if the cream is left in. Without the cream, there are no fat soluble vitamins —A, D, E—left in the milk unless it is fortified with them.

It should be noted also that for best absorption and utilization of calcium, some fat is needed. For adults this may be provided by butter or margarine or some other source of fat in the meal.

For infant and early childhood feeding, however, skim milk is inadequate and may be dangerous. The danger is two-fold: (1) because of lack of needed vitamins and essential fatty acids, and (2) the resultant high sugar content of the diet may be harmful.

Other Forms of Milk and Imitation Milk

Several terms used in the marketing of milk or milk substitutes may need clarification:

Two percent milk, often thought to have only half the Calories of whole milk, actually has only 13 to 30 Calories less per cupful (240 ml). With all of the cream removed, skim milk has only half the Calories of whole milk. Two percent milk has less than half the fat removed. (The average fat content of whole milk in the U.S.A. and Canada is 3.7 percent.) This leaves about 130 Calories per cupful of the 160 Calories originally there. With the cream gone, however, the milk loses "body," or a feel of richness. To improve the body, dry skim milk powder is often added. This has the advantage of adding protein, calcium, and other nutrients but also adds Calories that return the Calorie count to about 147 per cup or higher. This may be labeled "modified milk" or "with milk solids added."

Filled milk is skim milk with vegetable fat added. This additive is usually highly saturated coconut oil which is far more saturated than the cream that was removed.

Imitation milk is really not milk at all. It consists basically of water, sugar, vegetable fat (often a highly saturated one), sodium caseinate or isolated soy protein, artificial flavors and stabilizers. In no way does it equal milk nutritionally. All of the nutrients for which the use of milk is recommended are either missing entirely or present in inferior amounts and of inferior quality. While not on the market in Canada except as coffee whiteners or "creamers," it is on the U.S.A. market and often chosen by those who feel they are getting a bargain milk. Nutritionally it is no bargain!

Coffee whiteners or "creamers" are not the nutritional equivalents of milk or cream. The ingredients of a popular one are corn syrup solids, vegetable fat (usually coconut oil), sodium caseinate, dipotassium phosphate, emulsifiers, sodium silico-aluminate, and artificial flavor and colors. The product is advertised as having only 11 Calories per level teaspoonful (5 ml).

By contrast, dry skim milk has only five Calories in that amount of powder, and dry whole milk has only 11.

Whipped toppings rarely contain milk, although some do contain whey. Their fat is hydrogenated vegetable oil—often coconut oil made even more saturated by hydrogenation. They are far more saturated than cream and have the additional disadvantage of being almost entirely without the fat soluble vitamins A and D of the cream. They do decorate desserts with fewer Calories than the real thing. Whipped cream has about 25 Calories per tablespoonful (15 ml); whipped topping contains less than half that many. (There are some real cream toppings available with Calories and nutrients similar to home prepared whipped cream.)

Dry skim milk is easily made into a whipped topping that is low Calorie and inexpensive. It contains all of the nutrients of skim milk, no questionable additives except sugar (or honey), and no fat at all. It is little more trouble than mixing up an expensive one, and the product is tasty and stands up for hours. Here's how:

Fluffy Topping Recipe

Soften ½ tsp. (2½ml) plain gelatin in 1 Tbsp. (15 ml) cool water.
Melt the softened gelatin in 3 Tbsp. (45 ml) boiling water.
Add ¼ cup slush ice or very cold water and cool, but do not allow to set.
Add ½ cup (120 ml) dry, instant non-fat milk.
Beat at high speed until mixture stands in peaks.
Add slowly while beating, 2 Tbsp. (30 ml) sugar or honey (3 Tbsp. for very sweet).
Beat until thick.
Yields about 2½ cups, 9 to 10 Calories per tablespoonful (15 ml), and costs (at present prices) 8 to 9¢ a recipe.
(Note: tsp. = teaspoon. Tbsp. = tablespoon.)

The U.S.A. Department of Agriculture has warned the public that filled and/or imitation milk are not the nutritional equivalents of dairy milk and contain higher percentages of saturated fatty acids than milk from a cow.[14]

The Academy of Pediatrics Committee on Nutrition has warned parents not to substitute filled milk, imitation milk, or coffee whiteners for infant feeding, and has urged caution in using these products in feeding older children.[15] While filled milk does have all of the nutrients of skim milk, the others are inferior in all nutrients and cannot be considered a suitable replacement for milk in anybody's diet regardless of age. Coffee whiteners are especially low in protein, high in sodium, and lacking in other essential nutrients.

Lactose Intolerance

In recent years there has developed a supposition that milk should not be included in the dietaries of older children and adults of some, especially darkskinned, peoples because of a condition known as lactose intolerance. The milk sugar (lactose) is not properly digested, and may cause diarrhea, stomach pains, gas formation, or bloating. The problem is that there is a deficiency in the enzyme (lactase) needed to digest the sugar.

After careful study of the populations involved, the United Nation's committee studying the protein needs of these people has determined that there is good reason *not* to reduce the milk offered to these populations. Other nutrients of milk are valuable enough to justify modifications of the lactose, if necessary, to make it possible to use the milk without distress.

All people are born with the enzyme, lactase. It appears that 60 to 90 percent of non-Caucasian people (5 to 15 percent of the Caucasian) lose some of their lactase activity as they grow older. It is not clear whether this decrease may be associated with the practice of eliminating milk from the diet after weaning. It is clear, however, that there is still enough lactase activity in almost all people to utilize moderate amounts of milk—quantities of a pint (0.47 liter) or more at a time.[16]

Experience has shown that if milk is introduced gradually to those unaccustomed to it since weaning, there is rarely any problem with it. For those who do have some difficulty, the use of cultured forms like buttermilk or yogurt, in which lactose content has been reduced by bacterial action, makes the valuable nutrients of milk available without distress. Yeast lactase is also being utilized to reduce 90 percent of the lactose of regular milk to glucose and galactose without changing the flavor of the milk except to make it sweeter. Milk and whey so treated may then be used in fluid, concentrated, or dry form without causing discomfort.

Finally

Fortunate indeed are those people to whom milk is available in quantity. The nutrients the milk can supply contribute significantly to making good nutrition readily attainable. For those without it, by necessity or by choice, a real effort is required to supply the essential nutrients that milk supplies with ease.

---

1. National Academy of Sciences, *Recommended Dietary Allowances*, Eighth Edition, 1974, RDA Chart, and USDA *Composition of Foods*, Agriculture Handbook No. 8, 1963, by item.
2. L. Jean Bogert, George M. Briggs, Doris Howes Calloway, *Nutrition and Physical Fitness*, Ninth Edition, W. B. Saunders Co., Philadelphia, London, Toronto, 1973, pp. 128-131. For specific documentation see also "Dietary Causes of Congenital Abnormalities," *Borden's Review of Nutrition Research*, Vol. 5, No. 9, Nov. 1944, and "Clinical Studies on Prenatal Nutrition," *ibid.*, No. 10, Dec. 1944.
3. Bogert, *et al., op. cit.*, p. 245, and National Academy of Sciences, *op. cit.*, and USDA, *op. cit.*
4. Bogert, *et al., op. cit.*, pp. 132-133.
5. *Ibid.*, pp. 239-240.
6. *Ibid.*, pp. 240-241.
7. *Ibid.*, p. 243.
8. L. Earle Arnow, *Food Power, A Doctor's Guide to Commonsense Nutrition*, Nelson-Hall Co., Chicago, 1972, pp. 142-143.
9. Bogert, *et al., op. cit.*, p. 243, and *Dorland's Illustrated Medical Dictionary* by topic.
10. "Calcium Deficiency, Periodontal Disease and Loss of Teeth," *Journal of the American Dietetics Association*, Vol. 60, June 1972, p. 477.
11. Bogert, *et al., op. cit.*, 210. Also "New Requirement for Nutritional Content of White Bread," *Journal of the American Dietetics Association*, Vol. 60, Feb. 1972, p. 170.
12. Bogert, *et al., op. cit.*, p. 277. Also Alton L. Blakeslee, "Today's Health News," *Today's Health*, Feb. 1967.
13. National Academy of Sciences, *op. cit.*, and USDA, *op. cit.* (Calculated).
14. USDA Agriculture Information Bulletin No. 341, *Toward the New*, April 1970, p. 16.
15. "Today's Health News," *Today's Health*, Sept. 1972.
16. "Milk Intolerances," *Nutrition Reviews*, Vol 34, No. 2, Feb. 1976, pp. 35-37.

CHAPTER 7

Weight Control

All these to be used with prudence and thanksgiving.—Doctrine and Covenants 86:1a.

The Lord's instruction that we eat all foods with prudence and thanksgiving is continually validated in twentieth century world food situations. While for many people, getting enough food to sustain life is of major concern, for others reducing food consumption to maintain a reasonable weight is a problem.

For some in affluent countries, "reducing" has become an obsession with status. It is fashionable to be "on a diet," even though surplus pounds are really nonexistent or never yield to dieting. "Diet" is a conversation piece for those who have little of consequence to talk about and an attention-getter for some wherever food is served.

For others the obsession is of more serious consequence. The need to lose weight constantly haunts them, threatens their peace of mind, affects their relations with family, friends, and environment. Many are neurotic in their search for a slim figure that will, they feel certain, bring them the love, affection, respect, and success which they have never achieved and which they believe they are missing only because of excess avoirdupois. Indeed, with sveltness the fashion, it could be that success may elude the obese. There are, however, many who are obsessed with reducing who are not obese. Some afflicted with *anorexia nervousa* actually starve themselves to death still believing they are fat.[1]

All people who do weigh more than the mythical "normal" are not obese. Many athletes and other physically active persons weigh more than charts indicate is ideal for them. Their weight is not in excess fat but in well-developed muscles. Although "overweight," they have no excess fat to reduce.[2]

There are many overweight, or more properly over-fat, people, however, who do need to shed excess poundage for the sake of health. This condition has been termed the most widespread nutritional problem afflicting Western civilizations. A correlation has been shown between obesity and heart and circulatory disease, diabetes, high blood pressure, gall bladder malfunctioning, some forms of kidney and digestive diseases, and accidents. Certainly it is more painful for an obese arthritic to function than for one with less weight on sore joints. Some cancer seems to affect the obese more frequently than those of normal physique. Obesity makes one uncomfortable, less agile, and more susceptible to problems both of a social and physical nature.

Many times overweight is referred to as "overnutrition." This term is frequently inappropriate. Overweight is not always found in the upper economic strata of any nation nor among the well fed. Even nations with limited food supplies have their share of obesity, and frequently it is the very poor who are obese. Foods high in carbohydrates may be the only foods available to the poor or may be the ones chosen by the poorly informed. Efforts to satisfy hunger without adequate amounts of protein or fat can lead to the consumption of excess carbohydrates, which do stimulate fat production. At the same time, the underconsumption of fats and protein results in lack of other nutrients that are necessary to good health. Because victims feel lethargic, tired, and void of energy they reduce activity. The need for Calories diminishes, but their consumption remains high in an effort to satisfy hunger and to compensate for the mental depression that follows the lack of achievement apparent in the life and home of the obese one. The problem is not "over-nutrition" but malnutrition.

If overnutrition really does exist, however, it may be caused by a malfunction of the brain's mechanism that is to signal the time to stop or start eating, the "appestat" of the hypothalamus.[3] Normally it does a superb job of matching our food intake to our need for energy. In fact, if we had to count every calorie to keep our weight adjusted, it would be an impossible task. If we missed by only a few calories a day, we would soon be obese or emaciated. So, while our bodies take care of most of the task for us, some of us need to give more attention to the process than others. Some really are hungrier than others at the same level of activity and food consumption.*

A defective "appestat" is not the only reason for overeating, however. Out of habit some continue high food consumption past the time of need. When youthful growth stops and activity decreases, calorie need often decreases, too. Continuing youthful food habits results in overweight. Some eat excessively to relieve emotional stress. Food compensates for lost love, bad business deals, tension or boredom at home or at the office. Some people just have an inordinate appreciation of food, its taste, or its social value. Still others overeat because they are poorly informed concerning food values. Many for whom ice cream is taboo, for instance, will use ice milk copiously, unaware that the caloric value of a serving of one is similar to that of the other. Ice cream has more fat. Ice milk has more sugar, but the ice cream is enough lighter from whipped-in air that equal measures contain nearly equal calories. Hunger usually returns faster after eating ice milk.

I once helped an invalid friend plan a weight reducing regimen at her doctor's request. She did not lose weight, and her husband was unhappy with me for what he thought was a faulty plan.

One day I was in the home when the husband was preparing to leave for work. Before he left, he served his wife a glass of apple juice. I was immediately interested, for I knew that apple juice had not been mentioned when we drew up the plan.

"Does your wife drink apple juice frequently?" I inquired.

"Oh, yes!" was the enthusiastic reply. "She loves apple juice! I give her at least four glasses a day."

There was the answer to my friend's failure to lose a whole pound a week. She was getting 500 calories or more in apple juice daily in addition to the foods planned in her diet. The family was surprised to learn that fruit juice has many Calories.

Various factors must be evaluated to find the real cause of more than "normal" weight. Heredity, culture, stress, emotional trauma, physical inactivity, metabolic functions, to name a few, must be considered as well as the quantity and quality of food consumed. Whether from malnutrition or overnutrition, heredity, hormones, or boredom and sedentary life-style, genuine obesity

---

*Children with Prader-Willi syndrome have particularly bizarre insatiable appetites.

is often accompanied by, and either causes or aggravates, a number of malfunctions in the body. The condition is not a desirable one to allow to develop or to continue.

Some physicians are questioning the attitude that requires all people to be slender, however. Dr. C. Wesley Dupertuis and his wife and colleague, Helen, of Western Reserve University, Cleveland, Ohio, were pointing out dangers of reducing for some a number of years ago.[4] More recently Dr. Paul Scholten, a San Francisco obstetrician, wrote in the *American Medical News:*

> There is little firm evidence that a mild deposit of body fat shortens life. Even if it were to be proven true, it is debatable whether one would not be better off choosing 30 to 40 years of happy plumpness over the same span of selective starvation and guilt feelings in order to add one or two more years of hungry life at the end.... A moderately plump person can be in excellent health....[5]

Doctors Dupertuis and Scholten do agree that there are some persons who should reduce their weight. Dr. Scholten designates specifically those who are markedly obese and those excessively fat who have heart or kidney disease or diabetes.

Some fat is essential to support and protect vital organs, insulate the tissues against excessive heat loss, and to serve as reserve energy in times of stress or food deprivation. For some who are very thin, there is need to increase body fat; often they find it as difficult to add fat as the plump ones find it difficult to reduce body stores. If there is need to add body fat, basic nutrients must still be a paramount consideration. Additional calories may be taken in the form of less bulky foods, but they should be chosen from foods offering a complete team of nutrients.

Certainly all heart attack victims, kidney sufferers, and diabetics are not obese. Certainly, too, as Dr. Jean Mayer, Harvard nutritionist and authority on weight control, points out, one who is born a mesomorph (with heavy bones, prominent joints and massive, muscular chest) or an endomorph (with a large body, short arms and legs and a generally rounded contour, including a prominent abdomen) will never have an ectomorph profile (small slender body with long arms and legs, prized by many feminine fashion models) regardless of the weight he/she is able to maintain.[6] To dream of such an achievement is delusion, and efforts to accomplish it are doomed to failure and disappointment. The best one can do is to be a less fat endomorph or mesomorph, as the case may be, and it is wisdom to be happy with the achievement.

Since I cannot discuss all of the medical aspects of weight control, I will confine my concern to some measures that can be taken to keep weight under control. If there are special problems, the advice and care of a physician will be needed as well.

If one thinks he/she is obese (over fat), it might be advisable to get a good set of instructions from a doctor, public health or university extension service to help determine just what would be a desirable weight. There are new methods to determine fatness that may more accurately describe build, musculature, and desirable weight than the old charts. Just looking into the mirror will tell most people what they need to know—but not always. Many who are not fat see themselves as fat, and some who are fat would never admit it.

Characteristics of an Acceptable Reducing Diet

If there is to be weight reduction, whatever the motivation, it must be carried out knowledgeably and sensibly (with prudence), or more harm than good can result.[7] Mistaken notions about food values and physical activity are often responsible for unwise and frequently unsuccessful efforts to lose weight. Young people seem to have an especial tendency to make poor food choices at a time when optimum nutrition is crucial to them and to their progeny.

Diet for weight loss must, first of all, provide the nutrients needed by the body. If it is to be successful over a period of time, it will follow the basic food plans of nations as interpreted by the Scriptures. Bizarre diets designed for spectacular weight loss and those that may satisfy a neurotic tendency on the part of the dieter do not qualify as "prudent" according to the Lord's instruction.

Crash diets usually result in a rapid loss of weight and a rapid return of that weight. This yo-yo effect is more harmful healthwise than remaining fat in the first place, and it is psychologically traumatic as well. The victim is defeated, defensive, apologetic and often open to the next "miracle" diet proposed by friends or the media, which usually sends him/her on a similar round of concentrated effort, spectacular weight loss, and rapid weight gain. Even if the physiological damage and the psychological trauma is bearable for a time, the effect on the wardrobe is devastating! Even including the best of weight reducing regimens, the American Medical Association reports that 90 out of every 100 dieters regain their lost weight.[8]

That there are many diets which will take off pounds rapidly if adhered to strictly is apparent from the number of people who announce happily, "Look! I lost five pounds in four days!" What the happy dieter may not know is that about 3½ pounds (1.58 kg) of that weight loss is water and will return more quickly than it left when the special regimen is abandoned.

Water Balance and Weight Loss[9]

During the first three or four days of drastically reduced caloric intake, weight loss is about ⅔ water—even more if the diet is high in fat or low in carbohydrates. That the entire five pounds (2.25 kg) discarded cannot be fat is reasonable when one considers that a pound of fat represents approximately 3,500 Calories. If a woman who needs 2,200 Calories to maintain her life processes and activity cuts her food consumption to 1,200 Calories and gets the other 1,000 Calories from her own fatty tissues, it will take her about 3½ days to use up one pound of her fat. Only serious illness, ketosis, or a tremendous increase in physical activity could bring about more rapid fat reduction. (Increased requirement for basal metabolism[10] in cases of illness or injury is in the range of 10 to 20 percent for skeletal injuries, 25-50 percent for infections, and 40-100 percent for burns. Severely burned patients may need 4,000 Calories a day with large quantities of water, with the peak need coming about seven days after the burn.)

After the first few days, weight loss begins to slow down as water loss lessens. During the last half of the first week, water loss may account for about half of the weight loss. During the second week, water may account for only about one fifth of the weight lost. In other words, a two-pound loss during the second week may represent as much fat loss as the five-pound loss of the first week. During and after the third week, if the diet is well balanced, almost all of the weight loss is from fat.

Energy Consumption and Weight Loss

Recent studies of obesity in the U.S.A. and Canada have revealed that the obese do not always eat more than their normal weight counterparts. The difference often lies in their differing activity. To maintain a level of activity at least as high as that of the period before dieting is of especial importance to one wishing to lose weight. The tendency is to be less active as food consumption is reduced, either because one is more tired or because one is depressed, and the energy consumption plummets to match the food intake. The dieter declares he/she is eating like a bird and not losing a pound!

Actually, a brisk walk for half an hour daily, without increase in food consumption to compensate for it, can result in the loss of 10 pounds (4.5 kg) of fat in a year all by itself; and there is a small range of activity in which additional exercise does not seem to induce additional hunger. This amount of exercise may be within that range for most. Such exercise may develop some extra muscles that will not allow the scales to show the entire loss of fat, but the substitution of muscle for fat and the toning of other muscles will improve one's appearance as flabbiness is lost. The person stands more erect and generally feels better for it. The effect may be so beneficial psychologically that the need to eat excessively is curbed.

In addition to weight reduction without increasing hunger, and at no cost except for time, exercise may improve the functioning of the "appestat" so that it more adequately matches hunger with energy needs. For those who are sedentary (sit a lot) and for those who work to exhaustion, personal attention must be given to proper food intake without regard to hunger because of the malfunctioning of the mechanism intended to match hunger to our need. For the moderately active, the mechanism is generally effective.[11]

Half an hour's brisk walk, more specifically defined, means a rate of 2½ miles (4 kilometers) an hour, and a 150-pound (67.5 kg) person uses approximately 100 Calories doing it. Bicycling covering twice the distance in the same amount of time would use about the same number of Calories as the walk. Gardening, canoeing, lawn mowing (pushing the mower), swimming, or walking really fast—like 3¾ miles (6 km) per hour—increase the caloric need until the fast walk could mean a 15-pound (6.75 kg) loss in a year, all other conditions being kept under control. The more strenuous exercise also adds the increment of a higher rate of metabolism for some time after the exercise is completed.

It would also probably increase hunger.

Other exercise, sure to increase hunger but useful in using Calories, includes skiing at 10 miles (16 km) an hour or bicycling at 13 miles (20.8 km) an hour, each of which uses about 300 Calories in half an hour. Running at five miles (8 km) an hour uses up to 450 Calories in half an hour. At these daily rates for a theoretical 150-pounder, losses could total from 30 to 45 pounds (13.5 to 20.25 kg) in a year, except that as the weight is lost there would be fewer Calories used in each day's activities and the exerciser would get hungry.

For people who are forced to stay indoors most of the time, even toe-to-toe pacing while talking on the telephone can take a pound (0.45 kg) worth of Calories in a year if the telephone is used as much as thirty minutes a day. Knitting, mending, or whittling instead of sitting motionless while watching TV uses up 20 to 30 Calories an hour. For a two-hour show, that's the equivalent of at least a pound (0.45 kg) every ten weeks of the year.

Then there are the two exercises recommended by my physical education instructor friend at Iowa State University. One is an alternating sidewise rotation of the head when second helpings are offered. The other is to place the hands firmly on the table and push when a reasonable amount of food has been consumed.

Homeostasis, a Problem in Weight Reduction

Weight reduction, especially for the grossly obese, is complicated by the body's determination to survive. If the body determines that it is being deprived of the sustenance to which it has been accustomed, it begins to make adjustments designed to conserve its supplies and utilize its nutrients more efficiently. Homeostasis is the word for it.[12] After the body has lost about one fourth its original weight, this adjustment may have become effective enough that the body will operate on drastically reduced rations without further weight loss for an extended period of time. The fact that there has been a large weight reduction has decreased the number of Calories needed to move the body around and is in part responsible for the phenomena. The situation may be further complicated by a reversal in water balance that often occurs even with a well regulated regimen, causing a person who is still losing fat to regain weight. Poor diets that produce malnourishment can cause a body to increase its proportion of water from the normal 65 percent to 85 percent—a difference of 40 pounds (18 kg) for a 200-pound (90 kg) person.

Plateauing from homeostasis or water balance may occur many times before desired weight is achieved by an obese person and may be a source of discouragement to those attempting to acquire more acceptable proportions. For this reason, if for no other, these people may need the assistance of a knowledgeable physican, dietitian, or nutritionist to succeed. The support of a group is frequently helpful as well.

Even those who go on a complete fast, either by necessity or choice, are frequently appalled to see the weight return rapidly after only a small amount of food has been taken. The body's effort to maintain homeostasis accounts in part for the phenomenon, and its need for and use of protein is also involved.

We have seen that the body must have certain proteins daily even if it has to tear down its own tissues to get them. Some carbohydrates are also necessary daily, notably for the functioning of the brain and for metabolism of fat. After body stores are depleted these, too, must be made largely from proteins, although some fat may be used in the process. Much of the weight loss of a fasting person, then, is from protein of his/her muscles and organs and from water instead of just from fat.

When food is again available after fasting, the body sets itself to restore its lost protein tissues. With every pound (0.45 kg) of protein restored, there is a weight gain of four pounds (1.8 kg)—three fourths of it water, but a weight gain nonetheless and a persistent one that will continue even on low calorie intake until the muscles and organs are repaired. It is believed now that the actual fat lost in total fasting is no more than can be achieved with a well balanced diet providing 700 to 900 Calories.[13]

Irrespective of the fact that one may take advantage of the specific dynamic action of proteins or the body use of fats and carbohydrates for quick weight loss, the only safe way to really lose fat and to maintain that weight loss is to persistently eat a well-balanced diet of sufficiently few Calories that the energy used will be greater than the energy provided by food until the desired weight is achieved. Then just enough must be eaten to provide needed energy for the rest of life. The decision to reduce is futile or fateful unless it becomes permanently a new way of life. This may be either to decide to use more energy by changing work or recreational patterns while continuing present eating practices, to use a different type or quantity of food, or to adopt a combination of the two. In any case, it cannot be a sporadic venture if it is to provide acceptable results.

Fad Diets

For this reason, fad diets are useless or worse. There is no magic in grapefruit or safflower oil or protein or any of the other substances or combination of foods that are ardently recommended by enthusiastic bariatric physicians (weight specialists or diet doctors, many of whom are not qualified physicians),[14] well meaning friends, or misinformed journalists. Among the diets are several types:

Low carbohydrate diets must inevitably be high fat or high protein diets since carbohydrates are cut to a minimum, and they are a dangerous lot.[15] They give quick and encouraging weight losses by dehydrating the tissues and by surfeiting (making food disgusting by overindulgence), satisfying the appetite by slow digestion of fat, developing of ketones that depress the appetite, by malnutrition that produces anorexia (loss of appetite), and by sheer boredom.

Fortunately, low carbohydrate diets are often abandoned before long because of discomforts they induce and boredom with high fat-high protein meals. Unfortunately, with their cessation there comes rehydration of tissues and a shocking return of weight. They contribute heavily to the yo-yo effect previously mentioned.

Cutting carbohydrates from the diet deprives the brain of the chief food source of the type of energy it must have to function and the body of the necessary reagent it must have to safely metabolize fat. The body can produce glucose necessary for these functions from fats and protein, but it is difficult for it to keep up with the need.[16] As the energy needed for mental functions is reduced, along with the loss of body fluids and accompanying needed minerals, fatigue and mental depression frequently develop.

Postural hypotension is characteristic of those on very low carbohydrate diets. This is a dramatic drop in blood pressure that occurs when one changes position from reclining to sitting or standing upright. Sometimes it is manifest in a slight dizziness when arising from a chair or getting out of bed or out of the bathtub. Sometimes there is loss of consciousness and serious accidents occur.[17]

If the low carbohydrate diet emphasizes the use of fats, there will probably be the production of excessive amounts of ketones, producing a situation similar to the metabolic pattern of diabetics.[18] For complete utilization of fats, the body must have an adequate supply of carbohydrates. Ketones do dull the appetite. They also foul the breath and the feces, disturb the rhythm of the heartbeat, may damage unborn children, and can cause death. Any weight loss regimen designed to produce exessive amounts of ketones needs the direct supervision of a competent physician, if indeed it has a place at all in the sensible approach to treating obesity.

If the emphasis is on proteins, there must inevitably be a surplus of protein. The body will have no choice but to tear down the excess proteins and remake them into carbohydrates or fats, discarding portions that cannot be used. These protein metabolites must then be removed from the body, largely by the kidneys. Large amounts of liquids are required for the kidneys to handle these substances safely. Failure to supply needed water or already malfunctioning kidneys may result in an accumulation of substances that may aggravate painful diseases such as gout and arthritis.

Whether the emphasis is on fats or proteins, a low carbohydrate diet does not provide many of the nutrients essential to good health, nor does it have textures and flavors that promote its continuous use. Such a diet may be useful to a boxer or wrestler who cares more about weighing in at a figure below his normal weight than he cares about his health, but it is not recommended for people who care. If it is successful in reducing, it leaves a legacy of malnutrition. If it is not successful (and frequently it isn't) fats have two and a quarter times as many Calories as carbohydrates or proteins, weight for weight, and an increase in fat deposition is anything but helpful.

The American Medical Association's Council on Foods and Nutrition, while still extant, warned that the full impact of such a diet's effect on the health of its victims may not become apparent until long after the diet has been discontinued. The Council took the unprecedented action of specifically warning against two such diets, "Dr. Atkin's Diet Revolution" and Dr. Stillman's "Doctor's Quick Weight Loss Diet" and the books in which they are published.[19]

Currently the best-known and most popular of the low carbohydrate diets with emphasis on fat, and probably the most potentially dangerous, is Dr. Atkin's which, as of April 1974, according to *Today's Health*, had set an all-time record for the sale of any hardcover book of any kind, and paperback sales were into the millions. This high-fat diet has been around in many forms since William Banting, coffin maker for the Duke of Wellington, published his "Letter on Corpulence" more than a century ago. It has been dubbed the "Dupont Diet" of the 1940s, the "Air Force Diet," falsely ascribed to both the U.S. and Canadian forces, and the "Astronaut's Diet." In 1961, Herman Taller, M.D., revived the principle in his book, *Calories Don't Count*, distribution of which, with the sale of safflower oil, brought him a conviction for mail fraud in the U.S.A. The "Drinking Man's diet" compounds the errors of some of the other high fat diets by adding the empty calories of liquor to an already depleted regimen, as does the diet of Dr. Ernest Reinsh's *Eat, Drink and Get Thin*.

Dr. Atkin's own version of the diet appeared in *Harper's Bazaar* in 1966 and as *Vogue*'s "Super Diet" in 1970. Its exclusive feature—and one that earns it the epithet of "potentially most dangerous"—is his insistence on the production of ketones as a measure of the adequacy of the diet. When he uses it, apparently, he makes extensive tests to determine what is happening to blood levels of cholesterol, triglycerides, sugar, and uric acid. Among other treatments, he routinely prescribes a drug to prevent the formation of uric acid crystals.[20] Unfortunately, those who use his diet without medical monitoring have no safeguards against adverse physical developments and will never know if the uric acid level of their blood is high until they are ill from it.

Of the high protein diets currently popular, Dr. Stillman's— often called the "Water Diet" because it requires eight large glasses of water daily in addition to beverages used at mealtime—is best known. Stillman asserts that the specific dynamic action (energy required to metabolize protein) is so high with his diet that it brings weight reduction without concommitant reduction of calories. He claims a 275 Calorie benefit each day from the specific dynamic action of the protein.

If Stillman actually does get a 275 Calorie benefit from the protein, it would still take almost 13 days to lose a pound of fat from this action alone. Clearly, the tremendous weight losses are from the same sources as other low carbohydrate diet weight losses. The water drinking does help safeguard the kidneys, as they metabolize and excrete the protein wastes, and the high protein content with the water encourages frequent and copious urination. Calcium supplies would be seriously depleted by the nature of the diet, and when *Consumer's Guide* experts rated the diet, they found it inadequate in vitamins A, B_1, B_2, D, C, E, folacin, sodium, calcium, iron, copper, zinc, and flourine.[21]

Other low carbohydrate diets that emphasize protein include the "Hauser Does-It Diet," "Petrie's Lazy Lady Diet," and "deVille's Ratio Diet." Some others that emphasize fat include Dr. Frederick's six-meal-a-day diet that in *Consumer's Guide* is labeled a nibbler's version of the Taller Diet, the "Mayo Diet" (with which the Mayo Clinic at Rochester, Minnesota, had no part), and variations such as the egg diet, grapefruit diet, tomato juice diet, and lately an Oriental version promulgated by a Japanese doctor named Arai.[22]

One with knowledge of and faith in the Lord's instuction in the Word of Wisdom would immediately recognize the low carbohydrate-high fat or protein diet as not according to the Lord's wisdom. The initial premise of either rejects some of those foods the Lord says he ordained for our use and substitutes for the staff of life those foods the Lord instructed us to use sparingly.

On the other hand there are high carbohydrate diets also promoted to take off pounds and inches. Dr. Stillman of the high protein - quick weight loss fame is also the proponent of an "Inches Off Diet" which prohibits the use of high protein foods—no meat, poultry, seafood, milk, or cheese! Obviously it was intended to be a high bulk rather than high carbohydrate diet, and obviously Dr. Stillman knows it is nutritionally inadequate, for vitamin supplements are a must, and the diet is not to be used by growing children or pregnant or lactating mothers.[23]

The rice diet, originated as therapy for damaged kidneys,

has gained fame as a reducing diet. Dr. Kempner who originated it warns that in the hands of an amateur it can be ineffective or dangerous. It is the basis of a diet published by *Epicure* in 1973 and of several Stillman diets.[24]

A bananas and milk diet is frequently publicized. It is monotonous enough to cause one to lose weight, and get mighty tired of bananas. It is also severely deficient nutritionally.

Grapefruit diets are legion, and all with the erroneous information that there is some mysterious substance in the fruit that burns up fat. Grapefruit can help still hunger pains as any tart food can, and a 50-Calorie grapefruit half for dessert certainly promotes weight loss better than a 400-Calorie piece of pie or ice cream soda. The "Olympic Diet" is a version of the grapefruit diet combined with high fat - high protein designed to take weight down quickly but not permanently.

Some of the grapefruit diets are fairly well balanced, as is the "Redbook Wise Woman's Diet" and some of the computer diets, like the one offered by General Mills, which attempt to tailor the diet and excercise program to fit the individual or family involved. The "Amazing New You Diet" adds long daily walks and broadening social contacts to a basic 1,200 Calorie diet.[25]

Petrie's Miracle Diet starts with 1,200 Calories of supposedly nutritionally superior foods, to be eaten in six small meals daily. Other versions of the diet, called "Weight Shaker," "Weight Dissolver," and "Weight Blaster," graduate down to 600 Calories. With these low Calorie regimens, a doctor's supervision would be needed.[26]

McCall's "Snack Diet," also called the "Wisconsin Diet," and the "No Will Power" diet of *Ladies' Home Journal* are nibbling diets with Calories low, eating times frequent, a fairly good balance of carbohydrate, fat, and protein, but with too few Calories to be entirely safe without supplementation of some vitamins and minerals. Activities to distract the hungry are a part of the latter.[27]

Harper's Bazaar's "Nine-Day Wonder Diet" provides only 800 Calories or less and is not suitable for more than nine days, if it is suitable at all.[28] If used, a rapid return of most of the weight loss should be expected. For one needing 2,200 calories a day normally, only about four pounds of fat could be expected to be used up in this time. It is not recommended.

Reducing Diets that Maintain Health

There are hundreds of diets available that will take off pounds. For longtime benefit, however, a diet needs to take off pounds while providing all of the nutrients needed for bouyant health, and it needs to make provision for maintaining the weight loss. With a little time and effort dieters can tailor their own. Several have been planned by competent persons. They have the Calorie counting built in. By insistence on strict adherence to the plan, they keep dieters from making mistakes.

Dr. John Yudkin, London nutritionist and physician whose studies in heart disease have led him to believe the excessive use of sugar is implicated, has designed a well-balanced regimen that stresses the elimination of non-nutritious, refined foods. Ed. McMahon's "Thinking Man's Diet" has some of the same characteristics, with a gimmick for counting carbohydrate Calories still used.[29]

The late Dr. Norman Jolliffe designed a well-balanced plan for the public health obesity clinic in New York City, still in operation. With his diet, Jean Nidetch built the highly successful "Weight Watchers" organization. Dr. William H. Sebrell, former assistant surgeon general of the U.S.A. and one of the most trusted authorities in the history of nutrition research, is Weight Watcher's medical director. Recent updating of the diets has diversified the menus and included the use of less expensive foods (more in keeping with the Lord's instruction for use of luxury items) than once were allowed. Calorie restriction is obtained by the use of weighed amounts of food of predetermined caloric value. Hunger is allayed by the insistence upon the consumption of quantities of low calorie food. Other groups called "The Diet Workshop, Inc." and "Diet Watchers" have also adapted Dr. Jolliffe's regimen to their own commercial ventures.[30]

TOPS, acronym for *Take Off Pounds Sensibly*, and Overeaters Anonymous, patterned after Alcoholics Anonymous, are diet support groups that depend upon members working with the medical profession for dietary instruction and on the group for emotional support. Neither promotes a special dietary regimen.

Planning a Personal Weight Reducing Program

The weight reducing program that will be most effective is one that requires the least possible change in the dieter's normal eating pattern presuming that he/she is following a reasonable dietary. The foods used should be those of the basic food plans as previously discussed, with high calorie desserts and snacks eliminated or reduced to a very small amount. A program of regular exercise needs to be included, and attention should be given to handling emotional stress adequately.[31]

While calorie counting is unpopular, and actually ridiculous when one considers how inaccurate estimates are in comparison to the small amounts of miscalculation that could change the outcome of dieting, some understanding of caloric values of foods is necessary for intelligent choices to be made. A classic example of what happens when such knowledge is not available is lived out almost daily. Among the youth, there is the tendency to skip a meal to lose weight, then have a coke, a candy bar, and a bag of potato chips for a snack. Among adults, there may be a piece of pie, or some cake, ice cream, and a cup of coffee with sugar and cream to accompany a social visit or finish a meal, that just is not counted in the day's dietary. They do not realize that for the same number of calories as are provided in the snack or dessert, with minimal nutritive value other than calories, they could have an entire meal. And the meal could provide some foods from every basic group with several days' recommended daily allowance of some of the most often neglected nutrients. Consider the following comparison of three groups of foods, each with almost identical Calorie count:[32]

Snack—531 Cal.	**Meal—512 Cal.**	**Dessert—524 Cal.**
Coke, 10 oz. (300 ml)	Liver (beef), 3 oz. (84 g) with 1 tsp. (5 ml) fat	Apple pie, 1/6 of 9" pie
Candy bar, 1½ oz. (42g)*	Broccoli, 1 cup (240 ml)	Cheese, ½ oz. (14 g)
Potato chips, 1 oz. (28 g)	Potato, baked, 3½ oz. (100 g) *or* 1½ oz. (42 g) whole wheat bread with 1 tsp. (5 ml) butter	Coffee, 6 oz. (150 ml)
		Sugar, 2 tsp. (10 ml)
		Cream, 2 Tbsp. (30 ml)

*A chocolate-covered nut bar was chosen to give maximum nutritive value.

Snack—531 Cal.	Meal—512 Cal.	Dessert—524 Cal.
	Lettuce, 1/6 head with 1 tsp. (5 ml) Fr. dressing	or for 571 Cal. Ice cream, 1/6 U.S. quart (0.16 liter)
	Strawberries, ⅔ cup (180 ml) with 1 tsp. (5 ml) sugar	Iced cake (1/9 of 9" square cake)
	Tomato juice, ½ cup (120 ml)	Without beverage
	Milk, skim or buttermilk, 8 fl. oz. (240 ml)	

Nutrients in these food groups, unlike the Calories, vary widely. Note these differences in the meal and the snack in a few nutrients. See chart on page 157.

It is apparent that wise food choices can form the basis for a sensible weight reducing program. In fact, all that many persons really need to do is to eat good meals, eliminating high calorie snacks and desserts. Some may need only to reduce the size of the desserts and quantity of the snacks. Or those who are already free of snacks and desserts may need only reduce the type or quantity of some nutritious food being used in excessively large amounts. Our teen-age son found he could save 500 Calories a day just by changing from whole milk to skim milk. That one adjustment could reduce his weight by a pound (0.45 kg) a week—nearly 50 pounds (22.5 kg) a year if he kept it up and did not increase the intake of other foods to compensate for it.

Weight control requires consistent, continuous procedures. Cutting down on calories for a week and then going on an eating binge will never be satisfactory. Occasional treats may be included in the plan, however, if they are judiciously used and duly recorded so the frequency of their use is known.

Steps to More Serious Weight Losses

If more serious weight reduction is desirable, helpful steps may be taken:

1. Take inventory. Make a list of everything eaten for a few

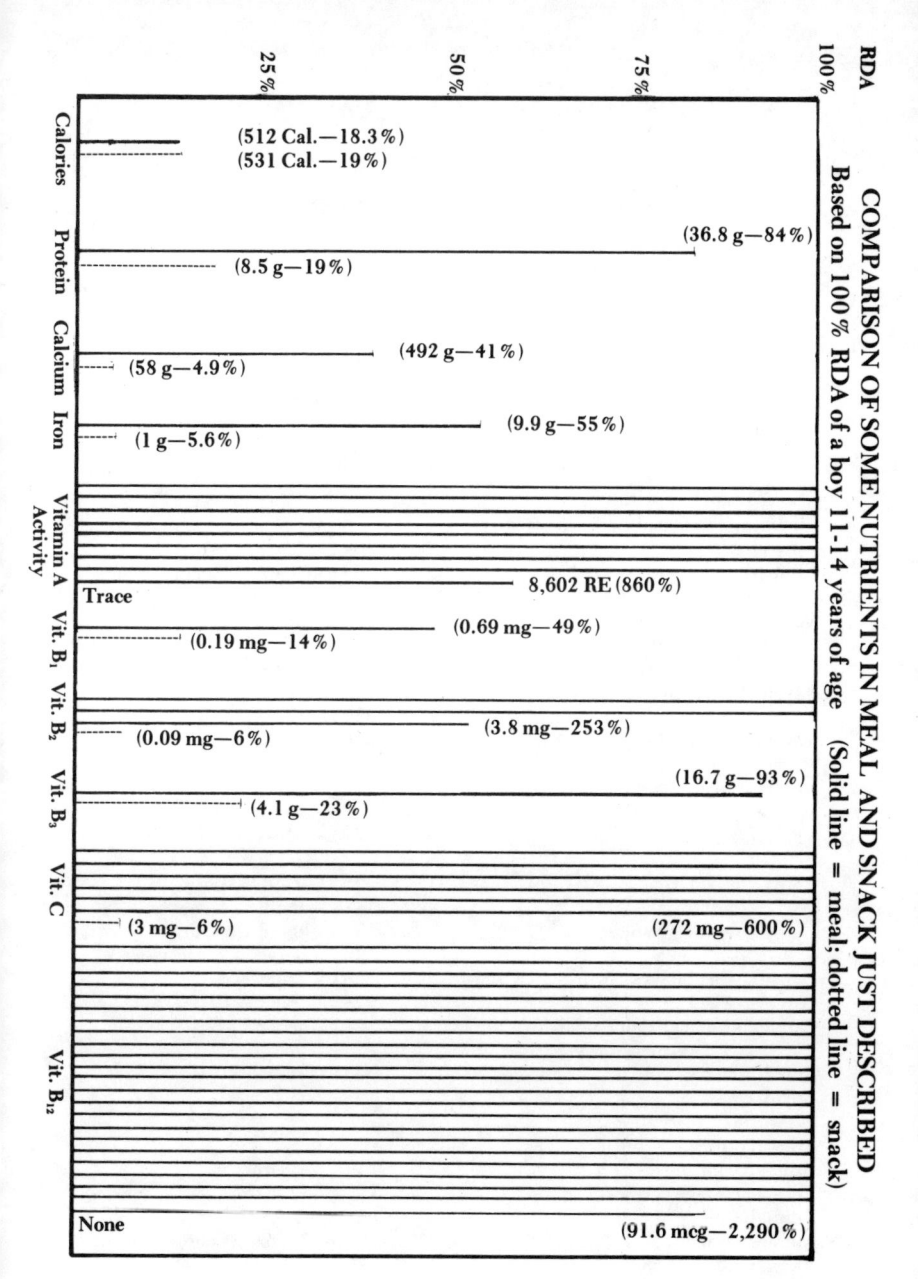

COMPARISON OF SOME NUTRIENTS IN MEAL AND SNACK JUST DESCRIBED
Based on 100% RDA of a boy 11-14 years of age (Solid line = meal; dotted line = snack)

Nutrient	Meal	Snack
Calories	512 Cal.—18.3%	531 Cal.—19%
Protein	36.8 g—84%	8.5 g—19%
Calcium	492 g—41%	58 g—4.9%
Iron	9.9 g—55%	1 g—5.6%
Vitamin A Activity	8,602 RE (860%)	Trace
Vit. B₁	0.69 mg—49%	0.19 mg—14%
Vit. B₂	3.8 mg—253%	0.09 mg—6%
Vit. B₃	16.7 g—93%	4.1 g—23%
Vit. C	272 mg—600%	3 mg—6%
Vit. B₁₂	91.6 mcg—2,290%	None

RDA scale: 25%, 50%, 75%, 100%

FOODS THAT PROVIDE EQUAL CALORIES

100 CALORIES FOOD	MEASURE
Milk, skim or buttermilk	288 ml (1-1/5 cups)
Milk, whole	160 ml (2/3 cup)
Milk, chocolate	80 ml (1/3 cup) to 120 ml (1/2 cup)
Cream, whipping (fluid)	30 ml (2 Tbsp.)
Cream, whipped	60 ml (4 Tbsp.)
Cream, artificial topping	115 ml (7 2/3 Tbsp.)
Juice, tomato	480 ml (2 cups)
Juice, orange	225 ml (15/16 cup)
Juice, apple	200 ml (5/6 cup)
Rhubarb, cooked plain	700 g—25 oz. (6 2/3 cups)
Rhubarb, sweetened with low calorie sweetener	504 g—18 oz. (5 cups)
Rhubarb, sweetened with sugar	168 g— 6 oz. (3/8 cup)
Vegetables, celery	794 g—28 oz.
Vegetables, lettuce	588 g—21 oz.
Vegetables, cabbage	454 g—16 oz.
Vegetables, green beans (frozen)	364 g—13 oz.
Vegetables, broccoli (frozen)	336 g—12 oz.
Vegetables, kale (frozen)	308 g—11 oz.
Vegetables, carrots	229 g— 8-1/6 oz.
Vegetables, potatoes	147 g— 5 1/4 oz.
Vegetables, peas (green)	140 g— 5 oz.
Vegetables, corn	121 g— 4 1/3 oz.
Cereals, rolled oats	25 g—scant 1/3 c. *dry*
	177 g—about 2/3 c. *cooked*
Cereals, wheat (ground)	28 g—about 1/6 c. *dry*
	140 g—rounded 1/2 c. cooked
Cereals, wheat flakes	28 g—about 2/3 c.
Cereals, wheat germ	28 g—about 1/3 c.
Cereals, granola (commercial)	21 g—about 3 Tbsp.
Bread, whole wheat	42 g—1 1/2 oz.
Bread, white	35 g—1 1/4 oz.
Animal proteins	
Animal, codfish	130 g—4 2/3 oz.
Animal, cottage cheese (plain)	117 g—4 1/6 oz.
Animal, liver	94.5 g—3-3/8 oz.
Animal, cottage cheese (creamed)	93 g—3 1/2 oz. (1/3 cup)
Animal, tuna in water	80 g—2-4/5 oz.

100 CALORIES FOOD	MEASURE
Animal, egg	61 g—1¼ large
Animal, mackerel	56 g—2 oz.
Animal, weiners (12 per pound)	42 g—1½ oz. (one wiener)
Animal, tuna in oil	34 g—1-1/5 oz.
Animal, hamburger (regular raw)	30.8 g—1.1 oz.
Animal, cheddar cheese	28 g—1 oz.
Animal, bacon (broiled)	16 g—4/7 oz.
Nuts, peanuts (shelled or butter)	18 g—0.63 oz. (1¼ T. butter)
Nuts, almonds (shelled)	16.5 g—0.6 oz. (2 T.)
Table fat, butter, margarine, or real mayonnaise	14 g—½ oz. (1 Tbsp.)
Table fat, mayonnaise type salad dressing	22g—¾ oz. (1½ Tbsp.)
Lard or vegetable oil	11.2 g—2/5 oz. (4/5 Tbsp.)
Fruit, grapefruit (pink or red, whole)	482 g—17 oz. (one large)
Fruit, grapefruit (pink or red, peeled)	378 g—13½ oz.
Fruit, orange (peeled)	301 g—10¾ oz.
Fruit, apple	182 g—6½ oz.
Fruit, banana	168 g—6 oz.
Fruit, raisins	35 g—1¼ oz. (¼ cup)
Sweets, honey	32.6 g—1-1/6 oz. (1½ Tbsp.)
Sweets, sugar (white or brown)	26.3 g—15/16 oz. (2 Tbsp.)
Desserts, candy bar	21 g—¾ oz.
Desserts, butter cakes, no icing	31 g—1.1 oz. (3" x 1" x 1½")
Desserts, cookies	20-28 g—5/7 to 1 oz. (1 small brownie to 3" oatmeal with nuts)
Desserts, pie (two crust)	1½" sector 9" pie

days. Be sure to include every snack, every taste of food being prepared, every sample picked up in the supermarket, every bite taken at "coffee break." Weigh and measure the amounts when possible.

Now get a good Calorie chart. (Most governments have free ones available at public health or extension offices.) Add up the Calories to see how many are really being eaten to maintain present overweight. Study the list to see where Calories could most easily be reduced without reducing needed nutrients appreciably. A rough estimate may be made by checking with the basic foods of the daily plan. For more specific values, a home economist, dietitian, or physician might be contacted.

2. Decide how much fat is to be lost each week. It should not be more than two to two and a half pounds (0.9 to 1.125 kg) unless one is very obese or has medical supervision. The idea is to keep the food intake high enough to provide nutrients needed for healthful living while fat stores are used up for energy. Most women should have 1,000 to 1,200 Calories of high quality foods for this purpose; men may require up to 1,500 or 1,800 Calories. On this amount of food, with similar physical activity, a very obese person should lose more pounds in a given time than a moderately overweight one, simply because the obese need more calories to keep functioning (have a higher basal metabolic rate) and to move around. Dr. Mayer reports, for example, that a 200-pound (90 kg) man requires one third more calories to play a game of tennis than his 150-pound (67.5 kg) opponent if they go about the game equally energetically.[33]

A pound (0.45 kg) of fat represents approximately 3,500 Calories. At two pounds a week, that would be about 7,000 Calories a week that one would need to eliminate from the dietary to shed two pounds. That represents about 1,000 Calories a day. For one who has been eating 2200 Calories to maintain overweight, reducing to 1200 Calories should bring about the two-pound reduction in weight. For one who has been eating 3000 Calories a similar cut to 1200 Calories should bring about a weight reduction of nearly 3.6 pounds a week. If only two pounds a week are to be lost, more Calories should be eaten—about 2000 in this case.

If one chooses to eliminate only 1000 Calories a day, the rate of loss will begin to decrease as weight is lost. Basic metabolic rate will decrease and fewer calories will be needed to move around. Dr. L. Earle Arnow estimates that with every 25 pounds (11.25 kg) weight loss, the need for Calories decreases by about 100.[34] What was a 1000-Calorie deficit at the beginning then becomes a 900-Calorie deficit after 25 pounds (11.25 kg) have been dropped, and only a 600-Calorie deficit after 100 pounds (45 kg) are gone. Thus for the very obese the diet needs to be periodically adjusted downward and the activity increased as weight is lost, or the beginning diet may show a larger deficit than the 1000 Calories of the moderately overweight. Always the basic food needs should be met.

Weight losses averaging only one pound a week, resulting from a daily reduction of only 500 Calories should be sufficient for most people, leaving them more comfortable and better able to function normally. That would total some 50 pounds (22.5 kg) in a year in a continuing program. Slow weight losses are not always practical, however, because most dieters are impatient to see results and may give up if dramatic losses are not experienced, and errors in calculating food values make it difficult to be sure of the deficit being maintained at that close a figure.

Lack of physical exercise may be largely responsible for "the shape we are in," and increased physical activity can help correct the situation.[35] To be effective, it must be specific and consistently followed.

3. Plan meals that are liked and that can be served to the rest of the family in modified form. Others may have regular salad dressing instead of a low calorie variety—which can save 50 to 100 Calories per tablespoonful (15 ml). They may season their vegetables with butter or bacon drippings, while the dieter has only salt, herbs, lemon juice, or a dash of vinegar—saving 35 Calories or more a teaspoonful (5 ml). The family may have fried eggs while the dieter's are poached or cooked in the shell—saving up to 100 Calories per serving. The rest may have gravy on their roast while the dieter eats roast plain with a bit of steak sauce or *au jus* (with drippings free of fat). They may have two pieces of toast dripping with butter; the dieter will have one with just the "smell" of butter.

The dieter will limit food choices largely to those recommended by government food plans (interpreted by the Scriptures), refusing high calorie desserts, many visible fats, and foods with few vitamins and minerals for the calories they offer. (Corn, for example, contains too many calories for the other nutrients it offers to be included in the reducing regimen.) Daily food choices will include roughly: two servings high quality protein foods; two servings vegetables, at least one of them leafy green; two servings fruit, at least one high in vitamin C; four servings whole grain, enriched breads, or cereals (if whole grains are not chosen, bran should be included); milk and milk products according to age and need, as in the case of pregnancy or lactation.

Dr. Mayer recommends that diets designed for weight reduction have a minimum of 14 percent of their calories from protein, with no more than 30 percent of them from fats, and the rest from carbohydrates with sugar (sucrose) kept to a minimum.[36] As the calories go lower in a good reducing diet, the *proportion* of protein will have to go higher, even though the quantity does not change. Protein needs are based on "ideal" body weight and do not fluctuate with actual weight. If the Calorie count is reduced to 1,000 for female adults, for example, about 22.5 percent of the Calories need to come from protein to meet RDA standards of the U.S.A. National Research Council. This is easily obtained from the basic foods previously listed. If the Calorie allowance is a more liberal 1,500, only 17 percent needs to be protein to meet the RDA of the same woman.

4. Choose beverages carefully. Many depend heavily on black coffee, plain tea, or other caffeine-containing drinks. Dr. Mayer does not recommend their use because of possible deleterious effects on health.[37] Others find their stimulation causes the secretion of hormones that may increase rather than decrease hunger. They also contain calories—coffee, tea, and some diet drinks, about one Calorie per ounce (30 ml), which seems negligible but equals the Calories of a whole tablespoon of sugar when ten five-ounce (150 ml) cups of coffee or five ten-oz. (300 ml) bottles of drink are consumed. Non-diet soft drinks average about 13 Calories per ounce—650 empty Calories for the amount previously noted.

Cereal-based warm beverages average one Calorie per ounce when made with fruit and two when made with molasses. They are without damaging drugs or stimulants to increase activity, but taken in place of stimulants may increase well-being enough to make activity pleasurable. The Lord recommends their use in the instruction to use barley and other grains for mild (non-alcoholic) drinks.

Here are some comparisons of other beverages that might be chosen:

Comparison of 8 ounces (240 ml) of beverage in Calories and nutrients

Beverage	Calories	Other nutritive values
Buttermilk or skim milk	85	Protein, calcium, riboflavin,

		vit. B_{12}, folacin, B_6, and many others
Lemonade	100	Some vitamin C, vitamins and minerals
Pineapple juice	116	Some vitamin C, vitamins and minerals
Apple juice	120	Some vitamin C, vitamins and minerals
Orange juice	110	Vitamin C, B_1, folacin, A, B_2, B_3, & others
Orange flavored crystals	115	Vitamin C only
Tomato juice	45	Vitamin C, A, B_1, B_2, B_3, iron, and others
Carrot juice	80	Vitamin A, iron, and others
Water	none	*Essential for life*

5. Determine the size of portions that can be consumed while using up fat stores. Even essential foods have calories, and one can get fat on any food but water if enough is eaten and reasonable health is maintained. Just as half an hour's brisk walk a day for a year could take off ten pounds (4.5 kg), three nice big carrots, half a pound (227 g), or one big apple a day over one's need can add ten pounds in the same amount of time.

Quantities should be weighed or measured at first until allowable amounts are memorized. Caloriewise, an apple is not just an apple. If it is small enough that there are three in a pound (0.45 kg), it has about 80 Calories. If it weighs half a pound (227 g) as many do, the Calorie count is close to 135. A small orange may have 50 Calories or less, a large one 125 or more (and the summer Valencias have more than the winter navels).

Choice, portioning, and preparation of protein foods is especially important to Calorie totals. It can be noted from the chart of 100-Calorie portions that one can have more than a quarter of a pound (112 grams) of codfish for 100 Calories but only 1.1 oz. (30.8 g) regular hamburger (about a third more if lean hamburger is chosen). Poultry and liver are also low in Calorie count compared with beef.

If regular hamburger is chosen and divided into five patties per pound. (0.45 kg) each patty may carry about 250 Calories if pan broiled in its own fat—perhaps 50 Calories less if it is broiler broiled until well done. If only three patties are made of the meat, however, each patty will start with over 400 Calories and vary with the method of preparation. If it is just the lean from a 16- ounce (454 g) steak that is eaten, the Calories will total 600 to 900. Well-marbled, "choice" meat is much higher in Calories and if the fat is also consumed, another 500 to 900 Calories must be added. If the meat is breaded and fried, the Calorie count soars.

Eggs, too, can vary from 80 Calories for a large egg cooked in the shell or poached without added fat to 96 for a "butter poached" one with one half teaspoon (2.5 ml) fat, to 113 if a teaspoon (5 ml) of fat is used to scramble it, to 180 or so if a tablespoon (15 ml) fat is used in frying it.

On the other hand, some foods have so few Calories and so many nutrients and so much bulk to satisfy hunger that they may be enjoyed almost any time. These include leafy green vegetables like parsley, kale, spinach, and others like celery, cucumbers, and radishes. Kept on hand for snacking at home, at the movies or on long motor trips, the dieter can avoid hunger without exceeding Calorie allotments. As a bonus there will be extra vitamins, minerals, and fiber for added vim and vitality. It must be remembered, though, that their Calories also count, and they need to be incorporated into the plan.

6. Distribute these foods throughout the day. If there is to be a food break midmorning and/or midafternoon, some chosen food should be used—with no extra drink being slipped in (unless it is water). A ten-ounce regular soda or lemonade will more than equal two slices of bread or a very large potato. And an ounce (28 g) bag of potato chips or sunflower seeds, a small candy bar, or a donut to go with the drink will cost more than three extra slices of bread or two large apples. One could save tomato or orange juice from breakfast for the midmorning break, though, and an apple or a pack of carrots from lunch for the afternoon one. If milk is not used at mealtime, a glass of skim or buttermilk at break time gives a bonus of protein, calcium, riboflavin, B_{12}, and other nutrients, all for the Calories of a small to medium apple.

If a snack at bedtime is to be continued, fewer foods should be eaten during the rest of the day. There are nearly 400 Calories in one sixth of a nine-inch cherry pie, and more than 400 Calories in one sixteenth of an iced chocolate cake. A cup of ordinary ice cream has 300 Calories and a cup of iced milk a few less.

A sandwich contains from 220 Calories up, depending on what is put into it. Two slices of bread and an ounce (28 g) of luncheon meat or cheese or a rounded tablespoon of peanut butter adds up to the 220 Calories. A teaspoon of butter and one of salad dressing adds 50 more (75 if real mayonnaise is used). If both meat and cheese are used another 100 Calories are added. Meat or cheese thick enough to equal eight slices to the pound (0.45 kg) instead of the sixteen commercial packers use, add another 100 Calories each. That could total nearly 600 Calories. On the other hand, if lettuce is used in place of the top slice of bread the basic 220-Calorie sandwich is reduced to approximately 160.

Perhaps the happiest choice for a bedtime snack would be a warm cereal beverage at five or ten Calories, an ounce (28 g) of carrot sticks at twelve, a whole wheat cracker at twenty-one, half a glass of skim or buttermilk at forty-two, or a piece of fresh fruit. If alcoholic beverages are considered here or at any time, it is wise to remember that an ounce and a half (45 ml) of 100 proof alcohol contains 130 Calories, provides no nutritive value, and can't even help metabolize its own Calories (see chapter on alcohol).

Calorie Bargain

Calorie bargains are helpful in planning. It's easy to learn to like eating vegetables without fatty seasonings. A dash of garlic and a sprinkling of salt make a green salad tasty without dressings. Minced onion and a dash of lemon juice or vinegar make greens more savory and the tartness tends to reduce hunger.

Liver is a bargain for all of the nutrients it provides on low calories and usually at low cost. Its use at least once a week during winter, periods of cold, famine, and special need is highly recommended. With the new nonstick pans, it can even be fried with just a trace of fat; smothered with onions steamed in the same pan it provides a low calorie, satisfying cuisine. It can be cooked with tomatoes or boullion or broiled with a few crisp bacon bits (meat or soya) for flavor and served up at a bargain.

Water is, of course, the best bargain in calories and money. It is the most essential dietary item. One can live longer without any other food than without water. In general there is no limit on the amount to be used (within reason), and a glass of water will often give the needed refreshment without adding a single Calorie. If one steps on the scale after drinking water, the weight of the water will register, but it does not contribute to the production of fat.

Some Nonnutritive Helps

A few simple practices calculated to cater to the psyche and raise the hunger threshold may be helpful. First of all, dieters should expect to be hungry. And even when they feel stuffed, there will be forbidden items for which they hunger. Burning one's own fat does not satisfy as eating food does, so there will be hunger for most people unless there is an appetite depressant in the form of a drug, ketosis, or malnutrition. No one of these is acceptable in a lifetime plan for weight control. Setting up distractions for those times when the hunger sensation becomes most persistent can help. Dieters should take on some interesting project that is far removed from food and keeps their minds occupied during the difficult times. They can get acquainted with the library, volunteer at the center for the mentally retarded, start a garden, paint the house, or visit shut-ins in the neighborhood. If they take a part-time job or long walks there will be double benefits. Maybe there will even be increased spiritual awareness and intellectual achievement. When distraction is not enough they can resort to low-calorie munching foods.

Mealtime beverages, except water, should be poured into small glasses, the measure of which is known. Allowable portions of foods should be served on small attractive plates—or, better still, larger plates filled with low calorie vegetables and salads. Eating slowly and chewing on bulky foods like celery may help, giving the satiety mechanism of the brain a chance to function. Eating in a social situation whenever possible may distract from the process of eating. (If, on the other hand, it develops envy and self-pity, the dieter should eat alone.) Eating should be avoided while one is watching an exciting TV program, since there is a tendency to eat mechanically in such a situation. For some, a full glass of water, a warm cereal beverage, or a nibble of salad or cracker before the meal may help. Brushing the teeth as soon as the meal is finished puts a touch of finality to the process.

Nibbling through the day on allowable foods seems to be helpful. Recent studies with rats[38] indicate that when food is concentrated in infrequent large feedings, the body metabolizes more of it into fat than if there is a more constant supply of food, even though the two supplies are equal in Calories. It is frequently observed, too, that the very obese are apt to skip a couple of meals a day and take their food in one large meal. The wise dieter will eat regular meals, at least three a day except when fasting, and more if it seems to help.

Those who fast for religious purposes should remember the Lord's instruction that, following the fast, food should be prepared "with singleness of heart"[39] that their fasting may be perfect. To eat imprudently to make up for the food missed during the fast vitiates the purpose of the fast and may be physically damaging.

Keeping socially active and interested in others helps. If food goes with the sociability, it should be planned in the day's regimen (or one can accept invitations only on condition that food restrictions will not disturb the party). Small helpings or none at all planned with the hostess before the party saves embarrassment for the dieter, disappointment for the hostess, and boredom for the other guests. If the temptation is too much and one does overeat, the ration for the next day may be lessened to compensate.

Weighing should take place at the same time of day and with the same amount of clothing. For some, weighing only once a week is helpful. Water balance fluctuations may not be so evident that way. A week's time should show encouraging progress. If weight does hit a high, eating activity should be checked. If the increase persists, professional help may be needed to get the water under control or to reevaluate the dietary.

It is wise to set up short-term goals and celebrate when they are reached, preferably with something other than food (a new shirt or dress, an evening out, or a visit to a friend). Penalties should be paid when goals are not reached; these should be declared to at least one person, since the dieter often carries through better that way. If 20 pounds (9 kg) need to be shed, it can be programmed in five-pound (2.25 kg) stints. This should give something to celebrate at least every three weeks if there is a 1,000-Calorie deficit in each day's food.

Record keeping is important. If it is on paper, there is no doubt about whether there is progress, and every success encourages continued effort. If there is failure, the record will help determine what went wrong so that errors can be corrected. Just knowing there is a record may be the factor that will inspire wise choices.

Maintaining Desired Weight

When the desired weight has been attained, the intake of food may be increased very gradually, but the basic pattern should be maintained. High Calorie desserts, beverages, and snacks will always be taboo. Increases should be in quantity of highly nutritious foods, not in empty Calories. Dieters should weigh every day. If even one pound is gained, they should cut back the food intake until the weight is stabilized. If there is no change in physical activity, this will be the level at which food intake will need to stay if the weight is to be maintained.

Once the body gets accustomed to the new weight, it will adjust its satiety mechanism to help keep it there if moderate activity is maintained (unless the mechanism has been damaged, making it necessary for one to control it consciously). Even with this help, however, there must be self-discipline for the rest of life if there is not always to be a battle of the bulge being fought unsuccessfully. A return to the habits that created overweight the first time will repeat the process.[40]

Organizations Offering Help

If dieters find that weight loss is more than they can handle alone, or even with a doctor's help, there are a number of groups they can join that provide moral support and motivation. Some prescribe rigid menus, weight goals, and continuous instruction to help take off the weight and keep it off. Some cost nothing but time. Others are quite expensive, both in time and designated foods. Those interested should examine the possibilities, ask the doctor for a recommendation, and select the organization best suited to the situation. There may be enough friends in the neighborhood to band together to form a new club or chapter of an existing one.

Proprietary Aids

Need for supplementation with vitamins and minerals during periods of weight loss depends on the quantity and quality of food used. If the Calorie count is not below 1,200, and basic foods make up the diet, it is possible to get the needed nutrients. If the diet is stringent and unbalanced, supplementation is a must.

Formula diets that come premeasured in a can or package may be helpful temporarily, but they do nothing to retrain the dieter for a lifetime of normal eating. Neither do the candies that carry vitamins and minerals and are designed to suppress the appetite. In this form, both candy and nutrients are expensive. The candy is carbohydrate, usually sucrose that may stimulate fat production and make water balance difficult to control, and every calorie of it counts![41]

Bulk-producing products on the market are designed to make one feel full and therefore satisfied with less than usual amounts of food. Cellulose may be helpful if it really stills hunger pangs and still allows enough food for good nutrition. The best sources are whole grains, vegetables, and fruits.[42] Some plastics imitate foods, but their value and safety are not yet certain.

Some Misconceptions About Food Values Corrected

"Dietetic" foods are not always low calorie. They are prepared for low salt diets, diabetic and other disease states. Often they offer as many or more calories than foods made from favorite recipes.

Margarine is not less calorific than butter. Diet margarine has fewer calories largely because emulsifiers allow more water to be whipped in. The same effect can be achieved—and for less money—by softening regular margarine or butter and spreading it thin.

Diet breads are usually little different from regular breads except that they are sliced thinner. Eating only a part of a slice or choosing regular breads that are sliced thin can bring the same results. Wood pulp breads are not recommended.

Sugarless products are not without calories. Sugarless gum may help reduce cavities, but the mannitol and sorbitol used to sweeten it are foods yielding about five Calories per stick instead of the usual eight. All sugar substitutes presently allowed in foods, except saccharin, contain some calories. They may help keep calories low, especially in beverages, cereals, and fruits. In baked goods they produce a lower yield of product of differing texture from the original recipe and may be less helpful.

From my cookie recipe that usually yielded five dozen crisp 90 Calorie cookies, I got four dozen and two 78 Calorie cookies the texture of muffins when I substituted a sweetener for half the sugar. Every one in the family took two for the usual one—156 Calories instead of 90—and enjoyed them less!

Two percent milk does not have half the calories of whole milk. The difference may be only 13 to 30 Calories in an eight-ounce (240 ml) glass (see chapter on milk for an explanation).

Salt intake does not affect the speed with which fat is reduced. Weight may be reduced more quickly with reduced salt but the difference is in water balance, not fat.

Night eating does not make fat more than other eating unless a disproportionate amount of food is taken. It may cause circulatory problems if the meal is high in fat, and easily gets out of hand.

Confining food to one meal a day is not helpful. It may lead to a higher proportion of fat manufacture. Food spaced throughout the day makes a more comfortable arrangement and can lead to lower consumption.

People who quit smoking do not always get fat. Many do gain (on the average, seven pounds [3.2 kg]) but by stepping up exercise and eating properly, they can keep their weight under control. Besides, a small amount of overweight is easier to correct than emphysema, lung cancer, heart disease, Buergers disease, or defective children—problems that have been linked to smoking.

Infants should not have unmodified skim milk formula to keep them thin. Fats are essential to their normal development (see chapter on Well Fed Infants).

Caution for Pregnant Mothers

Pregnancy is not the time to shed unwanted pounds unless it can be done simply by cutting out high calorie foods that offer few nutrients and by increasing physical exercise to a reasonable amount. Large numbers of babies enter this world having been malnourished in fetal life and so deprived of normal development of body or brain. Fetal malnourishment is a serious disease that should never be inflicted on a child by a mother trying to attain weight goals or retain her figure.[43]

That does not mean that a mother must sacrifice her figure to have her child. The recommended additional 300 Calories a day during pregnancy are to care for increased metabolic rate and to produce tissue, placenta, fetus, breast tissue, amniotic fluid, and additional blood, all of which are used up in producing and feeding the baby. With high quality foods, all the needs of both mother and child can be cared for without the production of excessive fat. The body does store some fat in preparation for the feeding of the baby. If artificial feeding is chosen instead, these stores may need to be reduced after the birth of the baby. If used as intended, they, too, are consumed naturally.

Finally

It really is not difficult to control weight simply by following the daily food plan recommended by the Lord and confirmed by modern nutrition once one is at peace with himself and the world and has some knowledge of food values. If one feels incapable of planning his/her own, a diet that follows these recommendations may be selected, with the help of a professional if necessary, and followed to provide a lifetime of happy, healthful living. It is the only safe way yet discovered to attain and maintain ideal weight. It has none of the trauma of heartbreaking gains following strenuous and sometimes dangerous deprivation. It is just "eating with prudence [cautious, practical wisdom, discretion, and good judgment] and thanksgiving [grateful acknowledgment of benefits received; true thanksgiving precludes waste or greediness]" as the Lord instructed long before it became fashionable to be "on a diet."

Epilogue: Lest it appear that I am one with a perfectly adjusted appestat that makes weight control easy, I want it to be known that I have been hungry since I was born. If I ate all I would like to eat, I would long ago have passed the 200-pound (90 kg) mark. As it is, I have always been too well rounded for my five feet four inches (160 cm). My problem is that, to date, I have not been motivated to eliminate unneeded desserts.

There was a period a few years ago which included two moves for the family, less than a year apart, with some stressful situations—nine months of schooling while I cared for the needs of my family in a new situation, adjusting to the culture of a foreign country, plus menopause. I gained 15 pounds (6.75 kg). Just a year ago, I took that weight off at two pounds (0.9 kg) a week regularly for just a little over seven weeks simply by using the foods on the daily food plan with no low nutrient snacks, no beverages except water, milk, and juices, and with a minimum of high calorie desserts. Those desserts were highly nutritious. I also elected to walk a number of places to which I had formerly ridden.

While working on this book, I found that my life was becoming more sedentary than formerly, my weight began to creep up, and I added just over a pound (0.45 kg). I reduced my desserts and visible fats, and the weight was gone in less than a week. Again I carry about the weight I have carried all of my adult life, and I am well aware that the mirror and charts tell me that it may be too much for best functioning. Perhaps one day I will find proper motivation for choosing a new and more pleasing profile.

---

1. Jean Mayer, *Overweight, Causes, Cost and Control*, Prentice-Hall, Inc., Englewood Cliffs, N.J., 1968, pp. 12, 130.
2. *Ibid.*, p. 28.
3. *Ibid.*, pp. 24-25. Also Roger J. Williams, *Nutrition Against Disease*, Pitman Pub. Co., N.Y., London, Toronto, Tel Aviv, 1971, pp. 100-102.
4. Wesley C. and Helen Dupertuis, quoted in "Who Should Be Fat," *Science Digest*, April 1968, p. 76.
5. Arthur J. Snider, "Fat Is Beautiful," *Science Digest*, Jan. 1974, p. 46.
6. Mayer, *op. cit.*, pp. 36-42.
7. Robert Sherrill, "Before You Believe Those Exercise and Diet Ads, Read This Report," *Today's Health*, Aug. 1971, pp. 34-36, 68-69.
8. Don A. Schanche, "Diet Books That Poison Your Mind...and Harm Your Body," *Today's Health*, April 1974, p. 59.
9. Miriam E. Lowenberg, E. Neige Todhunter, Eva D. Wilson, Moira Feeney, and Jane R. Savage, (all Ph.D.s), *Food and Man*, John Wiley and Sons, Inc., N.Y., London, Sydney, 1968, p. 163.
10. A. Fleck, "Protein Metabolism After Injury," *The Proceedings of the Nutrition Society*, Vol. 30, Sept. 1971, p. 152; and J.W.L. Davies, and S.O. Liljedahl, "The Effect of Environmental Temperature on the Metabolism and Nutrition of Burned Patients," *ibid.*, p. 165. Both are extracted in the *Journal of the American Dietetics Association*, Vol. 60, Jan. 1972, pp. 66-67.
11. Mayer, *op. cit.*, pp. 69-83.
12. *Ibid.*, pp. 12-14. Also Harry A. Jordan, M.D. (Dept. of Psychiatry, U. of Pennsylvania and Pennsylvania General Hospital), "In Defense of Body Weight," *Journal of the American Dietetics Association*, Vol. 62, No. 1, Jan. 1973, p. 17.
13. Seymour K. Fineberg, M.D., "The Realities of Obesity and Fad Diets," *Nutrition Today*, July/Aug., 1972. p. 25; Mayer, *op. cit.*, pp. 161-162. Also Phillip L. White, ScD. (Director American Medical Assn. Dept. of Foods and Nutrition), Comment on Allan Cott, M.D., *The Ultimate Diet, Total Fasting*, Bantam Books, Inc., 1975, *American Medical News*, Jan., 19, 1976, pp. 18-19.
14. Theodore Berland, and Editors of *Consumer Guide, Rating the Diets*, Rand McNally, April 1974, Chapter 7.
15. Fineberg, *op. cit.*, p. 24.
16. *Ibid.*, p. 25. Also R.B. McGandy, B. Hall, C. Ford, and F.J. Stare, "Dietary Carbohydrate and Work Capacity in Adolescent Males—A Pilot Study," *American Journal of Clinical Nutrition*, Vol. 25, Jan. 1972, p. 61, extracted in *Journal of the American Dietetics Association*, Vol. 60, April 1972, p. 331.

17. Schanche, *op. cit.*, p. 56.
18. *Ibid.*
19. *Ibid.*, pp. 56-61.
20. Berland, *et al.*, *op. cit.*, p. 261.
21. *Ibid.*, p. 235.
22. to 30. *Ibid.*, by diet title.
31. Frederick J. Stare, M.D., and Mary McSherry, "The Right Diet for You," *Reader's Digest* (Canadian), Feb. 1973, pp. 79-83.
32. Calculated from USDA *Composition of Foods*, Agriculture Handbook No. 8, by item.
33. Mayer, *op. cit.*, p. 71.
34. L. Earle Arnow, *Food Power, A Doctor's Guide to Commonsense Nutrition*, Nelson-Hall Co., Chicago, 1972, p. 49.
35. Mayer, *op. cit.*, pp. 69-83, 147-148, and 170-171.
36. *Ibid.*, p. 160.
37. *Ibid.*, pp. 162-163.
38. Gilbert A. Leveille, Ph.D., and Dale R. Romsos, Ph.D., "Meal Eating and Obesity," *Nutrition Today*, Nov./Dec., 1974, pp. 4-9.
39. Doctrine and Covenants 59:3.
40. Fineberg, *op. cit.*, pp. 23-26. Also Mort Weisinger, "How to Stick to Your Diet (helpful suggestions from Harvard's Dr. Frederick J. Stare, Manhattan psychologist Stephen Zaslow, and other authorities)," *Today's Health*, July, 1973, pp. 30-35.
41. Mayer, *op. cit.*, p. 161.
42. *Ibid.*, p. 162.
43. Howard N. Jacobson, M.D., "Nutrition and Pregnancy," *Journal of the American Dietetics Association*, Vol. 60, Jan. 1972, pp. 26-29.

CHAPTER 8

Well Born Children

All Saints who remember to keep and do these sayings, walking in obedience to the commandments, shall receive health in their navel.... —Doctrine and Covenants 86:3.

First of all the promises contained in the Word of Wisdom is one that there shall be health in the navel of those who follow the Lord's instructions. Clearly, this is assurance that our children will have a better chance of being born physically and mentally whole if we make wise choices. Under present circumstances we sometimes have little or no control over some factors such as inherited physical characteristics, accidental radiation, infections and environmental conditions, some of which we are not yet aware. Many of the factors affecting our children's birth we can directly determine by our choices, however, and thus avoid tragedies once thought to be acts of God.

To be well born, a child must be conceived from strong, undamaged sperm and egg, developed properly before birth, and delivered safely. Among factors necessary to achieve these essentials are the elimination of hazardous substances from the parents' lives (deleterious drugs, excessive radiation, infectious disease), the choice of properly nutritious foods, and preparation for safe delivery by proper exercise, rest, cleanliness, and mode of delivery.

Verification of the Promise

Scientific literature is replete with information indicating the damage that is done to sperm, eggs, and fetus by drugs, even socially accepted ones. Likewise it indicates clearly that food plays a significant role in the development of healthy babies. Dr. Roger J. Williams, University of Texas biochemist, discoverer of pantothenic acid, longtime researcher, and author in the field of nutrition, includes a chapter on "Stillborn, Deformed and Mentally Retarded Babies" in his book *Nutrition Against Disease*,[1] in which he documents his assertion that "we have evidence that the *prime* factor involved in reproductive failure is the inadequate nutritional environment furnished the cells of the developing embryos."[2] While this "inadequate nutritional environment" may result from factors other than food, dietary considerations significantly affect the incidence of spontaneous abortion (miscarriage), stillbirth, and the birth of premature, deformed, or otherwise defective children.

Every standard nutrition text cites animal experiments from which evidence of direct relationship between defects and dietary factors is abundant. In the early 1930s it was noted that pregnant pigs deprived of vitamin A gave birth to piglets without eyeballs, with cleft palates, harelips, accessory ears, and abnormalities of the kidneys, to name a few of the defects.[3] Zinc deficiencies in pregnant rats have been shown to result in failure of many fetuses to develop and in gross malformations in many of those that do survive.[4] Folic acid omitted from healthy pregnant rats' diets early in gestation results in no live births, as was noted in the chapter on herbs, and those young whose mothers have an insufficient supply of the nutrient are frequently born with abnormalities affecting skeleton, kidneys, lungs, heart, blood vessels, eyes, brains, sex organs, and other portions of the deprived animal's body.[5] Riboflavin removed from pregnant rats' diets during the time the bodies of the young are differentiating results in cleft palates, missing limbs or parts of limbs, club feet, abdomens that do not close and other abnormalities.[6] Every vitamin or mineral that has been shown to be needed by the animal being studied could be added to the list of those for which there is incontrovertible evidence that deficiency during fetal development results in defective young or reproductive failure.

We do not experiment with people as we do with animals; and it would rarely happen that one nutrient would suddenly be removed from a human mother's diet. Careful human studies have, however, provided abundant evidence that the human mother's choice of foods during the development of her child does significantly affect the state of well-being in which the child is born.[7]

Classic among human studies is one done by Dr. B. S. Burke and her associates at the Harvard School of Public Health, first reported in 1940 and still cited by the late Dr. L. Jean Bogert in the 1973 edition of her text *Nutrition and Physical Fitness*. After rating the diets of 216 pregnant mothers and studying them against the performance of the mothers and the ratings given their children by physicians who were not informed of the mother's nutritional status, Dr. Burke concluded:

> If the diet of the mother during pregnancy is poor to very poor, she will undoubtedly have an infant whose physical condition will be poor. In the 216 cases considered, all stillborn infants, all infants who died within a few days of birth except one, most infants who had marked congenital defects, all premature, and all functionally immature infants were born to mothers whose diets during pregnancy were very inadequate.
>
> If the mother's diet during pregnancy is good or excellent, her infant will in all probability be in good or excellent physical condition. Rarely it may happen otherwise.

Mothers as well as babies benefit from good diets during pregnancy. Of the mothers in Dr. Burke's study, two thirds of those on poor diets had complications during pregnancy and half of those on poor diets suffered preeclampsia, a condition characterized by high blood pressure, swollen feet, legs, and other tissues, and excretion of protein in the urine. Not one on a good diet experienced these symptoms, and fewer than one third of them had any problems at all.[8]

Dr. Burke's conclusions were corroborated by a study done at Toronto General Hospital by J. H. Ebbs and others reported in 1941 and 1942. By December, 1944 there was information to justify the *Borden Review of Nutrition Research* assertion:

> The combined results of prenatal studies here [U.S.A.] and abroad have pointed out two important facts: (1) The quality of the diet...markedly influences not only the course of the pregnancy and the health of the mother, but the condition of the infant at birth and its health at least six months thereafter; (2) the diet of a majority of expectant mothers falls short of meeting desirable nutrition goals during this critical period.[9]

Both these assertions have been validated in many subsequent studies and reaffirmed in recent nutrition surveys in the U.S.A. and Canada.

Specific Nutritional Problems in Reproduction

Among the conditions known to develop with deficiencies of specific nutrients are two endemic ones: they tend to occur in geographic areas in which the nutrients are in short supply in the soil. Cretinism occurs with lack of iodine and dwarfism with deficiency of zinc. (Cretinism may occur from other injury to the thyroid but is most often related to diet.)

Cretins exhibit stunted growth, peculiar facial conformation and skin texture, mental retardation, and other problems related to defective speech and hearing. If the condition is discovered soon enough after birth, the administration of thyroxine or iodine as needed can correct the situation. It may be largely prevented by the use of iodized salt.[10]

Dwarfism caused by lack of zinc is also treatable with zinc if the condition is discovered soon enough after birth. Mothers do not seem to transfer their own body stores to their children and must have adequate supplies in their current diet.

Our knowledge of the role of zinc in human nutrition is very new. The mineral was included in the Recommended Dietary Allowances of the U.S.A. for the first time in 1974. While data are not generally available indicating amounts contained in various foods, some known to provide zinc are seafoods, meats, eggs, legumes, and whole grain cereals. It seems to be more readily available from animal than from plant sources. I shall discuss it further in connection with infant feeding.[11]

Tooth development is a major consideration before birth. Even the permanent teeth begin to be formed during the fifth month of fetal life, and all the nutrients essential to life need to be present to make them strong. Calcium and phosphorus are of obvious significance, but these do not function without their teams including vitamins C, D, and B_6 and flouride must be present to make the enamel strong. Without iron, copper, protein, and a host of other nutrients there can be no supporting structure through which needed nutrients can be transported to the site of tooth formation and in which the teeth may stand. In spite of the fact that some genes seem to produce better teeth than others, and the child's nutrition and care of errupted teeth is significant in their development and maintenance, it is the mother's nutrition during pregnancy that determines whether they can ever be strong and whether she will have to give a tooth for every child, as was once believed. If the mother is well fed, there is no need either for the mother to lose her teeth or, in most cases, for the baby's teeth to be poorly formed.[12]

Protein-calorie deficiency, with attendant short supplies of vitamins and minerals, is probably the most widely suffered nutritional problem of pregnant mothers the world over. This deficiency persists in developing countries often because of the unavailability of food, among the poor because of lack of money and ignorance of food values, and among the more affluent because of poor food choices, sometimes because of ignorance and sometimes the mother's effort to maintain a slender figure. It results in full-term babies being born undersized and underdeveloped in many ways that are never fully corrected after birth. Prebirth malnutrition often followed by poor postnatal nutrition has also been identified as at least one of the possible factors in the growing number of apparently bright children who have learning difficulties because they do not see words and objects as the rest of the population sees them.[13]

Food Needs During Pregnancy

Being aware of the dangers of fetal malnutrition, the National Research Council Committee on Maternal Nutrition recommends that a pregnant mother never allow her intake to fall below 36 calories per kilogram (2.2 pounds) of pregnant weight.[14] For a 130-pound (59 kg) woman, that totals about 2,124 Calories and is the amount of energy found to be required for adequate protein utilization during pregnancy. It may require an additional 300 Calories a day over the diet of nonpregnant women and should result in a steady gain of from 0.25 to 0.45 kg (slightly over one half pound and slightly under one pound) per week, with a total gain of at least 11 kg (24.2 pounds). (The council recognizes the recommendation of other authorities that the gain should be more—12.5 kg [27.5 pounds].)

Extra foods are needed during pregnancy to meet these needs: the developing baby; the supporting tissues, including the placenta through which the child is fed in the uterus, the amniotic fluid in which the child rests, breast tissue and some reserve fat for milk production with which the infant is to be fed after birth; increased rate of metabolism that occurs as the infant develops; and energy to move the increased weight of mother, child, and supporting tissues.

Pregnant girls need additional Calories to provide for their own normal growth needs as well as those of their child. Undernourished women will also need to gain more than the average. Certainly pregnancy is not time to shed unwanted pounds unless it can be done by cutting out empty Calories and increasing activity to a reasonable amount.

On the other hand, pregnancy is no excuse for becoming obese either.[15] The need is to concentrate on eating wholesome naturally nutritious foods indicated in the basic food plan and eliminating high calorie foods that contribute little of the essential nutrients. No food essential is to be eliminated, and fat is one of the essentials. Diets low in essential fatty acids often result in excessive hemorrhaging of the mother at delivery and damage to the developing child.

Protein is of critical importance during pregnancy. The recommended increase is almost half again the normal requirement. For those already on generous protein intakes, this may not require any additional consumption. An overload of protein is not helpful either. For those now using the recommended amount, the additional will provide about half of the extra 300 Calories a day. In fact, since protein comes in combination with fats and carbohydrates, foods containing the protein needed will probably supply the entire extra calorie allowance.

The need for most vitamins and minerals also increases during pregnancy—some of them dramatically, as is indicated by reviewing the RDAs of the various nutrients. Vitamin D alone remains the same throughout. Most of the others are increased by one fourth to one third of the RDA of adult women. Calcium, phosphorus, and magnesium RDAs are increased by one half of the normal for women, and folacin and iron are recommended to be about double that recommended for the nonpregnant female.[16]

It is wisdom to supply these needs as much as possible from food. This can be done by using whole grains, milk, green and leafy vegetables, lean meats, fish, legumes, eggs, liver and fruits. Supplements may be used as recommended by a physician, but to depend on a supplement may mean that there will be some nutrients not yet known or not included in that particular supplement that may be missing, and an excess of some nutrients that may cause trouble.

Excess vitamin D, for example, has been found to damage the hearts of the unborn. Blood flow to the child's developing cells is restricted, causing poor development that frequently affects the brain. In one study 58 children of mothers taking large doses of vitamin D were found to have heart damage associated with the use of the vitamin, and half of those with heart damage were also mentally retarded. Elfin-like appearance is also characteristic of this sort of damage.[17]

Special Problems for Teen-age Mothers

Very young mothers produce proportionately two times as many premature babies as older mothers, even including smoking mothers in both groups. Two factors seem to be involved: the mother's body is itself immature and so has a high demand for nutrients also needed by the baby, and many teen-age diets are poorly chosen and lacking in the nutrients needed.[18]

In one study of teen-age families it was noted that teen-age mothers and fathers frequently ate diets low in milk, vegetables, and fruits. Their babies, on the other hand, were given too much milk with too little eggs, meats, vegetables, and fruits.[19] Consistently, studies of teen-age diets indicate that up to two thirds of them show less than desirable consumption of vitamins C and A, calcium and iron—deficiencies related to the neglect of milk, green leafy vegetables, and fruits.[20] Those who choose to produce children early in life should show more concern for giving those children a chance to enter the world healthy.

Every woman, teen-ager or adult, who has any possibility of becoming pregnant should be consciously prepared at all times to give her child a chance to be formed and born normally by being constantly well nourished herself and free of deleterious drugs. Many mothers are not aware of their pregnancy during the first few weeks—the critical time when body structures are differentiated—so congenital malformations may occur before the women are aware that they need to change their habits if they have not chosen a good way of life from the beginning. Fortunately, an infant can draw from its mother's stores for most of its needs for a time, but that time is limited and withdrawal from her stores leaves the mother less able to face the rigors of pregnancy with ease and equanimity than if she had provided enough for herself and her child from the first. For greatest satisfaction, there should also be conscious preparation for the child's birth by the formation of adequate skeletal structures and musculature to permit normal delivery. This requires adequate nutrition from one generation to another as well as present attention to good nutrition and exercise.

Special Problems for Those Taking Oral Contraceptives

For those who have been taking oral contraceptives, there is special need to be concerned with nutrition.[21] While such contraceptives are in use, the need for many nutrients is greatly increased. Already we know there is increased need for vitamins B_6, B_{12}, E, folacin, and zinc, each of which can be crucial in the development of the fetus. We know other requirements are also increased, and there is need for further research.

After five months on an oral contraceptive, some women have a vitamin B_{12} level of blood which is indistinguishable from that of a person with pernicious anemia unless additional B_{12} is taken. The folate level of the blood falls when "the pill" is taken, and the deficiency is sometimes apparent in blotchy pigmentation similar to that which occurs in tropical sprue or during pregnancy when the diet is folacin deficient. Vitamin B_6 deficiencies have been confirmed repeatedly in those who use these contraceptives, some of them so severe that they require massive doses of the vitamin to bring about amelioration. In one study normal concentration of vitamin C could not be maintained in 126 women taking oral contraceptives even with vitamin supplementation. There have been more than fifty metabolic changes related to nutrition noted in women using oral contraceptives, according to a review of the subject published in the *Journal of the American Dietetics Association.*[22]

These "pill" oriented deficiencies can, of course, be responsible for a number of health problems with both physical and mental manifestations. Severe anemias can result, and with a variety of trace mineral or vitamin deficiencies they may be responsible for much of the depression and other personality changes noted in up to 50 percent of the patients who use "the pill," according to Canada's Food and Drug Directorate.[23]

If these increased nutritional needs have not been cared for during the period the prospective mother has been on the contraceptive, such a woman is poorly prepared for pregnancy. If pregnancy after the discontinuance of the contraceptive is to be wholly successful, these nutritional needs must be met. For the sake of the woman involved, they should be met from the time "the pill" is first taken. For the sake of the unborn child, they ought to be met before pregnancy occurs.

Finally

The birth of defective babies is a tragic fact in the lives of a vast number of twentieth century parents. It ought not to be so. While there are hereditary and environmental factors that we are not yet knowledgeable enough to control, there are many defects related to the use of deleterious drugs and to faulty nutrition that we can avert. It is God's purpose that we have healthy children. It is our stewardship as prospective parents to make choices that will help to make it possible.

---

1. Roger J. Williams, University of Texas, *Nutrition Against Disease*, Pitman Publishing Corporation, N.Y., Toronto, London, Tel Aviv, 1971, p. 51.
2. *Ibid.*, p. 52.
3. "Dietary Causes of Congenital Abnormalities," *Borden's Review of Nutrition Research*, Vol. 5, No. 9, Nov. 1944, pp. 1-2.
4. Williams, *op. cit.*, p. 58, documented p. 235.
5. *Ibid.*, pp. 59-60, documented pp. 235-236.
6. "Dietary Causes of Congenital Abnormalities," *op. cit.*, pp. 6-9.
7. Williams, *op. cit.*, pp. 51-66, documentation pp. 231-237.
8. L. Jean Bogert, George M. Briggs, Doris Howes Calloway, *Nutrition and Physical Fitness*, Ninth Edition, W. B. Saunders Co., Philadelphia and London, 1973, pp. 443-444.
9. "Clinical Studies on Prenatal Nutrition," *Borden's Review of Nutrition Research*, Vol. 5, No. 10, Dec. 1944, pp. 5-10.
10. National Academy of Sciences, *Recommended Dietary Allowances*, Eighth Edition, 1974, pp. 96-97. Also L. Earle Arnow, Ph.D., M.D., *Food Power, a Doctor's Guide to Commonsense Nutrition*, Nelson-Hall Co., Chicago, 1972, pp. 64, 154-155.
11. National Academy of Sciences, *ibid.*, pp. 99-101 (also H. H. Sandstead, "Zinc Nutrition in the United States," *The Am. J. of Clinical Nutrition*, Vol. 26, Oct., 1973, p. 1251.
12. Williams, *op. cit.*, pp. 114-118.
13. Bacon F. Chow, Ph.D., R. Quentin Blackwell, Ph.D., Roger W. Sherwin, M.B., "Nutrition and Development," *Borden's Review of Nutrition Research*, Vol. 29, Third Quarter, 1968, pp. 25-37. Also Grace A. Goldsmith, M.D., "Nutrition and World Health," *Journal of the American Dietetics Assn.*, Vol. 63, Nov. 1973, pp. 513-518.
14. National Academy of Sciences, *Recommended Dietary Allowances*, Eighth Edition, 1974, p. 31.
15. Jean Mayer, *Overweight Causes, Cost and Control*, Prentice-Hall, Inc., Englewood Cliffs, N.J., 1968, p. 113.
16. National Academy of Sciences, *op. cit.*, chart.
17. Alton L. Blakeslee, "Today's Health News," *Today's Health*, Feb. 1967, p. 9.
18. Ted Berland, "Giving More of Our Infants the Lives They Deserve," *Today's Health*, Aug. 1971, pp. 16-19, 70-72.
19. M. S. Van de Mark, V. R. S. Underwood, "Dietary Habits and Food Consumption Patterns of Teenage Families," *Journal of the American Home Economics Association*, Vol. 63, Oct. 1971, p. 540, abstracted in *Journal of the American Dietetics Association*, Vol. 60, Jan. 1972, p. 63. Also M. Markham, "Developmental Nutrition and the Facts of Life," *What's New in Home Economics*, Vol. 36, Jan. 1972, p. 31, abstracted in the *Journal of the American Dietetics Association*, Vol. 36, April 1972, p. 354.
20. B. C. Schorr, D. Sanjur, and E. C. Erickson, "Teenage Food Habits," *Journal of the American Dietetics Association*, Vol. 61, Oct. 1972, pp. 415-420.
21. "Requirements of Vitamin B_6 During Pregnancy," *Nutrition Reviews*, Vol. 34, No. 1, Jan. 1976, pp. 15-16; Myron Winick, M.D., "Nutritional Disorders of American Women," *Nutrition Today*, Vol. 10, Numbers 5 and 6, Sept. Oct./Nov. Dec., 1975, pp. 26-28.
22. C. E. Butterworth, Jr., M.D., "Interactions of Nutrients with Oral Contraceptives and Other Drugs," *Journal of the American Dietetics Association*, Vol. 62, May, 1973, pp. 510-514.
23. Food and Drug Directorate (Canada), R_x *Bulletin: Oral Contraceptives*, Dec. 1970, p. 25.

CHAPTER 9

Well Fed Infants

Opportunity to give children the best possible start in life does not stop with good birth. Their emotional and spiritual nurturing, cleanliness, immunizations, rest, education, and food are the responsibility of parents for a number of years. Generous amounts of love and judicious fondling, regular but not too frequent bathing, clothing and covers that are loose enough and light enough to permit freedom of movement, a chance to rest in quiet, well-ventilated quarters, and immunizations as they appear advisable all promote health.

Of prime importance to the child's physical well-being, however, is the food with which he/she is nourished. If it is adequate, some deficiencies in other areas may be overcome. If food is inadequate, however, the child has no chance to build a healthy body or mind.

Mother's Milk, Baby's Best First Food

The best food for a newborn baby is human milk. True, many a child has grown to "healthy" adulthood, by commonly accepted standards, on artificial feeding, and some artificial feeding may be necessary. Grave concern is being expressed by World Health Organization personnel over a trend toward artificial feeding among mothers of developing countries, however, and increasing encouragement is being given to return to breast feeding among those of more affluent nations.

It is easy to understand the concern for breast feeding in those areas in which equipment, food supplies, and sanitation necessary to safe artificial feeding are not available. Advantages of breast feeding in more developed areas of the world may not be so apparent. Breast fed babies do, however, have a higher degree of immunity to many diseases, less indigestion, fewer allergies, fewer early deaths, and if they do acquire severe infections, they overcome them more readily than artificially fed babies do.[1]

Breast fed babies frequently seem more emotionally secure than others, but studies indicate that it is the close physical contact rather than the kind of milk that is most responsible. A similar element can be introduced into the bottle fed baby's life if it is held during feedings and cuddled frequently instead of being shunted off to a propped-up bottle while its parents tend to less important duties.

The nutritional quality of mother's milk has never been duplicated for artificial feeding, however. The quality of the product is good reason for continued emphasis on the desirability of breast feeding, not only in developing countries where it can be crucial to the very life of the child, but everywhere children are born to whom parents wish to give a maximum opportunity for health and well-being. A comparison of some characteristics of mother's milk with that available for artificial feeding will give some indication of the nutritional reasons for breast feeding being the best feeding for a baby.

Colostrum—Characteristics and Values

Colostrum, that protein-rich secretion that precedes the secretion of milk, has no counterpart in artificial feeding. Not only is it richer in protein than the milk that follows but the protein is very like the gamma globulin of blood, which plays a significant part in the production of immunity to disease.

Colostrum is also mineral rich and fat and sugar poor. The mineral content accounts, at least in part, for the natural laxative quality of the substance, which helps the infant dispose of the mucous that is in its digestive tract at birth. With early satisfaction of the strong sucking instinct present at birth and the colostrum, the digestive tract of the infant early begins to operate in the right direction, avoiding the problems attendant upon the infant's regurgitation and sometimes aspirating (breathing) the mucous.

Colostrum is richly endowed with vitamins, especially A and E. At one week, the breast fed infant has as much as five times the amount of vitamin E in its body as does its bottle fed counterpart whose formula has not been enriched with this important nutrient.[2]

Infant Need vs. Human Milk and Artificial Formula

When the actual milk flow is established, it is exactly suited to the metabolic equipment of the newborn. Cow's milk, usually substituted for it, must be modified to be usable at all. It has to be diluted to produce the concentration of protein and calcium that the infant digestive system can handle. It must be heated to form a soft enough protein curd to be digested, kill harmful bacteria that may have invaded the milk, and keep it from irritating the intestines. It must be reinforced with carbohydrates or fats (sugar is usually used) to provide energy for the infant's needs, and it must be fortified with a number of vitamins and minerals to meet those needs.

Protein of mother's milk is largely lactalbumin. It forms a soft, flocculent, easily digested curd in the baby's stomach. Protein of cow's milk is principally casein, which must be heated to make a curd that the child can digest. Protein of mother's milk has a good supply of cystine, an amino acid suited to the digestive enzymes of the infant and needed for rapid growth. Protein of cow's milk is rich in methionine, an amino acid for which the newborn is not at first equipped.[3]

The result of these differences is that human milk protein is utilized almost 100 percent by the infant, about twice as efficiently as the cow's milk protein.[4] Consequently, for the baby to get needed protein, the formula fed must have many more ounces (milliliters) of food and additional water must be supplied to dilute the protein wastes so the kidneys can handle them without damage.

Mother's milk has nearly half of its calories in the form of fat, about 10.6 percent of which is essential linoleic acid. Cow's milk has only 2.1 percent linoleic acid before dilution. Both milks contain palmitic acid. That in mother's milk does not interfere with calcium absorption. Some of that in cow's milk combines with calcium and is excreted with loss of both calcium and fat.[5]

Cholesterol is also present in mother's milk in generous supply, to the advantage of the breast fed, it is believed. Laboratory animals introduced to cholesterol in mother's milk tend to grow into adults equipped to handle dietary cholesterol effectively. Some researchers suggest that one of the significant factors in the increase in serum cholesterol in some persons may be related to the use of cow's milk formula for infant feeding and early weaning of those who are breast fed.[6]

Fatty acids are essential for developing infants. They are the source of energy the infant body prefers to support its rapid growth. More importantly, fatty acids are essential for normal development of many tissues including those of the brain. They are essential for myelinization (covering with a fatty sheath) of the brain, a process that takes at least three years.[7] This need should be kept in mind by those who propose feeding infants nonfat (skim) milk in the hope of reducing obesity.* It would hardly be profitable to produce a generation of slender people with defective brains. Breast milk provides essential fatty acids abundantly, yet a wholly breast fed baby is rarely obese.[8]

The carbohydrate of mother's milk is lactose, for which the baby is supplied with enzymes and which does not irritate the infant's digestive system. It also has a particularly beneficial effect on the flora (microorganisms) of the intestines. As the lactose is digested, an acid medium is formed in which many putrefactive and harmful bacteria cannot grow. The bacteria most prevalent are *Lactobacillus bifidus*, a safe and protective culture that helps the child resist disease. It seems to specifically interfere with the activity of the influenza virus.[9] Bacteria are favored that produce additional supplies of B vitamins and vitamin K.[10]

Lactose is sometimes used in formula, and some formula is made with lactic acid or cultured milk. Frequently, however, sucrose is used for convenience and economy. Sucrose is irritating to the tissues and produces an alkaline medium in the intestines in which many unacceptable bacteria flourish. A foul smelling stool reflects their presence. Breast fed children usually have innocuous stools until other foods are added.[11]

When sugar is used to provide needed energy to formula, the proportion is much higher than in mother's milk. This practice is being questioned because it may cause formation of excessive numbers of fat cells, develop tastes for sweet foods that foster obesity, and have deleterious effect on teeth.[12]

The possibility of tooth decay is increased if faulty feeding

---

*Other considerations with respect to nonfat milk feeding for infants include the following: Fats must be present for calcium to be absorbed properly; without fats, eczemas develop; fat soluble vitamins must be supplied as supplement. Vitamins A and D frequently are added to nonfat milk. Vitamin E rarely is.

practices are followed. Certainly leaving the bottle in a child's mouth while it sleeps, whether it contains sweet formula or a fruit juice promotes decay of newly erupted teeth.

If a mother eats an adequate diet, her milk provides everything known to be needed by an infant during its first few weeks or even months of life, with the possible exception of vitamin D.[13] This may be added to the mother's diet, or the child may be exposed to the sun daily so it can manufacture its own vitamin D. Since both these procedures may be inconvenient or uncertain, most doctors prefer to prescribe some supplement early in life whether the child is breast or formula fed. (Such supplementation is imperative for the formula fed, not only for vitamin D but for a number of other nutrients.)

The well nourished, full-term baby is born with a store of iron that will last from two to six months when supplemented with mother's milk. This should care for the child's need until foods rich in iron can be introduced. Cow's milk, however, has only traces of iron even before dilution. If it is not properly heated it can cause gastrointestinal bleeding that further increases the need for iron. It is wise to give supplemental iron to one so fed to prevent an iron deficiency anemia. When iron is added, it is recommended that copper be added, too. One cannot work effectively without the other.[14]

A macrocytic anemia that does not respond to iron therapy affects some children.[15] In fact, additional iron makes it worse. This is caused by lack of vitamin E and occurs most frequently in infants of low birth weight or those whose mothers have been on high polyunsaturated fat diets. Normally human milk provides the needed vitamin E, but cow's milk does not. The American Academy of Pediatrics recommended in 1969 that vitamin E be included in all infant formula.

Vitamin A is a nutrient well known to be essential for growth and development. Mother's milk provides generous amounts of it. Whole cow's milk diluted for formula has about one third as much of the vitamin. Without additional supplies, the formula fed are susceptible to serious ills that affect their growth, sight, and general health. On the other hand, excessive amounts are dangerous. Only those amounts recommended by reliable sources should be given.

Closely related to the use of vitamin A is the supply of zinc available to the infant. Since vitamin A cannot be withdrawn from storage in the liver without zinc, if the mineral is not in good supply the child is susceptible to many conditions that are similar to those related to lack of vitamin A. Inadequate amounts of zinc also produce impairment of taste and smell acuity (hypogeusia) which makes eating less enjoyable. Eight percent of 150 children in middle income families in Denver, Colorado, recently showed this response to low zinc intake.[16]

Fortification or supplementation with zinc, if needed, must be done skillfully because of its relation to other nutrients, especially copper,[17] and its toxicity in large amounts. Using mother's milk eliminates the necessity for such supplementation. The National Research Council (U.S.A.) recommends the fortification of formula with iodine to meet the RDA[18] and notes that chromium, tin, vanadium, nickel, flourine, silicone are other minerals known to be needed for which RDAs have not yet been established.[19]

Vitamin C must be provided daily for infants from very early in their life. Mother's milk contains the vitamin, and the amount may be maximized by the mother's consumption of a high vitamin C food half an hour before the baby is fed. Formula fed must have a supplement. Usually it is combined with vitamins A and D in drops given almost from birth. Infants born to mothers who have been taking massive doses of the nutrient have been reported to have an increased need for the vitamin.[20]

Lactoferrin, a protein containing iron that offers protection from some infections, characterizes breast milk. It protects especially from *Escherchia coli* enteritis, a debilitating intestinal infection occurring most frequently among infants exposed to unsanitary conditions. Its presence is one more reason for concern that mothers in developing countries continue to breast feed their children.[21]

Underfed mothers produce surprisingly good quality milk. In areas of general undernutrition, breast fed babies generally develop similarly to their counterparts in more fortunate areas of the world for about the first six months of life. One exception is that those mothers who subsist principally on polished rice frequently have babies with infantile beriberi.[22]

On the negative side, a mother may do her baby a disservice

if she introduces deleterious drugs into his/her formative body through her milk. Alcohol, nicotine, morphine, opium, heroin, and similar drugs are in the milk as well as in the placental blood of the drug-using mother, and no child should be subjected to them. Some laxatives, tetracycline, penicillin, and other therapeutic drugs also pass into the milk. Some pediatricians feel that antihistamines and oral contraceptives should not be used during breast feeding.[23]*

Non-nutritive Reasons for Choosing to Breast Feed

Breast feeding is convenient. The nursing mother is ready to feed her baby at any place at any time. She has no need to carry huge amounts of paraphernalia with her, for she does not have to mix formula or sterilize either the formula or equipment. Strange water is of no concern to her, nor is temperature, either with respect to preserving the food or having it at a temperature acceptable to the child when it is needed. True she must be near her baby and be the one free when it needs food. For many mothers, this is a pleasure.[24]

Breast feeding affects the mother's health in at least three beneficial ways.[25] (1) She is less likely to develop breast cancer. The mechanism of protection is not understood, but the statistics indicate it incontrovertibly. (2) The sucking of the baby exerts a powerful contracting influence on the uterus, assisting to expel the placenta if the child is permitted at the breast immediately after birth, reducing the probability of excessive bleeding and causing the uterus to return to its normal quiescent size more quickly than is possible without the stimulus. (3). Breast feeding *may* reduce the likelihood of another pregnancy soon after the birth. This possibility is related to the level of the pituitary hormone, prolactin, induced by the nursing of the baby. If it is kept high, it triggers the production of progesterone which in turn prevents the release of an egg. If there is no egg, there can be no pregnancy. Partial breast feeding may not provide needed stimulation to keep the hormone level high enough to prevent the release of an egg, however, and with early introduction of other foods, most Western babies are only partially fed. When

---

*Jaundice sometimes associated with breast feeding is usually temporary and harmless. All jaundice should be checked by a physician, however. See LaLeche League International, Inc., *Information Sheet* #10, "Breastfeeding and Jaundice," Sept. 1971, for information.

there is not adequate stimulation to prevent it, the menstrual cycle will resume and with it the possibility of another pregnancy.[26]

Considering the benefits available to all concerned, members of the symposium to which reference has been frequently made in this chapter concluded, "Breast feeding is cheaper, more available, easier and more convenient than bottle feeding; it is better in every way for both the baby and the mother."

Biology of Breast Feeding

Breast feeding is dependent on two biological mechanisms—the production of milk and the release of that milk for expulsion from the breast.[27] Milk production is automatic when the proper hormones are present in the proper concentration in the body of the mother. As pregnancy is terminated, the level of prolactin (also called lactogen) secreted by the pituitary gland is high, and the breasts that have been prepared for the event during pregnancy fill, first with colostrum and then with true milk. To maintain production, the breasts must be emptied. In fact, even though the period of high prolactin at the close of pregnancy may have passed without needed stimulation from emptying the breast to maintain milk flow, the level of the hormone can be raised again by putting a child to the breast and receiving the stimulation of sucking.

To empty the breast, a reflex that is triggered by another pituitary enzyme, oxytocin, must be operative. Normally it is a simple physical response to the baby's touch on the nipple as it searches for food. The response is, however, extremely sensitive to the mother's emotions. Any disturbances, especially in the early stages of lactation, can prevent production of the hormone, the ducts through which the milk should flow remain constricted, the milk cannot be emptied from the basket cells into the larger sinuses just below the nipple, and even a powerful breast pump can remove only a small portion of the milk that has been produced.

Blocking the let-down reflex may come from embarrassment over exposing the breast for the feeding, from anxiety over whether there will be enough for the baby or whether the husband-father will approve the procedure (if this has not been decided in previous preparation or by mature judgment), or how the doctor bill will be paid or if the other children are well, or from simple irritations, interruptions, or a fear of pain. Even the presence of a brusque, unsympathetic doctor or nurse can stop the flow.

If the emotions are such that a good let-down reflex is not operative, the child is deprived of the richest of the milk. First milk at each feeding is thin (lacking in fat). The richest milk is held in the alveoli until the last one third of the feeding. Unless all the milk is released, and the breast emptied, production dwindles. Emptying the breast stimulates further production.

If the mother, therefore, allows something in her environment to prevent her letting down her milk, her supply dwindles and there is not enough—not because she cannot produce an adequate supply of excellent quality food but because she has not learned to relax enough that her child can be fed. It is this situation that has led some practitioners to recommend the dubious practice of giving the mother a glass of wine or a bottle of beer or another tranquillizer while she is getting accustomed to breast feeding. Mothers who want to feed their children and have the peace that can come through the Christ have no need for a sedative.

Successful Breast Feeding

Mothers who are awake at the birth of their children respond most readily immediately after birth to the impulse to feed the baby. If they are allowed that privilege, and the process progresses from these early moments of life together, many of the problems that presently beset new mothers never arise.[28] There are no painfully engorged breasts, no struggling frustrations with "lazy" babies that refuse to nurse simply because they are already filled with some sugar solution or formula from the nursery. There are no painful emotional upheavals that go with inadequate supply from lack of stimulation, fewer problems with let-down reflexes in a confident mother. The modern physician sees that the baby nurses at the earliest possible opportunity after birth—within the hour if possible—to insure successful breast feeding.

Almost every mother who is normally healthy can breast feed if she wants to do it. She can even produce an excellent quality food for her child without having an adequate diet herself, as is demonstrated daily by mothers in developing countries. This food production is, of course, at the expense of the mother's body. For superior food for the baby and continued good health herself, the breast feeding mother must eat a sufficient quantity of well-balanced foods daily. Special foods are not needed—just more of those she is already charged to eat.

More calories probably may be eaten during lactation than at any other time. It takes energy to produce milk, and a child wholly breast fed for the first few months takes up to a liter (1.06 quart) a day. Since most people introduce other foods before that amount of milk is needed, however, the 1974 RDAs call for only about 500 extra Calories a day for the lactating mother (1968 RDA called for 1,000 extra). If these are not enough to keep up production, prevent undesirable weight loss for the mother, and give acceptable satisfaction of hunger, more should be taken. One should just make sure the extra calories are going into milk production and not into fat. If there is no breast feeding, there is no after birth calorie splurge. In fact, there is need to reduce even the fat reserves set up for breast feeding.

For milk production, there is not quite as much protein or folacin needed as during pregnancy. There are increased needs for vitamin A (an extra 1,000 IU—200 RE), vitamin C (20 mg more), riboflavin (up 0.2 mg), niacin (up 2 mg), iodine (up 25 micrograms), zinc (up 5 mg), and all the rest of the nutrient RDAs remain as for pregnancy for the present.[29] This simply means more emphasis on fruits, vegetables, and whole grains, continued use of milk and iodized salt. Fluids are needed, of course, and caffeine-containing beverages are not good choices. They are diuretics and flush water from the system.[30]

Nursing mothers can eat any food they normally eat without distress. Most of the problems that come from eating a food believed to be taboo is the mother's anxiety over having broken the taboo. Babies may be startled at a new flavor that comes through their milk, but a mother's cheerful acceptance of their reaction and her assurance that the milk is still hers is usually enough to satisfy the child and help him/her to return to a satisfying meal. One writer has suggested that if garlic is a flavor the family enjoys, the baby had just as well get accustomed to it.

To breast feed most successfully, then, requires that a mother must want to do it, should nurse her child soon after birth and frequently during the first few days, must live a healthy, well-adjusted life free from excessively disrupting emotional conflicts or anxieties, and should eat enough good food to care for her needs and the baby's. She will need a physician and hospital that will cooperate. And an understanding, helpful husband may be the key person in the entire situation.

A father who understands that breast feeding can be a rich experience for the family, that mother and child will benefit by it healthwise, and that it will contribute to his wife's beauty can set the stage for successful breast feeding.[31] First of all, he can be of real help in convincing the physician that breast feeding is really the plan of the family and in choosing a hospital that will cooperate. Then he can be the instigator of a happy, relaxed atmosphere in the home, and a constant source of encouragement toward good food, proper exercise, rest, and happy experience conducive to good lactation.

We inadvertently demonstrated that a mother can breast feed her child even under adverse circumstances when I fed our first child. Our son was four days old when the doctor told me I would have to bottle feed him. I was shocked. I was sure I had lots of milk, but the doctor said that was an illusion. The baby had never received more than one fourth ounce (7½ ml) from me at a feeding. I knew the nurses had said I had inverted nipples and had had trouble keeping him awake to nurse, but there was no hint that I was not feeding him.

Having some knowledge of the physiology of lactation and knowing the nutritional and psychological advantages of breast feeding, I protested that I was going to feed our baby. As a nutritionist who had advocated breast feeding vocally, by radio and press, to have done otherwise would have been devastating to my ego and to my reputation. Besides, I was determined to give our children the best possible chance for a healthy life.

Gently the doctor reminded me that I was not physically equipped for the task, and that after four days I was already drying up. It was impossible!

It was then I learned that the baby had been bottle fed in the nursery from the start, and when he was brought to me he was never hungry enough to make the effort to get food from my recalcitrant nipples. I was angry and demanded that the doctor give me a chance by ordering all bottle feeding stopped immediately and that the baby be brought to me when he was hungry.

The doctor countered that the baby would lose weight. Since he was full term and weighed nine pounds at birth, I was certain that would not be a serious problem. I was sure he would soon have all the food he needed if I just had a chance. The doctor agreed that a modest weight loss would not be detrimental to his health and reluctantly ordered the feedings stopped.

The doctor's insistence that I could never feed the child shook my confidence a little, and I asked for God's help to see us through.

When they brought our son to me again, there was no need for nurses to try to keep him awake. He was hungry enough to work at getting his food and strong enough to make his efforts effective.

We went home that day without the formula the doctor insisted I should take. After my milk flow was established, I did supplement it a little to be certain the baby was not hungry. Supplements were soon refused, however, by a contented breast fed baby.

The doctor would not believe that the baby was breast fed until my testimony was corroborated by his nurse, who was my sister-in-law. When he was finally convinced, he remarked, "If that is true, Mrs. Smith has convinced me that with a little time and effort I could breast feed a baby!"

The necessary milk flow continued until the baby was weaned at nine months. Bottles offered then were refused with indignation.

Our second son was born in the same hospital with the same physician attending. When I reminded him, before the baby's birth, that I would be breast feeding, he smiled, recalled our first experience, then assured me that the child would not be given even water in the nursery. I told him I did not mind the water, but he ordered that nothing be given the child except mother's milk. There were no problems at all with feeding him or our three subsequent children, none of whom had supplementation except for other foods that were introduced into their dietaries as their physicians designated.

Mine was not an isolated case.[32] For healthy mothers, breast feeding is not only advisable but almost always possible. Even those who are completely dried up can return to production if they are willing to make the effort. (For additional assistance in successful breast feeding, contact the La Leche League International, Inc., 9616 Minneapolis Avenue, Franklin Park, Illinois, or one of its branches.)

The attitude of the person feeding the child can be more important to its emotional development and the establishment of good food habits than whether the milk is the mother's or a cow's.[33] If feedings are approached in a relaxed, happy, and confident manner, the child is likely to respond in a relaxed, confident, and trusting manner, not only to his/her food but to life in general. If the task is approached in a tense, resentful, unhappy way, the child will often fret, cry, fail to eat enough to satisfy his/her need even when food is available. With breast feeding, such a negative attitude can easily reduce the supply.

Adding Foods to the Growing Child's Dietary

Since mother's milk is not a perfect food for long, other foods must be added as the digestive system develops to handle them. Feeding during this period is still crucial from the standpoint of obtaining foods to support rapid growth and development and of developing good food habits for the rest of life.

Development of the brain and nervous system is still of especial importance to the child for the first three years or more. While the most rapid growth in these areas normally occurs just before birth and during the first two years, rapid development continues so that by four years, the child's brain is about 80 percent of its adult size. Children severely malnourished during this period of most rapid development, before or after birth, frequently suffer deprivation all of their lives. Their brains never attain normal size or weight, intellectual development is permanently impaired, their brain waves show abnormal encephalograms, and as they grow, their visual perception is abnormal, resulting in impaired learning. They have a poor grasp of the concept of time and a low level of ability to organize materials with which they work or play.[34]

Although good nutrition is still important after brains are well developed, temporarily being without food then will never have the devastating effect on the mental capabilities and the nervous system of the person involved that it has on the infant. Temporary impairment may result in the poorly fed adult, but the effects are largely reversible.[35]

Not only the brain grows rapidly in early infancy. After a preliminary adjustment during which as much as 10 percent of birth weight may be lost, the well nourished, full term infant doubles his/her weight in four to five months and triples it in a year. His/her length extends from 20 to 22 inches or so to 30 to 32 inches. Though this rapid growth requires more energy per unit of body weight than will ever be needed again,[36] because he/she is so tiny, it does not add up to a lot of food. Many an anxious mother insists on providing more than is needed and so develops eating habits that may create obesity later. Overfeeding of supplemental vitamins and minerals may be particularly dangerous. Only prescribed amounts should be given.

Generally physicians' recommendations are followed in offering new foods to children. For the breast fed child, solid foods may not be needed until four months or more.

Cereals are usually the first additional food offered, with the possible exception of orange juice and cod liver oil, because cereals provide iron and babies generally like them. They may be offered the formula fed at one month to six weeks or these may be delayed until much later, especially if there is a history of obesity in the family. Fruits and vegetables follow, maybe when the baby is three months old.[37] Thoroughly cooked and sieved egg yolk and meats may be introduced about a month later. Too early feeding of complicated foods, especially proteins, may result in the development of allergies. Some children cannot cope with even the protein of cow's milk and must have alternate formula. As the digestive system develops, the child is less likely to become allergic or to aspirate the food causing choking and lung irritation.

Developing Good Eating Habits

Feeding an increasingly wide variety of nutritious foods to a hungry but happy baby in quantities that can be taken in a relaxed manner forms the beginning of good food habits that foster good health through a happy childhood and a vigorous adulthood.[38]

Early emphasis on good food habits is important, for they often continue a lifetime. Foods eaten in childhood are likely to have memories and emotional responses attached to them that will tend to protract their use into adulthood or strike them forever from the approved list. Little Johnny spits out his carrots. Mother decides he does not like carrots and says so every time they are served. Big Johnny stoutly maintains that he does not like carrots, and unless he is trapped into trying them or makes an intelligent decision to try them as a result of later education, he goes through life refusing a very good and useful food.

On the other hand, Jackie spits out his broccoli. Mother removes the serving to avoid a mess. The next time broccoli is served, Jackie receives a small serving along with the rest of the family. Any comments made are general and to the effect that we taste all foods. There is no scene, no high pressure coaxing, no bribing or threatening. Gradually Jackie's portion increases as he learns to like broccoli and to try all new foods. Big Jack is a good eater of all wholesome foods.

Actually, in all probability, Johnny (or Jackie) was not spitting out his food because he did not like it. He had been accustomed to getting food by sucking. When he tried to suck the soft mass deposited in his mouth it just went the wrong way. When the child is first learning to eat from a spoon, it will help if the spoon is rested on the baby's tongue long enough for him to suck off the food and then removed for him to work with the food in motions that will eventually become chewing.

Finally

The best beginning food for most children is breast milk. It needs to be followed by a variety of foods offered in a manner designed to establish good food habits that help to assure good nutrition throughout life. Baby's food needs are measured in teaspoonfuls and ounces, milliliters and grams. Adult needs are measured in tablespoonfuls and cupfuls, portions of kilograms and liters. Basically, they are the same needs, and they fit into the plan enunciated by scientists and the Lord. Every child deserves to be well fed.

---

1. Symposium, "The Uniqueness of Human Milk," *American Journal of Clinical Nutrition*, Vol. 24, No. 9, Sept. 1971, pp. 970-1005. Extracted in the *Journal of the American Dietetics Association*, Vol. 59, Dec. 1971, pp. 599-600.
2. Karen Pryor, *Nursing Your Baby*, Harper and Row, N.Y., Evanston and London, 1963, pp. 60, 75. Also Alice Gerard, *Please Breast-Feed Your Baby*, Hawthorne Books, Inc., N.Y., 1970, p. 52.
3. Symposium, *op. cit.*, György, "Biochemical Aspects."
4. Pryor, *op. cit.*, p. 49. Also Symposium, *op. cit.*
5. Symposium, *op. cit.*
6. R. Reiser, and Z. Sidelman, "Control of Serum Cholesterol Homeostasis by Cholesterol in the Milk of the Suckling Rat," *Journal of Nutrition*, Vol. 102, Aug. 1972, pp. 1009-1016. Abstracted in

Journal of the American Dietetics Association, Vol. 61, Nov. 1972, p. 585.
7. Symposium, *op. cit.*
8. Sally Wendkos Olds, "Breast-Feeding Is Nature's Way of Saying Mother Knows Best," *Today's Health*, Vol. 54, No. 3, March 1976, pp. 47-49. Also Myron Winick, M.D., "Childhood Obesity," *Nutrition Today*, May/June, 1974, pp. 6-12.
9. Pryor, *op. cit.*, pp. 51-52. Also Symposium, *op. cit.*
10. Olds, *op. cit.*, p. 48.
11. Pryor and Symposium, both *op. cit.*
12. Olds and Winick, both *op. cit.*
13. Pryor, *op. cit.*, p. 55.
14. National Academy of Sciences, *Recommended Dietary Allowances*, Eighth Edition, 1974, pg. 95. Also J.R. Seeley, "Copper Deficiency in a Premature Infant Fed an Iron Fortified Formula," *New England Journal of Medicine*, Vol. 286, Jan. 13, 1972, p. 109. Extracted in *Journal of the American Dietetics Association*, Vol. 60, April 1972, p. 345.
15. "Vitamin E Therapy in Premature Babies," *Nutrition Reviews*, Vol. 33, No. 7, July 1975, pp. 206-208. Also J.G. Bieri, Ph. D., "Vitamin E," *Nutrition Reviews*, Vol. 33, No. 6, pp. 161-167. Also Pryor, *op. cit.*, p. 53.
16. National Academy of Sciences, *op. cit.*, pp. 99-100.
17. L.M. Klevay, "Hypercholesterolemia in Rats Produced by an Increase in the Ratio of Zinc to Copper Ingested," *The American Journal of Clinical Nutrition*, Vol. 26, Oct. 1973, p. 1060. Extracted in *Journal of the American Dietetics Association*, Vol. 64, Feb. 1974, p. 202.
18. National Academy of Sciences, *op. cit.*, p. 97.
19. *Ibid.*, pp. 101-102. Also "Trace Minerals and Iron," *Journal of the American Dietetics Association*, Vol. 64, Feb. 1974, p. 163.
20. W.J. Rhead and G.N. Schrauzer, "Risk of Long-Term Ascorbic Acid Overdose," *Nutrition Reviews*, Vol. 29, 1971, p. 262.
21. "Lactoferrin—A Bacteriostatic Protein in Human Milk," *Nutrition Reviews*, Vol. 30, Sept., 1972, p. 225. Extracted in *Journal of the American Dietetics Association*, Vol. 62, Jan. 1973, p. 106.
22. Pryor, *op. cit.*, p. 55.
23. Health Protection Branch, Department of National Health and Welfare (Canada), *RX Bulletin*, Vol. 6, No. 1, Jan./Mar. 1975, pp. 8-9.
24. Symposium, *op. cit.*, M. Thompson, "The Convenience of Breast-Feeding," p. 991.
25. Olds, *op. cit.*, Also Symposium, *op. cit.*, M. Newton, "Mammary Effects of Lactation," p. 993.
26. Pryor, *op. cit.*, p. 26. Also Derrick B. Jelliffe, and E. F. Patrice Jelliffe, "Choice of Contraceptives," Letter to the *British Medical Journal*, Vol. 4(594s) Dec. 14, 1974, p. 658.
27. Pryor, *op. cit.*, pp. 32-41. Also D.B. Jelliffe, and E.F.P. Jelliffe, "Approaches to Village Level Infant Feeding. V. How Breast Feeding Really Works (Facts vs. Medical Folklore)," *The Journal of Tropical Pediatrics and Environmental Child Health*, Vol. 17, June 1971, p. 62. Extracted in *Journal of the American Dietetics Association*, Vol. 60, Jan. 1972, p. 64. Also Jelliffe and Jelliffe, "Confidence and the Science of Lactation," *Journal of Pediatrics*, Vol. 84, March 1974, p. 462. Abstracted in *Journal of the American Dietetics Association*, Vol. 64, June 1974, p. 698.
28. Pryor, *op. cit.*, pp. 73-74.
29. National Academy of Sciences, *op. cit.*, Chart.
30. Gerard, *op. cit.*, p. 7.
31. Olds, *op. cit.*
32. *Ibid.*
33. Symposium, *op. cit.*
34. Alton L. Blakeslee, "Today's Health News," *Today's Health*, June 1967, p. 7. Also Williams, *op. cit.*, p. 59, with documentation pp. 232-237.
35. L. Earle Arnow, Ph.D., M.D., *Food Power, a Doctor's Guide to Commonsense Nutrition*, Nelson-Hall Co., Chicago, 1972, pp. 70-71.
36. Robert S. Goodhart, M.D., D.M.S., and Maurice E. Shils, M.D., Sc.D., editors of *Modern Nutrition in Health and Disease, Dietotherapy*, Fifth Edition, Lea and Febiger, Philadelphia, 1974, pp. 659-660.
37. American Academy of Pediatrics members of Today's Health "Committee of 100," "Growing Pains," *Today's Health*, Jan. 1973, p. 22.
38. Goodhart, *et al.*, *op. cit.*, p. 675.

CHAPTER 10

Alcohol

I have warned you, and forewarn you... that inasmuch as any man drinketh wine or strong drink among you, behold, it is not good, neither meet in the sight of your Father, only in assembling yourselves together, to offer up your sacraments before him.

And behold, this should be wine; yea, pure wine of the grape of the vine, of your own make. And again, strong drinks are not for the belly, but for the washing of your bodies.—Doctrine and Covenants 86:1a-c.

Drinking of alcoholic beverages has become so prevalent that among large segments of the world's people there is no longer a question of whether a person drinks but only whether a person is a "good" drinker. While there is much literature available that cautions against the "misuse" of alcohol and alcoholism, the use of alcohol is generally represented as innocuous and desirable for those who handle it properly.

In the Lord's instruction there is no equivocation. He does not say it is not good to get drunk or to become an alcoholic. He says it is not good to *drink* wine or strong drink. The only exception that he indicates as acceptable to him is use in the sacrament of Communion; and that must be wine made new by the group that uses it, not the strongly alcoholic or fortified wine of commerce.*

For those who have faith in the Lord's instructions and are committed to his purposes in the Restoration, abstinence is the chosen way of life. That this is the expectation of the Lord was

---

*See discussion of the Lord's instruction on the use of meat for further information concerning this exception.

reiterated in the revelation of 1976: "Some have been overcome by the grosser sins of the world—the spirit of revelry, wanton living, use of drugs, drinking and fornication—and fallen away."[1] The prophet, President W. Wallace Smith, emphasized the expectation in his 1976 Conference sermon when he said, "I am very disappointed to learn that it seems to be in vogue in some members' homes and on the part of some of the priesthood to drink dinner wines at times. Where this practice is known to exist, the administrative officers should take considerate but firm action to end it."[2]

For those deeply committed to a religious faith that requires it, abstinence has been a way of life for multitudes of people—Muslims, Buddhists, the Brahmin caste of India, and some denominations of Christianity.[3] For those not choosing abstinence because of their religious faith or whose religious-cultural orientation does not regulate their drinking as Judaism does, there seems an urgency in understanding facts about alcohol to promote responsible decision making.[4] For those who want to understand the custom of social drinking, problem drinking, and alcoholism, such information is likewise significant.[5]

Some Facts About Beverage Alcohol[6]

Beverage alcohol is ethyl alcohol. Other common alcohols such as methyl and isopropyl are immediately toxic and must not be drunk.

Ethyl alcohol is produced by the fermentation of sugars. Beer and whiskey are made from malted (germinated) grains, wine largely from grapes and berries, and rum from molasses.

Hard liquors result from the distillation of the alcohol produced by fermentation to concentrate the alcoholic content of the beverage. Whiskey, scotch, gin, vodka, and other liquors are distilled beverages.

Any two drinks that contain the same amount of alcohol will have a similar effect on the drinker when taken under the same circumstances. The same amount of alcohol is contained in approximately 12 ounces (360 ml) of beer, three ounces (90 ml) fortified wine, four ounces (120 ml) natural wine, and 1½ ounce (45 ml) of whiskey. This is the quantity that will be referred to as a drink in this discussion.

Alcohol is technically a food because it provides calories.*
It has no nutritional value except as energy, however. To
metabolize alcohol requires nutrients that must be provided by
other foods if health is to be maintained. Those interested in
nutritional implications of alcohol consumption may find Chapter
11 of Roger J. Williams' *Nutrition Against Disease* (Pitman Publishing Company, New York, 1971) of interest.

Alcohol is a mood-changing *drug*. As such it is every bit as
active in the body as prescription drugs, usually taken in carefully
regulated doses, and its misuse constitutes the most serious drug
problem faced by many nations.

Some Characteristic Responses to Alcohol

Alcohol's primary effect is on the brain, although the whole
body is affected. Since it does not have to be digested as most
foods, moments after it is consumed it reaches the brain, and every
other tissue, organ, and secretion of the body.[7]

Alcohol is a depressant, not the stimulant that many believe it
to be. Although people vary widely in their response to the drug,
some general observations have been made.

At low levels of alcohol in the blood, such as might result
from one drink taken in an hour, there may be a mild
tranquilizing effect. Higher blood levels depress brain activity
further to a point that memory, muscular coordination, and
balance may be temporarily impaired. Still higher levels, resulting
from larger intake or more rapid drinking, depress deeper
parts of the brain causing loss of control, severely affecting
judgment, and dulling sensory perception. If blood levels continue
to increase, eventually the deepest levels of the brain will be
anesthetized and coma or death may result.

Alcohol may seem to stimulate at first. This illusion occurs
because its first effects are on the part of the brain in which

---

Calories Provided by Alcoholic Beverages

Beverage	Quantity	Calories
Distilled liquors, 80 to 100 proof	1½ oz. (45 ml)	100 to 125
Natural wine	3½ oz. (105 ml)	86
Fortified wine	3½ oz. (105 ml)	140
Natural beer	12 oz. (360 ml)	140
Cocktail: 1½ oz. (45 ml) 100 proof liquor, 3 oz. (90 ml) mix	4½ oz. (135 ml)	165 to 175

Source—USDA Home and Gardens Bulletin No. 72, *Nutritive Value of Foods*

learned behavior patterns such as self-control are stored. After a drink or two this learned behavior may temporarily disappear, making the drinker lose inhibitions. One may talk more freely, feel more confident, more aggressive. Or one may feel more depressed.[8]

The first consistent and sizable changes in mood and behavior appear at blood levels of approximately 0.05 percent (1 part alcohol to 2,000 parts blood).[9] Concentration, thought, judgment, and restraint may be affected, especially for one who has not built up tolerance for the drug by long use.[10] At this concentration many drinkers feel carefree, released from many ordinary tensions and inhibitions.

At 0.10 percent blood alcohol concentration (1 part in 1,000), voluntary motor actions, hand and arm movements, walking, and sometimes speech may become plainly clumsy. At 0.20 percent (1 part in 500) the entire area of the brain that controls motor activity and the emotions is measurably impaired. The person may stagger or want to lie down. He may be easily angered or boisterous or weep. At 0.30 percent concentration the areas of the brain concerned with stimulus and understanding are dulled. Although he may be aware of his surroundings, he understands little of what he sees or hears and may lapse into a stupor.[11]

Coma results for most drinkers if blood alcohol concentrations of 0.40 to 0.50 are achieved. Higher concentrations block the centers of the brain that control breathing and heartbeat. Death ensues.[12]

Circumstances That Modify Effects

The rapidity with which blood alcohol concentrations are increased and the extent of the increase may be modified by a number of circumstances.[13]

How much one weighs. Alcohol is quickly distributed evenly throughout the circulatory system. With the same amount of alcohol the lighter weight individual with less blood will naturally have a higher blood alcohol concentration (BAC) than his heavier counterpart with more blood.

How fast one is drinking. Alcohol is metabolized at a rate approximating one drink per hour. Limiting drinks to one per hour may prevent extensive buildup of blood alcohol concentration

(BAC). Gulping a drink may produce immediate intoxicating effects and depression of deeper brain centers.

Whether the stomach is full or empty. Eating before and with drinking slows down absorption and gives a more even response to alcohol.

Dilution and nature of the drink. Wine, beer, and distilled beverages diluted with a liquid such as water are generally absorbed a little more slowly than distilled beverages taken straight. Dilution with carbonated beverages can increase the rate of absorption.

The setting or circumstance. If the drinker is comfortably seated and relaxed with a friend, alcohol will have less effect than when he is standing and drinking as at a cocktail party. On the other hand, alcohol may have a stronger effect than normal on one who is emotionally upset, under stress, or tired. Expectations also affect the response. If one expects to become drunk, the ease and speed with which he feels intoxicated is increased.

Chronic heavy drinking. Drinking large amounts of alcohol over long periods of time seems to change the sensitivity of the brain to the effects of alcohol. Larger amounts of alcohol are required to produce the same effects. This adaptation is called "tolerance" and is believed to be the basis for addiction or dependence on alcohol as for all other addictive drugs.

The alcohol-dependent person with increased tolerance must take relatively huge amounts of alcohol to produce the changes in feelings and behavior that were previously attained with smaller quantities. And such a one has the capacity to drink prodigious amounts without losing control of his actions, although he may have no memory of what transpired. Over some period of time, the alcoholic person may be able to drink a fifth of whiskey a day without showing signs of drunkenness. He may perform complex tasks accurately at blood levels several times those that would incapacitate moderate to heavy drinkers. Later, during chronic stages of alcoholism, however, tolerance decreases. The victim then becomes drunk on relatively small amounts of the drug.

Practices That Cannot Modify Effects

Alcohol's effects can be controlled only by the circumstances (rate and concentration) under which it is taken into the body. Once it is in the bloodstream, nothing can be done to remove it except to wait for the body to metabolize it. Most of the work must be done by the liver, though 2 to 5 percent of it may be excreted unchanged through the breath, sweat, and urine. Metabolism in the liver proceeds at a nearly constant rate, and as a general rule it will take as many hours to sober up as the number of drinks consumed.[14]

One cannot sober up by drinking black coffee, taking a cold shower, or breathing pure oxygen. These practices merely produce a wide-awake, potentially dangerous drunk.[15]

Neither is there scientific evidence to support claims for coffee, vitamins, drugs, and a number of specific foods as cures for hangovers. A hangover is the body's reaction to too much alcohol taken at a time when the drinker is tired or under stress. Individuals vary in the associated miseries they experience—nausea, gastritis, anxiety, headache—but a universal characteristic of all hangovers is extreme fatigue. To avoid a hangover, susceptible people must avoid intoxication. For recovery, doctors usually prescribe aspirin, rest, and solid food.[16]

Taking several drinks before bedtime has been found to decrease the amount of rapid eye movement (REM) or dreaming sleep. The consequences of being deprived of REM sleep are impaired concentration and memory, anxiety, tiredness, and irritability.[17]

Some Dangers Accompanying the Use of Alcohol

All substances that affect the brain have the potential for being dangerous. Alcohol affects the brain, organs, and other tissues. Just how dangerous its use is is not fully known. The Alcoholism Commission of Saskatchewan (Canada) makes this statement: "A majority of drinkers seem to use alcohol without damage to job, family life, or mental and physical health. Risk of damage to bodily organs is known to exist, however, if an average of about six drinks per day [as defined above—i.e. a 12 oz. (360 ml) bottle of beer, 1½ oz. (45 ml) spirits, 5 oz. (150 ml) table wine, or 3 oz. (90 ml) fortified wine] is taken regularly over a long period. Nevertheless, it cannot be assumed that use of smaller quantities is safe."[18] The Alcohol, Drug Abuse and Mental Health Administration of the U.S. Department of Health, Education and Welfare says of alcohol's long-term effects: "Drinking alcohol in moderation apparently does little permanent harm. But when taken in large doses over long periods of time, alcohol can prove disastrous, reducing both the quality and length of life. Damage to heart, brain, liver, and other major organs may result."[19]

The extent of some of the dangers quite obviously may depend on factors such as the person using alcohol, and the time, place, quantity and reason for its use. The relation between alcohol usage and traffic safety is a dramatic example.

Alcohol starts to be a factor in fatal motor vehicle crashes at blood alcohol concentrations (BAC) as low as 0.05 percent. This level of concentration may be reached by a 160-pound (72.2 kg) person consuming two one-ounce drinks of 86 proof spirits, or two small glasses of wine, or two 12-ounce (360 ml) bottles of beer in one hour with little or no food in his/her stomach. If the alcohol is taken within two hours of eating an average meal, the 0.05 percent BAC would occur after approximately three drinks.[20] If the drinker is a smaller person or if the beverage is drunk more quickly, less alcohol is required to produce the same BAC. And since small amounts of alcohol can impair judgment before it impairs driving skills, the U.S.A. Department of Transportation, National Traffic Safety Administration, warns young drivers that even at 0.05 percent BAC, they are probably in greater danger of having a fatal accident than more experienced drivers.[21] The less experience a person has with either drinking or driving, the less alcohol it takes to impair driving performance.[22]

As blood alcohol concentration (BAC) increases with increased consumption or more rapid consumption, the danger of having a fatal accident multiplies dramatically. At 0.10 percent BAC a person is seven times as likely to have a fatal crash as when sober. At 0.15 percent BAC that person is 25 times as likely to have a fatal crash as when sober. At 0.18 percent BAC the chances rise to 60 times more likely, and at 0.20 percent BAC one would be 100 times more likely to be responsible for a fatal crash than if he/she had not been drinking at all.[23]

A drinker does not have to be involved in an accident to be declared legally impaired. Blood alcohol concentrations declared to be legal evidence of impairment vary with political jurisdictions. In some European countries, especially Scandinavian, a BAC of 0.05 percent is considered legal evidence of impairment.

In Canada 0.08 percent BAC is defined as legal evidence of impairment. In the U.S.A. the standard varies from 0.08 percent to 0.15 percent with 0.10 percent the BAC most frequently established as denoting legal impairment. For one to drive with the BAC specified as legal evidence of impairment is illegal and may result in arrest and conviction.[24]

Alcohol plays a role in half of all traffic fatalities in the U.S.A. now totaling about 60,000 yearly. (An additional 500,000 or more are injured yearly in alcohol related accidents.) An estimated two-thirds of the alcohol related fatalities involve problem drinkers, i.e. heavy escape drinkers, compulsive drinkers, or outright alcoholics. The other one-third of the alcohol related accidents, however, involve social drinkers, particularly heavy social drinkers driving after a spree and young drivers who are learning to drink at the same time they are learning to drive.[25]

The U.S. Department of Transportation states the problem among youth this way:

> About 50 young Americans will be killed today. Nearly 250 will be maimed or disfigured. Not from drugs or disease. But from alcohol. About 50 will die on America's highways. Half of them because someone was drunk. Not a 40-year-old drunk. Not someone with a red nose and a pot belly. But someone like you. Someone who, just this once, is drunk out of his mind and behind the wheel of a car. He might kill his best friend. He might kill a stranger. Or he might just kill himself. But either way, someone young and alive is suddenly young and dead.
>
> Nearly 8,000 young Americans are killed in one year in drunk-driving accidents. That's more than war. More than drugs, or suicide, or disease. And most are killed by people their own age. In fact, the number one killer of young Americans is young Americans. It doesn't make any sense.
>
> You're young. Just beginning to really live. You see things wrong in the world and want to change them. You march against war, protest against pollution because you want a better life for everyone. Yet the thing that cripples and kills more young Americans than anything else, you do nothing about.... It just doesn't make any sense.[26]

Extensive studies of alcohol and highway safety are reported in the U.S. Department of Health, Education and Welfare, National Institute on Alcohol Abuse and Alcoholism's *Second Special Report to the U.S. Congress on Alcohol and Health*, June 1974.[27] They reveal the following facts: At any given time it can be expected that 80 to 90 percent of all motor vehicle drivers will have no alcohol in their blood; 5 to 10 percent may have from 0.01 to 0.049 percent BAC, 3 to 10 percent may have 0.05 to 0.099 percent BAC, 0.5 to 3 percent may have BACs ranging from 0.10 to 0.149, and only 1 percent or less have BACs over 0.15 or over. It is this small percentage of the drivers in the last three categories who are responsible for over half the fatal traffic accidents.

• Of the clear record drivers tested, 98 percent had no alcohol in their blood. The other 2 percent had 0.01 to 0.049 percent.

• A large proportion of high blood alcohol driver fatalities occur in single car crashes.

• About one-third of fatally injured adult pedestrians have BACs of 0.10 or higher. Those making the study concluded that if there is alcohol in the blood of a pedestrian who has been killed, it is likely that the driver is innocent.

• Men represent two-thirds of the licensed drivers but 90 percent of the fatally injured drivers and 98 percent of those convicted of driving while intoxicated.

• Ninety percent of women drivers do not drive after drinking at night. Women who do drink and drive at night are more likely than men to be involved in crashes and at low BACs—0.05 percent.

• Married drivers are proportionately less involved in drinking-driving problems than single, divorced, separated, or widowed drivers.

• Divorced and separated men are especially overinvolved in drinking-driving problems.

• People in lower occupational levels have proportionately more drinking-driving problems.

• High BACs frequently are associated with heavy consumption of beer.

• A surprisingly large proportion of very young drivers can be classified as heavy and frequent drinkers.

Teen-agers are of particular immediate concern. A recent study[28] in the U.S.A. indicates that high school students are in contact with alcohol-related situations almost as often as adults, and that a major proportion of high school youth participate regularly in unsupervised drinking with their peers. Approximately half the young people say that once a month or more they are part of social occasions in which alcohol is served without adult supervision. Of this group 45 percent say they drink once a week or more. They also drink heavily and often get drunk. Thirty-nine percent studied said that the most they had consumed on any one day was between one and three drinks, 29 percent said they had four to eight, and 14 percent said nine or more. Sixty-one percent of the youth considered that they had been "pretty drunk" at least once in the month preceding the study, and 15 percent had been drunk four or more times.

Many of these young people drive when they are "really pretty drunk." One quarter of them said they had driven once or twice while intoxicated, and an additional quarter of them said they had driven three or more times when drunk. Altogether, 66 percent said they had driven while drunk.

It should be remembered that the group being studied was not composed of drop-out, alienated, or underachieving students. They reported the same range of activities as students not involved in social drinking situations and all levels of scholastic achievement. Although most were older, 25 percent of them were 15 years of age or younger. Four out of ten of them were female.

Compared with other high school students, those frequently involved in alcohol-related situations did display more impulsive, risk-taking personalities. They were motivated more by peer pressure than by respect for authority, and were not very concerned with dangers of driving while intoxicated. Seven percent actually thought they could drive better under the influence. Only 8 percent thought their ability to drive was "much worse." And only 19 percent of them thought there was any likelihood of drunk teen-age drivers being involved in an accident resulting in death or crippling injury. When they had the opportunity to do so, only about a third of them stopped another drunken teen from driving.

A large proportion of youth who drink display the same misconceptions about alcohol that adult drinkers have. For example, although beer is the beverage they drink most often, many do not understand that beer is as intoxicating as distilled spirits. Forty-two percent of those queried thought they could drink five to seven cans of beer within two hours without risking intoxication, and 15 percent of them thought they could consume eight cans or more. Seventy percent thought a cold shower would sober them up, while 62 percent thought black coffee would be effective.

Mixing Other Drugs with Alcohol

Of this danger the U.S. Alcohol, Drug Abuse, and Mental Health Administration has issued a warning that among the hundreds of new drugs introduced in recent years to induce sleep, tranquillize, sedate, relieve pain, motion sickness, headache, cold, or allergy symptoms, many are dangerous when taken with alcohol. There are narcotics, barbiturates, and other hypnotic-sedative drugs, tranquillizers, antihistamines, and volatile solvents, some of which act on the same brain areas as alcohol does. "When used simultaneously with alcohol, these drugs can grossly exaggerate the usual response expected from alcohol or from the drug alone," the warning reads.

"The use of any drug that has a depressant effect on the central nervous system in combination with alcohol represents an extra hazard to health and safety, and, in some cases, to life itself." Alcohol and barbiturates taken in close order are particularly dangerous and may result in death.[29] Darvon with liquor may bring death. Seconal and alcohol can produce unconsciousness.

On the other hand, stimulants can offset sleepiness without counteracting other effects of alcohol thus canceling the body's natural defense against fatal BACs and other destructive behavior. Alcohol taken with aspirin increases the danger of excessive bleeding. For those interested *The Medical Letter* of February 1975 offers an extensive list of specific drugs and their effect when taken with alcohol.[30]

Alcohol and Crime

For some drinkers, alcohol releases violent behavior that might be unlikely or even unthinkable in their sober state. Half of all homicides and one-third of all suicides are alcohol related—accounting for about 11,700 deaths yearly in the U.S.A. alone,[31] according to the National Institute on Alcohol Abuse and Alcoholism. Alcoholics have a suicide rate 58 times that of nonalcoholics.[32] Alcohol is frequently involved in assaults and offenses against children and in less violent criminal behavior. Almost half of the 5½ million arrests yearly in the U.S.A. are related to the misuse of alcohol.[33]

Some Other Long-Term Health Hazards

(1) *Cancer.*[34] Heavy drinking increases the risk of cancer of the mouth, throat, esophagus, and other sites having direct contact with strong solutions of alcohol, particularly in prolonged heavy drinking. It also seems implicated in primary liver cell cancer and a number of others. The risk is multiplied if heavy drinking is combined with heavy smoking, which is frequently the case, and the frequency of the combination makes it difficult to distinguish which drug is responsible for specific symptoms.

(2) *Heart and other muscles.*[35] Drinking apparently does not cause coronary heart disease, but it is associated with another disease of the heart called cardiomyopathy. Recent research indicates that it may be toxic to heart and lungs. It is known to be connected with various muscle diseases and tremors.

(3) *Liver.*[36] Previously it had been thought that malnutrition was responsible for liver damage among those who drank heavily. Recent studies show that very large amounts of alcohol can cause liver damage even in well-fed individuals. Cirrhosis of the liver occurs eight times as often in alcoholics as among nonalcoholics.

(4) *Gastrointestinal System.*[37] Nausea, vomiting, and diarrhea are mild indications of irritation. Gastritis, ulcers, and pancreatitis often occur in alcoholics.

(5) *Infectious Disease.*[38] Heavy drinkers have lowered resistance to pneumonia and other infectious diseases, not only because of malnutrition but because of direct interference with immunity mechanisms. In those with BACs of 0.15-0.25 percent, the reduction of white blood cell mobilization is as great as that found in severe shock.

(6) *Brain and Personality.*[39] Heavy drinking over many years may result in serious mental disorders. There may be irreversible damage to the brain or peripheral nervous system. Mental functions such as memory, judgment, and learning ability can deteriorate severely. Personality structure and grasp on reality may also disintegrate.

(7) *Damage to the Unborn.*[40] A woman who indulges in heavy drinking during pregnancy can adversely affect the unborn child, both through malnutrition and by the direct effect of the alcohol. With respect to nutrition, the NIAAA reports: "Since actively alcoholic women tend to be malnourished, infants born to them

are less healthy, less alert, and less well developed than other newborns." Of the direct effect of alcohol on the fetus, there have been a number of reports of an increased rate of birth of maldeveloped or malformed infants to alcoholic mothers. The exact causes are under intensive study.

Whether such damage results, the NIAAA reports that an unquestionable effect of heavy drinking by the pregnant mother is that as she becomes intoxicated, so does the fetus. The BAC of the fetus is approximately the same as the mother's. When the mother is deprived of alcohol in the hospital before the baby's birth, if she has been on a bout, she is likely to suffer withdrawal symptoms, sometimes even delirium tremens.

> Since the fetus underwent the same severity and duration of alcohol intoxication as the mother, the newborn too will show symptoms of an alcohol withdrawal syndrome and will require appropriate treatment just as the mother does. This observation...opens up the possibility, based on the view that addiction is defined by withdrawal phenomena, that such infants are in fact born alcohol addicts; or, that the prenatal addiction may establish a permanent addictive liability in the newborn child's central nervous system.

(8) *Alcoholism.* A disease suffered by an estimated 9,000,000 of the approximately 100,000,000 persons age 15 or over who drink in the U.S.A.[41] and by an increasing number of those throughout the world where alcohol has been accepted as a "recreational drug," as the U.S.A. Clearing House for Drug Abuse designates legal drugs used for "fun" or to get away from the stresses and strains of life.[42]

Alcoholism is a complex, progressive illness that, if not treated, ends in permanent mental damage, physical incapacity, or early death. It ranks among the major diseases along with cancer, mental illness, and heart disease. It is recognized as the most serious drug problem in terms of the number of victims, cost to society, physical damage, and the number of fatalities resulting from withdrawal symptoms.[43]

Contrary to popular opinion, the typical alcoholic is not a skid-row derelict. Only about 5 percent of the alcoholics are in this group. Most alcoholics are employed or employable, family-centered people. The NIAAA says that more than 70 percent of the problem drinkers live in respectable neighborhoods with their families, performing more or less effectively as businessmen, executives, housewives, farmers, salespersons, industrial workers, clerical workers, teachers, clergymen, physicians—representing all ranges of employment, social strata, and professional status.[44]

The costs of alcoholism are staggering. Some economic costs of the disease to the U.S.A. were computed in 1971 at more than $25 billions—10 billions in work time lost, $9 billions in health and welfare services to the alcoholics and their families, and nearly $6.5 billions in motor vehicle accident costs.[45] Human costs cannot be calculated.

Many costs to individuals and to society have already been noted. In addition, life expectancy of the alcoholic is ten to twelve years shorter than that of the general public. Alcoholism appears as the cause of death on more than 13,000 U.S.A. death certificates yearly, and the NIAAA believes it contributes to many deaths attributed to other causes.[46]

Families of alcoholics suffer unhappy marriages, broken homes, desertion, divorce, impoverishment, displaced or deprived children. Altogether about 36,000,000 Americans alone are represented in alcoholic families. Alcoholism accounts directly or indirectly for 40 percent of the problems brought to U.S. family courts.[47]

One of the disturbing facts about alcoholism is that children of alcoholics are much more apt to become problem drinkers themselves and to suffer developmental problems than the general population. All the reasons are not known, but the NIAAA reports that it is increasingly clear that "familial learning" is an important factor.[48]

Fortunately, alcoholism is a treatable disease. Education, early detection, and community treatment facilities are the greatest forces at work to control and reduce it. Identification of the disease is an essential.[49]

Although there is no definition that completely satisfies all those who work with alcoholism, all agree that the alcoholic is addicted to the use of the drug and has lost control over his/her alcohol intake. Professionals agree that there is no exact dividing line applicable in all cases separating the alcoholic from the nonalcoholic. A consistent pattern of drinking problems indicates a loss of control over one's drinking, however. The NIAAA suggests that one has a drinking problem who (1) must drink to function or "cope" with life; (2) frequently, by his/her definition or that of family and friends, drinks to intoxication; (3) goes to work while intoxicated; (4) drives a car while intoxicated; (5) sustains bodily injury that requires medical attention while intoxicated; (6) comes into conflict with the law as a consequence of being intoxicated; (7) under the influence of alcohol does something he vows he would never do without alcohol.[50]

Familiar signs that give early warning of developing alcoholism overlap these criteria. Those noted by NIAAA include:[51]

- Gulping drinks for the effect that rapid drinking produces.
- Starting the day with a drink.
- Drinking alone, to escape reality, boredom, or loneliness.
- Alcohol-taking behavior criticized by an employer, spouse, or others, and absenteeism or impaired job performance because of drinking.
- Rationalization about drinking behavior, characterized by such comments as "I just need one more to relax" or "How about one for the road?"
- Marked personality and behavioral changes after taking one or more drinks.
- Frequent overdosing with alcohol, or drunkenness.
- Experiencing "blackouts"—alcohol-induced amnesia. (Such drinkers do not pass out. They walk, talk, perform in a full state of consciousness, but later cannot remember what transpired.)
- Drinking to relieve hangovers, thereby perpetuating a vicious cycle: the more one drinks, the worse one feels, the more one drinks.
- Requiring medical or hospital attention, or having frequent minor accidents or physical complaints, as a result of drinking.

A special list of danger signals for women drinkers has recently been published by the National Council on Alcoholism,[52] written by Marty Mann, who believes there may be nearly as many women as men who are alcoholic. The first danger noted is careless drinking. She says careless drinkers become dependent drinkers. Specific symptoms listed are (1) gulping drinks; (2) making promises to do better next time if her behavior causes comment or worries her; (3) lying about drinking—concealing the number of drinks taken or denying drinking at all; (4) taking a drink before a party or appointment at which there will be drinking; (5) finding it necessary to have drinks at certain times; (6) insistence on a certain span of time for drinks before meals regardless of inconvenience to others; (7) insistence on drinks with every special event; (8) needing three or four drinks before entertaining the boss, meeting a difficult client, or introducing a speaker; (9) requiring a drink for nerves caused by a shattering day at the office or a frantic day with the children; (10) drinking when "blue" to forget worries or problems.

The AA (Alcoholics Anonymous) World Library also describes signs of developing alcoholism intended to alert alcoholics or potential alcoholics and their families to the need to get help. One excellent publication is their book *Am I Drinking Too Much?*[53]

Without alcohol, alcoholism would be impossible. All who drink alcohol do not become alcoholics, however. Alcoholism, then, is a symptom of more than just a drinking problem. Although its specific causes are still not precisely defined, there appear to be physiological, psychological, and sociological factors involved.[54]

Effective treatment must reach all the areas involved in the development of the problem and its consequences in the life of the drinker, his/her family, employer, and community. It may require the services of all the health professions, the church, welfare agencies, social services, industry, government, and volunteer agencies.[55] With proper treatment, between one- and two-thirds of those who seek treatment recover.[56]

Alcoholics Anonymous is probably the best known agency offering help to alcoholics. It provides a spiritually based, self-help, group support program. Its related organizations, Al-Anon and Alateen, offer similar assistance to families and relatives of problem drinkers and alcoholics.[57]

Local affiliates of the National Council on Alcoholism exist in many communities in the U.S.A. Many communities and government jurisdictions have official programs where help can be found or sources of treatment recommended. The National Institute on Alcohol Abuse and Alcoholism (NIAAA) of the U.S. Department of Health, Education and Welfare provides research, literature, and support for community services that will be increasingly available in that country. Many churches offer counseling and referral services.* And a great many other

---

*Charles L. Massie's *Family Ministry in Alcoholism, Which Will It Be, A Light of Understanding or a Shadow of Confusion*, is a valuable resource.)

agencies are involved in the "helping network" described in the NIAAA booklet, *Facts About Alcohol and Alcoholism*, some of which extend world wide.[58]

Although alcohol alone may not cause alcoholism, alcoholism cannot develop or be maintained without the drug. The NIAAA believes that there will always be people who cannot "sustain safe drinking practices" regardless of how intense social and other pressures are on them to do so. Most alcoholics are in this group, as are many whose alcoholism is not yet detected. For these persons, abstinence must be a way of life if health and well-being are to be maintained. It is widely recognized that the disease cannot be cured; it can only be arrested. The truly alcoholic must refrain from using alcoholic beverages for the rest of life if they wish to live without dependence.[59]

Preventing Alcohol Problems

Problems with alcohol cannot be averted by treating the casualties. The NIAAA suggests that there must be[60] (1) full respect for and acceptance of an individual's choice not to drink whether for moral, health, economic, religious, or any other reason; (2) development of responsible attitudes and behavior concerning the use of alcohol by those who choose to use it; (3) early identification and treatment of problems.

Attitudes that accompany responsible and irresponsible drinking behavior in cultures have been identified. Overt drinking problems are rare in societies where drinking is practiced only as an adjunct to other activities, where guidelines for drinking are strictly adherred to, and where drunkenness is severely censured. On the other hand, where drinking is accepted as a way to avoid reality or where drunkenness is condoned or tolerated there is a high incidence of problems.[61]

It is essential that there be universal agreement that drunkenness is not sanctioned by the group. NIAAA finds this principle particularly important. Being drunk is not funny, and the drunk should not be represented as a comic character in a society attempting to deal with alcohol problems. Excessive drinking does not indicate adult status, virility, or masculinity, and is not a solution to problems. Drunkenness is a condition in which a person is overdosed with a drug and is particularly liable to poor judgment and dangerous actions.[62]

Programs of education about alcohol are under way. The aim is to prevent problems with alcohol by developing public awareness of the facts about alcohol, its properties and effects, its potential for harm, and its responsible and irresponsible uses. NIAAA stresses that alcohol education should be one phase of education about living, coping with life, and developing self-respect—not just alcoholism education.[63] The basic issue in any meaningful discussion of the use of alcohol must be "How can that behavior be promoted which enhances well-being and human dignity?"[64]

In the development of attitudes toward drinking and decision-making on the part of the young, it is becoming increasingly apparent that families have a decisive role. The most influential teachers are parents or the most prestigious persons in a youth's environment. Children tend to follow the patterns established by their family and their social group.[65]

In his effort to enhance well-being and promote human dignity, the Lord recommends total abstinence for all. If his advice is followed, there is no consequence of drinking to be experienced: no damage to self or others, no drinking problems or alcoholism developed, no possibility of being the person whose example may cause another to suffer damage from the use of alcohol.

1. Doctrine and Covenants, 152:4b.
2. President W. Wallace Smith, 1976 Conference Sermon, "Let Us Walk in the Light," Reorganized Church of Jesus Christ of Latter Day Saints, *World Conference Bulletin*, Monday, March 29, 1976, p. 220.
3. National Institute of Alcohol Abuse and Alcoholism (NIAAA), Alcohol, Drug Abuse and Mental Health Administration (ADM), U.S. Department of Health, Education and Welfare (DHEW), 5600 Fishers Lane, Rockville, Maryland, *First Special Report to the U.S. Congress on Alcohol and Health*, Dec. 1971, p. 6. (DHEW Pub. No. [ADM] 74-68, reprinted in 1974.)
4. NIAAA, ADM, DHEW, *Young People and Alcohol*; reprinted from *Alcohol Health and Research World*, summer 1975; distributed by U.S. Department of Transportation, National Traffic Safety Administration, Washington, D.C., p. 2.
5. Leonard C. Hall (for the NIAAA), *Facts About Alcohol and Alcoholism*, (U.S. DHEW Pub., No. [ADM] 75-31), 1975, p. 6.
6. *Ibid.*, pp. 1-6; NIAAA, ADM, DHEW, *Alcohol, Some Questions and Answers*, (DHEW Pub. No. [ADM] 76-312), 1976, pp. 1-2; NIAAA, ADM, DHEW, *First Special Report, etc., op. cit.*, pp. 6-7.
7. NIAAA, ADM, DHEW, *Alcohol, Some Questions and Answers, op. cit.*, pp. 2-3.
8. *Ibid.*
9. Hall, *op. cit.*, p. 7.
10. *Ibid.*, p. 8.
11. *Ibid.*, pp. 7-8.
12. *Ibid.*
13. *Ibid.*, pp. 7-10. Also NIAAA et al., *Alcohol, Some Questions and Answers* pp. 3-4.
14. Hall, *ibid.*, pp. 11-12; *Questions and Answers*, pp. 6-7.
15. *Ibid.* Also R.M. Gilbert, "Caffeine Beverages and Their Effects," *Addiction*, Vol. 21, No. 1, Spring 1974, Addiction Research Foundation of Ontario, Toronto, p. 80.
16. NIAAA, *Questions and Answers*, p. 7.
17. Hall, *ibid.*, pp. 10-11.

18. Educational Division of the Addiction Research Foundation of Ontario, *Facts About Alcohol*, June 1971, distributed by Alcoholism Commission of Saskatchewan, Regina, Sask.
19. Hall *op. cit.* p. 13.
20. NIAAA, *Questions and Answers*, p. 6.
21. U.S. Department of Transportation, National Highway Traffic Safety Administration, *Young Americans. Drinking, Driving, Dying*, pp. 9-10.
22. Ed. Div. of the Addiction Research Foundation of Ontario, *op. cit.*, p. 2.
23. NIAAA, ADM, DHEW, *op. cit.*, *Second Special Report to the U.S. Congress on Alcohol and Health, New Knowledge*, June, 1974, p. 102.
24. *Ibid.*, pp. 97-98, and Ed. Div. Addiction Research Foundation of Ontario, *op. cit.*, p. 4.
25. Hall, *op. cit.*, pp. 16-17. Also U.S. Department of Transportation, National Highway Traffic Safety Administration, Washington, D.C., *Communications Strategies on Alcohol and Highway Safety, Vol. II, High School Youth, Synopsis*, 1975, Introduction. (Full report available.)
26. U.S. Dept. of Transportation, Nat'l Highway Traffic Safety Adm., *Young Americans. Drinking, Driving, Dying*, p. 2.
27. NIAAA, ADM, DHEW, *op. cit.* (*Second Special Report to the U.S. Congress on Alcohol and Health, New Knowledge*), pp. 97-110.
28. Dept. of Transportation, etc., *Communications Strategies, etc., op. cit.* Also NIAAA, ADM, DHEW, *Young People and Alcohol, op. cit.*
29. Hall, *op. cit.*, p. 11. Also James H. Coleman, William E. Evans, (both Pharm. D.), "Drug Interaction with Alcohol," NIAAA *Alcohol Health and Research World*, Winter, 1975-1976, 16-19.
30. *Medical Letter*, Vol. 17, No. 5, Feb. 28, 1975, p. 17 plus.
31. Hall, *op. cit.*, p. 17.
32. National Council on Alcoholism, Kansas City Area, Inc. *Facts on Alcoholism* (Pub. 361-5900).
33. Hall, *op. cit.*, p. 17.
34. NIAAA, ADM, DHEW, *op. cit.*, *Second Report, etc., op. cit.*, pp. 53-67.
35. *Ibid.*, pp. 68-72. Also Hall, *op. cit.*, p. 13.
36. *Ibid.*, pp. 73-78. Also Hall, *ibid.*
37. Hall, *ibid.*
38. *Ibid.*
39. *Ibid.*
40. NIAAA, ADM, DHEW, *op. cit.*, *Second Report, etc., op. cit.*, pp. 45-50.
41. Hall, *op. cit.*, p. 14, and National Council on Alcoholism, *op. cit.*
42. National Clearinghouse for Drug Abuse Information (5600 Fishers Lane, Rockville, Maryland), *Resource Book for Drug Abuse Education*, Second Edition, pp. 26-27.
43. National Council on Alcoholism, *op. cit.*
44. Hall, *op. cit.*, pp. 15-16.
45. *Ibid.*, p. 18.
46. *Ibid.*, p. 16.
47. *Ibid.*, and National Council on Alcoholism, *op. cit.*
48. NIAAA, etc., *Second Report, etc.*, pp. 112 and 151.
49. National Council on Alcoholism, *op. cit.*; NIAAA, ADM, DHEW, *op. cit.*, *Second Report, etc., op. cit.*, pp. 111-127. *Ibid.*, *Alcohol, Some Questions etc., op. cit.*, pp. 9-10.
50. Hall, *op. cit.*, pp. 14-15.
51. NIAAA, etc., *Second Report, etc.*, p. 164. Also see Hall, *ibid.*, and NIAA, etc. *Alcohol, Some Questions, etc.*, p. 8.
52. Marty Mann, *Danger Signals for Women Drinkers*, National Council on Alcoholism, 2 Park Ave., N.Y. (L31-25M-3/75).
53. Doyle F. Lindley, and Robert T. Dorris, *Am I Drinking Too Much?*, AA World Library, No. 122, copyright 1970, published quarterly by A.A. World Publishing Corp.
54. Hall, *op. cit.*, pp. 19-22. Also NIAAA, etc., *Alcohol, Some Questions and Answers*, p. 9.
55. NIAAA, etc., *Second Report, etc.*, pp. 111-139. Also Hall, *ibid.*, pp. 23-31.
56. NIAAA, etc., *Alcohol, Some Questions, etc.*, p. 10.
57. Hall, *op. cit.*, p. 36.
58. Hall, *op. cit.*, pp. 36-42.
59. NIAAA, etc., *Second Report, etc.*, p. 164.
60. NIAAA, etc., *Alcohol, Some Questions, etc.*, p. 10.
61. *Ibid.*, p. 11.
62. Hall, *op. cit.*, pp. 33-34.
63. *Ibid.*
64. NIAAA, etc., *Second Report, etc.*, p. 151.
65. Hall, *op. cit.*, pp. 32-33, and NIAAA, etc., *First Special Report, etc., op. cit.*, p. 101.

CHAPTER 11

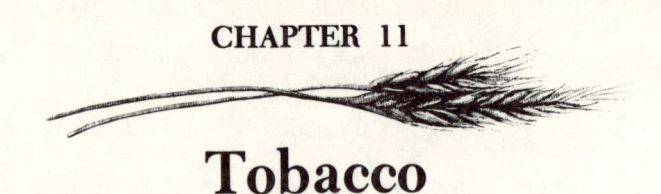

Tobacco

I have warned you, and forewarn you,... tobacco is not for the body, neither for the belly, and is not good for man.... Doctrine and Covenants 86:1.

The use of tobacco, like alcohol, constitutes a health hazard and in many ways presents the same problems because of the acceptance and advertising that accompany the use of alcoholic beverages. As more is known of its dangers, however, more intelligent resistance to its use is being exhibited. No longer does one who desires to honor the Lord's advice that tobacco is not good for man find himself standing alone.

Extensive campaigns have been instituted at public expense in the U.S.A., Canada, Britain, and many other nations in which cigarette smoking has become prevalent, to inform the public of the dangers of smoking and to try to influence people away from the practice. The American Cancer Society estimates that at least 29,000,000 adults—about one of every four who tried—stopped smoking between 1965 and 1969. It is reported that by 1969, more than 100,000 doctors in the U.S.A. and a comparable 10,000 in Canada had stopped smoking. Only one doctor in four of those studied in the U.S.A. still smoked in 1969. Of those who operated on lung cancer only one in seven smoked. Of those who still smoked, 89 percent said they did so against their better judgment.[1]

Unfortunately, women and youth have not been as responsive as men and doctors. While those who start smoking early could quit early more easily than established smokers, they frequently do not. One British researcher has found that 70 percent of the teen-agers who smoke even one cigarette will smoke for the next forty years if they survive that long.[2] Of women of child-bearing age who thought they had successfully stopped smoking in 1966, one in four had begun again four years later.[3]

Special Hazards When Women Smoke

For a time it did seem that women were fairly immune to the dangers of smoking, but it is becoming apparent that they are more than equalling men in this area. Not only are women succumbing to the same diseases smoking men have suffered (i.e. lung and other related cancers, coronary heart disease, chronic bronchitis, and emphysema) but they and their young suffer additional loss during pregnancy and lactation.

"There is strong evidence," Jesse L. Steinfeld, Surgeon General of the U.S.A., stated in a report to the American Congress in January 1971, "to support the view that smoking mothers have a significant greater number of unsuccessful pregnancies due to stillbirth [dead at birth] and neonatal death [death soon after birth] as compared to nonsmoking mothers."[4]

The fetus of smoking mothers is harmed by the carbon monoxide, nicotine, and other noxious substances from tobacco smoke that pass across the placenta from the mother's blood. The nicotine constricts the baby's blood vessels, reducing both the nourishment and the oxygen available to the developing child. Carbon monoxide further reduces the oxygen available, according to the American Lung Association, until the child experiences almost chronic carbon monoxide intoxication. A mother who smokes two packs a day blocks off approximately 40 percent of her child's oxygen supply.[5]

In studies made in the U.S.A. and in England, the damages have been documented. Of 7,500 pregnancies followed in the U.S.A., the incidence of spontaneous abortions and premature births was twice as high among smoking as among nonsmoking mothers. For the surviving children and the 17,000 studied in Britain, birth weights were markedly lower, averaging 170 grams (about 6 ounces), less in the U.S. study. Neonatal deaths occurred more frequently among both groups if the mother smoked—30 percent more frequently among those in the British study. These children of smoking mothers had a double risk of congenital heart defects and a persistent lag in the surviving children's learning abilities.[6] Both studies corroborated the U.S.A. Surgeon General's assertion that not only are babies born to smoking mothers being lost but many of those who live are handicapped.

Children of smoking mothers are frequently born with an addiction to nicotine. Their withdrawal symptoms may not be overcome for about three months. During this time, even after convulsions and other acute symptoms subside, the child may be restless, sleep fitfully, and constantly demand attention. If the smoking mother breast feeds her child, she prolongs the addiction.[7]

Smoking by Teen-agers

Knowledge of damage to the developing fetus and danger of drug addiction even before birth are of special importance to teen-agers who are adopting the practice of smoking in spite of the information available to them.

Young men are influential in determining whether young women smoke. Cigarette smoking is "contagious as the measles," Dr. Donald R. Chadwick, director of the National Center for Chronic Disease Control (U.S.A.), asserts.[8] Both parents are responsible for the atmosphere in which their child is conceived, born, and lives. Children who live in smoke-filled houses suffer many more respiratory diseases than those not so exposed. If a child is to be born free of handicaps that result from smoking and to breathe unpolluted air, the parents must support each other in their efforts to be free of the addiction and to keep others from contaminating the home atmosphere.

Parents are also important factors in determining whether their children will smoke. As with alcohol, the example of the prestigious persons influences greatly the behavior of the young. One U.S.A. study revealed that only 4.2 percent of the teen-agers became regular smokers who lived in households where neither parent nor older brothers or sisters smoked. If one parent or an older sibling smoked, 24.9 percent of the teen-agers became victims of the addiction. If both parents smoked, teen-age addiction was increasingly a fact of life.

Those young who choose to smoke suffer early consequences. One school study in the U.S.A. indicated that among regular smokers 14 to 19 years of age, respiratory ills were nine times as common as among nonsmokers. Even occasional smokers suffered such ills 2.6 times as often. In 1971 Yale Medical School physicians documented lung damage in the young. With cessation of smoking the irritation is remedied, but they believe that smoking may prematurely arrest lung development, which normally continues in young men even after other growth stops, and so permanently damage the smoker.[9] Many surgeons are reporting lung cancer in patients under twenty years of age, some of whom do not survive. And it is 50 percent more likely that those who began smoking before the age of fifteen will die of lung cancer than those who started smoking after their twenty-fifth year.[10]

Knowledge of the early damage from smoking is particularly important in areas in which children are adopting the addiction. The Ontario Home and School Association found that throughout Canadian schools in 1972, 9 percent of the children were regular smokers by the age of 11; most boys began their addiction at ages 13-14; and girls waited just a little longer. By 16 years of age, more than 50 percent of all Canadian school children were regular smokers.[11] Dr. H. Medovy of Children's Hospital, Winnipeg, recommends education to prevent smoking in grades one to four in Canada if it is to be effective. This information was confirmed for much of the world at the Ninth International Cancer Congress in 1966.[12]

According to U.S.A. National Clearinghouse for Drug Abuse information, teen-age smoking in the U.S.A. was on the decline at the turn of this decade. While still on the increase after adult percentages declined, an estimated 42 percent of the U.S.A. fellows and 28 percent of the girls were smoking in 1971. Those most successful in their studies, who are leaders in their schools or choose to go to college, are less likely to smoke.[13] In 1942, 42 percent of college freshmen there smoked. In 1966 only 9 percent of that group were addicted.[14]

Hazards of Other Uses of Tobacco

Since educational campaigns center on reduction of cigarette smoking, many believe other forms of tobacco use are safe. Not so. Back in 1859 the French physician, Bouisson, first discovered cancer related to the use of tobacco in 67 patients who smoked cigars or a pipe and one who chewed tobacco—long before cigarettes were invented. Each cancer was at the site where tobacco or its smoke came into contact with the tissues.

Recent studies show that cancers of the lips, tongue, pharynx, and other oral tissues occur ten times as frequently in cigarette smokers as in non-tobacco users. For pipe and cigar smokers and those who chew tobacco or use snuff, the rate is five times that of the nonuser. Cancer of oral tissue is common in South India where snuff is mixed with a ground nut, wrapped in a lemon-leaf, and held in the mouth for hours.[15]

Death rates from these oral cancers are correspondingly high, ten times the nontobacco user rate for the cigarette smoker and five times that rate for other tobacco users. Of those who develop oral cancers, an average of 20 percent survive five years or more after the discovery of the disease. Early detection and treatment can raise the survival rate to 65 percent. If treatment is delayed until the cancer is well established, that rate plummets to 2 to 5 percent.[16]

Lung cancer rates for pipe and cigar smokers, while far below that for cigarette smokers, is still twice that of persons who do not smoke at all. Their bronchial tubes show cell changes characteristic of developing cancer. Their emphysema rate is 1.4 times higher than that for those who abstain from smoking.[17]

Specific Hazards of Cigarette Smoking

Excluding problems created by the use of tobacco in other forms, the Surgeon General of the U.S.A. rates cigarette smoking as "the greatest preventable cause of illness, disability, and premature death" in his country. New York State's State Commissioner of Health is quoted as saying, "Bullets, germs, and viruses are killers; but for Americans cigarettes are more deadly than any of them." The American Cancer Society says, "Cigarette smoking is the major known cause of cancer deaths." The American Heart Association says, "Cigarette smoking is a major factor in coronary heart disease," and "The use of tobacco in all forms is a cause of peripheral vascular disease...that is spasms of and thrombus [clot] formation in the arteries of the legs and arms."

The American Lung Association has concluded that "the risk of chronic bronchitis, emphysema, and certain other diseases is much greater among cigarette smokers." The American Public Health Association states, "The health hazard of smoking is an accepted medical fact.... Immediate remedial action is essential to prevent thousands of unnecessary deaths." Representatives of many other nations at a world conference on smoking and health reported similar concerns. Dr. Diehl, who compiled the statements for his book, *Tobacco and Your Health: The Smoking Controversy*, 1969, declares that no medical or health association in the world disagrees.

Death by smoking has become epidemic in many areas of the world. Substances in cigarette smoke are considered to be the primary contributory cause of 350,000 known deaths in the U.S.A. and Canada yearly; and these do not include the many cardiovascular deaths believed by Dr. Alton Oschner, eminent lung cancer surgeon and researcher of Oschner Clinic, New Orleans, to be related to smoking but not so recorded. Canadian officials declare that smoking kills eleven times as many people as road accidents there. Britain's Royal College of Physicians says, "Cigarette smoking is now as important a cause of death as were the great epidemic diseases such as typhoid and cholera and tuberculosis that affected previous generations in this country."[18] Three diseases in particular claim disproportionately large numbers of cigarette smokers:[19]

Disease	Numbers Who Die Nonsmokers	Smokers U.S.A.	Smokers Canadian
Lung cancer	10	110	130
Emphysema and chronic bronchitis	10	60	120-150
Heart disease	10	17	20

Some researchers have estimated that for every minute of smoking one is likely to give up a minute of life. Dr. Linus Pauling calculates lost life at 14.4 minutes per cigarette. Others have suggested that if a man 25 years of age looks over 100 of his friends, if none of them smoke, there will probably be about 78 of them alive to celebrate their sixty-fifth birthdays. If they all smoke a little (no more than nine cigarettes a day) there may be about 66 alive for that day. If they are average smokers (20 to 39 cigarettes a day) 61 may live that long. If they smoke more heavily, only 54 can be expected to live those forty years. In fact, if smokers use even less than one pack a day, the chances that they will be dead before the age of 50 are 70 percent greater than for those who refrain. For heavy smokers the chances of dying before 50 are 160 percent greater than for their nonsmoking counterparts.[20]

The immediate effect of smoking is to reduce the appetite, dull sense of taste and smell, put stains on teeth and fingers, and establish malodorous breath. The nervous system frequently reacts with headaches, sleeplessness, and irritability, especially if the next smoke is delayed. Eventually disease states develop that may include damaged eyesight and hearing in addition to the more deadly cardiopulmonary hazards with which smoking has been identified.

Nicotine addiction is the factor that keeps people smoking when they would rather not. It is a nerve poison so powerful that one drop injected into the bloodstream would cause nearly instant death; yet many heavy smokers inhale this amount daily, with varying results. Nicotine poisoning brings dizziness, faintness, rapid pulse, clammy skin, nausea, and sometimes vomiting and diarrhea to the beginning smoker. Habitual smokers experience increased heartbeat, reduced skin temperature, and occasionally other obnoxious effects, but with increased dependence on the drug, they tend to ignore the undesirable effects.

When nicotine enters the bloodstream with the first puff of tobacco smoke, the body is stimulated to get rid of the dangerous drug. The heart speeds up an average of 20 beats a minute. The adrenals secrete adrenalin and other hormonal substances, some of which are related to a number of disease states in the body.[21] The blood sugar level rises. More oxygen is delivered to the brain, and more energy to body cells to fight the invader. The smoker gets a "lift." Soon, however, the sugar is used up, and fatigue follows. The body settles into a kind of depression called "smoker's tension" unless another smoke provides nicotine for another round of stimulation.[22] Relief from nervous tension sought by most smokers comes only from satisfying the addiction. Otherwise smoking is not a tranquillizer.

Smoking one cigarette, whether the smoker is experienced or a novice, constricts peripheral blood vessels, reducing the temperature of fingers and toes by an average 5.3 degrees Fahrenheit (about 3 degrees Celsius) and may reduce it as much as 15.5 degrees F. (8.7 Celsius). With increased pressure from faster heartbeat, some people, especially those of Jewish descent, develop spasms of small arteries in these extremities followed by clotting. Blood flow is reduced or stopped completely. Tissues die. Gangrene may develop with resultant progressive amputations. This is termed Buergers Disease.[23]

In addition to its adverse effects on heart, adrenals, and the circulatory system, nicotine interacts with irritants from the smoke to gradually destroy lung elasticity and lung tissue, preparing the way for emphysema and cancer.

There are seven known and many suspected carcinogens in tobacco smoke, and there are phenols that help them lodge in the lungs. The phenols destroy the protective action of the cilia, those hairlike structures that normally sweep the respiratory tract clean, preventing the entry or lodging of destructive substances. With the cilia out of order, lungs and bronchial structures become clogged with debris of the smoke and other pollutants that are in the air. Chronic coughing develops but cannot clear the passages of tars and other destructive materials. Bronchitis is a common development, and for many there is cancer. Although the primary lesion (place where the cancer first forms) may be the lungs, cancer cells may be carried by the blood (metastasize) to other parts of the body. The brain seems especially vulnerable for such attack, although bladder, kidneys, pancreas and other organs may also be affected.

The likelihood of an early death from lung cancer can be reduced sharply by giving up smoking early. For those who have stopped smoking for five years, the death rate by lung cancer is only half that of those who continue to smoke. After ten years of desisting, those who survive have a death rate which is comparable to that of the rest of the population.[24]

Death by emphysema is increasing in cigarette smokers at a rate far in excess of that of lung cancer. In this disease, the lungs expand abnormally but do not have the ability to contract to fulfill their function. Alveoli—tiny air sacs from which carbon dioxide is exchanged for oxygen by the blood—are clogged or destroyed, so the body can neither obtain needed oxygen nor rid itself of surplus carbon dioxide. Shortness of breath inevitably results, and breathing becomes laborious. Eventually it becomes painful for the victim to cross a room without resting, and to climb a short flight of stairs is frequently impossible. This constitutes disability for about 14,000 additional persons yearly in the U.S.A. An estimated 100,000 deaths now occur yearly and 20,000,000 workers are disabled by it. As a crippler, emphysema ranks second only to heart disease.

Coronary heart disease has become the number one killer of the Western world. Addiction to smoking is estimated to cause a twofold increase because of the stress it puts on the heart. It speeds the heartbeat while it constricts blood vessels. Its interference with blood flow and oxygen exchange in the lungs and the reduced oxygen carrying ability of the blood because of other substances there also deprive the heart of an adequate blood supply. The American Heart Association estimates that in the U.S.A. more than 100,000 deaths from heart disease yearly result from smoking. The Canadian figure is set at 10,000 yearly.

Accidents, too, are frequently related to smoking. In one year in the U.S.A. there were 163,000 smoking-linked fires doing $80,000,000 worth of damage and claiming 1,800 lives. Auto accidents occur four times as frequently among smoking drivers because of three circumstances inherent in the situation.

(1) Reflexes are reduced sharply within a minute after one starts to smoke. On a high nicotine cigarette, this reduction may reach 67 percent in four minutes of smoking. It takes 20 minutes after the cessation of smoking for the reflexes to return to normal.[25]

(2) Carbon monoxide causes drowsiness. This gas, frequently the cause of death when accidentally inhaled from auto exhausts or improperly functioning heaters, is present in cigarette smoke in concentrations at least 400 times the allowable environmental level where pollution controls are in effect.[26] In a room of smokers or a closed car, it can easily pollute all the air at a rate twice that allowable even in industry. Its presence in the blood reduces the oxygen carrying capacity of that substance; cells are deprived and shortness of breath occurs as the body struggles to get needed oxygen, resulting in increased inhalation of carbon monoxide-laden air. The gas is not completely eliminated from the blood in less than six hours of refraining from smoking. For some, there is no more than a 30 percent reduction overnight. Other noxious gasses are also present in high concentration. (Hydrogen cyanide, the gas of the execution chamber, is present in cigarette smoke at a rate of 1600 parts per million, 160 times the 10 parts per million considered the maximum for safety in industry. Among other harmful gasses identified in tobacco smoke are nitrogen dioxide, hydrogen sulfide, acrolein, ammonia, and acetone.[27])

(3) The distraction of the cigarette takes attention away from the road, driving, and traffic dangers.

The Surgeon General of the U.S.A. estimates that U.S. cigarette smokers experience more chronic illnesses—12,000,000 more—than nonsmokers of the same age; they also spend 88,000,000 more days in bed and 306,000,000 additional days in restricted activity each year from illnesses associated with smoking.[28] In Canada men 40 to 69 years of age who smoke are hospitalized 50 percent more often than nonsmokers; and 46 percent of the heavy smokers among 500 Toronto women studied had chronic bronchitis, more chest abnormalities, and less chest capacity than their nonsmoking counterparts. Even the light smokers showed impaired elasticity in their lungs and the presence of obstructions to proper oxygenization of blood.[29]

Of nutritional interest is the recent discovery that smokers need almost double the quantity of vitamin C to maintain the same blood level of the nutrient as nonsmokers. Absorption is somehow inhibited by smoking. This fact coupled with the role of vitamin C in maintaining tissue integrity may help to explain why smokers are twice as likely to be toothless between the ages of 30 and 59 as their nonsmoking counterparts.[30] This might be a factor in the facial wrinkling that occurs in many smokers, even some who smoke heavily only in their youth before wrinkling normally occurs.[31]

Of concern is the way in which the chemicals of tobacco smoke react with other chemicals in the environment to endanger health. These synergists are found in alcoholic beverages, asbestos, and even some foods.[32]

Smoking and Nonsmokers

Damage is also inflicted on those who do not choose to smoke but are forced to inhale air laden with the noxious substances of tobacco smoke simply by being in the vicinity of smokers. Burning tobacco pollutes the air with all the objectionable substances of tobacco smoke. No filter decreases the amount of nicotine, tars, or toxic gasses emitted from an idling cigarette, pipe, or cigar. Only the smoker recieves any benefit from even the best of filters, and that for only the approximately twenty-four seconds that he/she inhales from each cigarette. The rest of the twelve minutes that the average cigarette burns (pipes and cigars idle much longer), the noxious substances pour into the air unrestrained. As ashes accumulate and butts grow shorter, there is an increase in the amount of cadmium released into the air, increasing the danger to those unfortunate enough to have to breathe the polluted air. The idling cigarette, pipe, or cigar gives off smoke containing almost twice the tar and nicotine of inhaled smoke, which is filtered in part by the body of the smoker. It is danger from this smoke that is causing a change in attitude toward the "right" of a smoker to satisfy his/her addiction in public places.

There was a time when smoking any place at any time was considered acceptable. That day is past. Now the right of the nonsmoker to breathe unpolluted air has begun to be recognized. This recognition has caused many commercial institutions to provide services free from the irritants of smoke. Airlines designate seating for nonsmokers. Restaurants reserve areas for those who choose to eat without inhaling the pollutants. Buses are returning to the practice of restricting smoking to rear seats if it is permitted at all. In some progressive cities, smoking in retail stores and restaurants is forbidden.

There is an organization dedicated to eliminating smoking in public places; its services are available to those who wish to bring relief from involuntary second-hand smoking to their areas. It goes by the initials ASH (Action on Smoking and Health); the address is 2000 H Street, Northwest, Washington, D.C. 20006.[33] Only parents in a home, however, can bring relief to children in their care.

Deciding About Tobacco

One who is deciding whether to use tobacco can consider all of the available facts or refrain simply because the Lord advised this is the intelligent way to go. If the facts are to be considered, one must weigh the reasons for wanting to smoke against the facts that show smoking is a major cause of illness, disability, and premature death. It is also a financial burden that requires the addicted to spend many thousands of dollars over even a shortened lifetime just to pay for the tobacco (to say nothing of the doctor bills and lost working time). It damages all and offends many of those with whom the smoker's smoke comes in contact. It leaves a legacy of handicapped infancy and often chronic illness for the children of smokers. It can crease skin with the premature marks of age. Those who are really interested in the health and happiness of others, most of all the Creator, advise against using it.

Quitting Tobacco

Quitting is not easy because the use of tobacco is not just a habit; it is an addiction to a powerful drug, and withdrawal brings suffering. Time, willpower, and discomfort are involved in quitting in all but a fortunate few. Most are uncomfortable, unhappy, and their craving may interfere with their thinking, interrupt their work, make them careless, cross, and irritable. But it can be done, as millions have demonstrated.

While quitting tobacco, some people experience mild to severe restlessness, insomnia, anxiety, tremor, amnesia, and drowsiness. All these will pass, authorities say. They may be relieved in part by available drugs, group therapy, and counseling. Personal prayer and ministry through the laying on of the hands of the elders help those who have faith to receive divine healing of their addiction. Authorities say there are three formidable enemies of the newly resolved ex-smoker—tension, frustration, and boredom. These need to be guarded against by careful planning of busy, happy days during the time in which the addiction is being terminated.

The Canadian Cancer Society and other authorities have offered suggestions to help those who wish to stop smoking.[34] Some of these are as follows:

1. Set a Q (quit) day no more than two weeks away and either taper to it or quit cold on that day.

2. Avoid situations associated with smoking. This may mean avoiding unsympathetic friends for the withdrawal period.

3. Collect interesting reading material, games, puzzles, or handwork with which to fill rest periods and work breaks.

4. Start a bank account with the money being saved by not smoking, and make a definite plan to spend it for something special. (Bishop Ed Ford calculated at one time that the Saints were building churches on the money saved by not using tobacco. Canadians alone spent $1,200,000,000 for cigarettes in 1970. The average U.S.A. smoker, where tobacco is much less expensive

than in Canada, easily spends $15,000 on tobacco in a lifetime at pre-1970 prices—much more with inflation.)

5. Practice breathing deeply when the urge to smoke develops.

6. Do not allow unlimited weight gains to accompany nonsmoking. This will be difficult since food tastes better and metabolism improves some 5 to 15 percent without nicotine. And since smoking is a nervous habit that requires the oral satisfaction of having something in the mouth, food often becomes a substitute. For some, gaining may be desirable. For most a weight problem is not as serious as tobacco addiction but neither is it desirable. One heart specialist suggests that it would take a weight gain of 80 pounds (36 kg) to a 160-pound (72 kg) man or a 60-pound (27 kg) gain for a 100-pound (45 kg) woman to equal the health risk of smoking. To prevent unwanted gain:

(1) Stock up on fresh fruits and vegetables—low calorie snacks—and gum for oral satisfaction.

(2) Increase physical activity. Walk to work, paint the house, play an extra game of tennis daily. Provide distraction from the need to smoke while helping control the weight. (See chapter on weight control.)

7. Don't expect it to be easy. Those who experience no difficulty have been richly blessed.

8. Do be assured that the rewards will be worth all of the effort. As soon as smoking ceases the body will go to work to repair the damage smoking has done. Unless some lethal disease has established itself irrevocably, coughing will diminish and may cease. Breathing will be easier, circulation will improve, and energy will increase. Olfactory perception will be more acute.

9. Do not try to sneak just one smoke after quitting. The addiction is easily revived. Fewer than 2 percent of those who try become occasional smokers.

Finally

Clever advertisements would lead one to believe that tobacco will make the user happy, relaxed, popular, attractive, appealing. Misleading pseudoscientific propaganda from the tobacco industry continues to feed public skepticism about the dangers of indulging.[35] The Lord said that it was for this very reason—to combat the evils and designs that did exist in the hearts of conspiring men in 1833 and would still abound in 1976 and beyond—that he revealed the truth about tobacco. It was never meant to be used inside the human body. Intelligent response to the environment demands that the drug with its pollutants, irritants, carcinogens, and noxious gas be eliminated from human consumption except as an "herb for bruises," as he intended.

---

1. Harold S. Diehl, and others, Health and Safety for You, McGraw Hill Book Co., New York, 1969, pp. 78-82.
2. Harold S. Diehl, Tobacco and Your Health: The Smoking Controversy, McGraw Hill Book Co., New York, 1969. (Dr. Harold S. Diehl, Dean of Medical Science and Professor of Public Health, U. of Minn., 1935-1958. After retirement, Senior Vice-President for Research and Medical Affairs and Deputy Executive Vice-President of the American Cancer Society. Served on the National Advisory Council of the U.S. Public Health Service and as a member of the U.S.A. delegation to three World Health Assemblies.)
3. National Tuberculosis and Respiratory Association, U.S.A., 10 Million Women Have Quit Smoking, "Pregnant Women Who Smoke," p. 3.
4. American Medical News, Jan. 18, 1971.
5. Nat'l T.B. and Respiratory Ass'n, U.S.A., op. cit.
6. Diehl, Tobacco and Your Health, op. cit., p. 96.
7. Nat'l T.B. and Resp. Ass'n, U.S.A., op. cit.
8. Today's Health, "News," Nov. 1967.
9. Dr. Janet E. Seely, Eugenija Suskin, Arend Bouhuys, John B. Pierce Foundation, Dept. of Medicine, Yale University School of Medicine, New Haven, Conn., Science, V. 172; #3984, May 14, 1971, pp. 741-743.
10. Diehl, et al., Health and Safety for You, op. cit., p. 80.
11. Study by the Ontario Federation of Home and School Associations released at Canadian Home and School and Parent Teachers Federation meeting in Regina, Saskatchewan, May 1972.
12. Proceedings of the Ninth International Cancer Congress, 1966, p. 169. Also "Education on Smoking for Grades 1-4?", Star Phoenix, June 7, 1972, p. 6.
13. National Clearinghouse for Drug Abuse Information, U.S.A. Dept. of Health, Education and Welfare, Cigarette Smoking, Some Questions and Answers, 1971.
14. Diehl, et al., op cit., p. 77.
15. U.S. Dept. of Health, Education and Welfare, National Institute of Alcohol Abuse and Alcoholism, Second Special Report to the U.S. Congress on Alcohol and Health, June, 1974, pp. 54-55. Also Diehl, op. cit., pp. 17, 79-81.
16. Data from University of Saskatchewan Medical Exhibit, Oct. 1973.
17. Health Education and Information Branch, Saskatchewan Dept. of Public Health, Why Smoke, pamphlet, 1973.
18. S.S. Field, "Nicotine: Profile of Peril," Reader's Digest (Canadian), Sept. 1973.
19. Diehl, et al., op. cit., p. 79 for U.S.A. figures; University of Saskatchewan medical exhibit, Oct. 1973, for Canadian figures.
20. Diehl, et al., p. 81.
21. Dr. Alfred Kershbaum, et al., Philadelphia General Hospital, published in the Journal of the American Medical Association and reported in Today's Health, "News," Nov. 1967, p. 9.
22. Canadian Cancer Society, Help for Smokers (pamphlet).
23. Diehl, op. cit., p. 68, and Canadian Cancer Society, Help for Smokers.
24. Diehl, et al., op. cit., p. 80. Also Saskatchewan School of Medicine exhibit, Oct. 1973.
25. Diehl, op. cit., p. 98.
26. Field, op. cit. Also Diehl, et al., op. cit., p. 77.
27. Saskatchewan Department of Public Health, Why Smoke? op. cit.
28. Diehl, op. cit., pp. 80-81.
29. Canadian Tuberculosis and Respiratory Disease Association, Me Quit Smoking? Why? (pamphlet)
30. Omer Pelletier, "Cigarette Smoking and Vitamin C," Nutrition Today, Autumn 1970, pp. 12-15.
31. Dr. Harry W. Daniell, published in Annals of Internal Medicine, reported in "Today's Health

News," *Today's Health*, May 1972, p. 7. Also "A New Wrinkle on Smoking," *10 Million Women Have Quit Smoking*, *op. cit.*, p. 2.
32. Nicholas Gonzalez, "Preventing Cancer," *Family Health/Today's Health*, May, 1976, p. 32.
33. John Banzhaf III, "Please Put Your Cigarette Out; The Smoke Is Killing Me!" *Today's Health*, Apr. 1972, pp. 38-41.
34. Canadian Cancer Society, *op. cit.* Also Nat'l T.B. and Respiratory Association, *op. cit.* Also many other pamphlets from cancer societies and public health departments.
35. Diehl, *op. cit.*, pp. X and XI (Preface). Also Nat'l T.B. and Respiratory Association, *op. cit.*, p. 4, "Ad Target Women."

CHAPTER 12

Hot Drinks and Strong Drinks

And again, strong drinks are not for the belly.... And again hot drinks are not for the body or belly.—Doctrine and Covenants 86:1.

While the Lord mentioned only one beverage by name (wine) when he warned us about those substances not intended for our bodies, he did speak of strong drinks and hot drinks. That hot drinks are harmful has been abundantly substantiated in modern research. For a quarter of a century the American Cancer Society and the American Medical Association have been publishing data indicating that any beverage drunk at temperatures hotter than 120 degrees Fahrenheit (49 degrees Celsius) can cause damage to tissues of the mouth, esophagus, and stomach. About twenty-five years ago there was a news report that Russian scientists placed the safe limit at 118 degrees F. (48 degrees C.). "Hot" drinks may thus be identified as those with temperatures that exceed the safe limit, which is far from boiling (212 degrees F., 100 degrees C. at sea level).

"Strong drinks" associated with wine are also easily identified as additional alcoholic beverages, but it is not so easy to identify other "strong drinks" that are harmful. The late prophet-president of the Reorganized Church of Jesus Christ of Latter Day Saints, Israel A. Smith, writing in the *Saints' Herald*, expressed his conviction that tea and coffee, while not listed in the revelation by name, frequently qualify as "strong drinks." He said, "I am convinced that tea and coffee are harmful and injurious because of their constituent elements, and those who share in such conviction have overlooked and do mainly now overlook their most valid objection, in my opinion, which is that they are, generally speaking, *strong drinks*"[1] (emphasis is

President Smith's) (though I concede they might be so diluted that the term *strong* could hardly be applied).

"With this argument there is a double phase: tea and coffee, if *hot* drinks are taboo by the plain, simple, and unequivocal terms of the Word; and even if *not* hot or heated, they are or *may be* strong drinks," Brother Israel concluded.

That the Word of Wisdom was early understood to contain a warning against tea and coffee is evident from an article printed in *Times and Seasons*, publication of the early church.[2] The article, signed "Omega" at a time when Joseph Smith, Jr., the prophet through whom the instruction was given, was editor of that paper, reports a sermon by Presiding Patriarch Hyrum Smith, brother of the prophet and formerly a member of the First Presidency. Hyrum preached at length about the Word of Wisdom, the article says, and answered the question of the people of that day concerning the intent of the revelation: "I say it does mean tea and coffee." Then he discussed some of the possible ill effects of using the beverages.

That caffeine-containing beverages may well qualify as "strong drinks" is increasingly validated in modern research. Caffeine is a habit-forming, psychoactive drug.[3] The United States National Clearinghouse for Drug Abuse lists it with alcohol and tobacco as one of the "recreational drugs" made legal as a way to have "fun" and to get away from the stresses and strains of life, not because they are safe but because they are socially accepted.[4] (Incidentally, in this situation many alienated youth find inconsistency, hypocrisy, and justification for their flouting of the law.)

Among the stimulants used the world over, caffeine may be the least noxious, so far as we are presently aware. Certainly cocaine of the coca leaves[5]* and the amphetamines and methamphetamines (speed, crystal, meth) of the present drug culture produce serious effects more readily and have well earned their illegal status.[6]** To make intelligent choices about the care of our

---

*Coca leaf chewing is not illegal in the Andes Mountains where the leaves are part of the wages of the poorly clothed, undernourished, and overworked Indians who use the drug to relieve hunger and fatigue. Coca leaves from which the cocaine has been extracted are used in the production of cola beverages. Originally the cocaine was also included.

**Amphetamines were described with caffeine as causing relatively benign effects (with amphetamines less costly in side effects than caffeine) as recently as 1962. It was not then anticipated that they would be taken in the quantity in which they became used for nonmedical purposes.[7]

bodies, however, we need to be informed about the effects of this stimulant that occurs in many foods and over-the-counter medications. Caffeine is present in coffee, tea, cola, and "pepper" beverages, mate, chocolate beverages and confections, "stay-awake" preparations, headache and other pain relievers,[8] and guarana (long used by the natives of the Amazon River countries and now the basis of a popular Brazilian beverage. It contains three times as much caffeine as a similar weight of coffee).[9]

Effects of Caffeine

Caffeine and two other xanthines that sometimes occur with it, theophylline in tea and theobromine in chocolate, all stimulate the central nervous system, act as diuretics on the kidneys (increase the flow of urine), stimulate heart muscle and relax smooth muscle (particularly bronchial muscle). Caffeine, however, has the most powerful effect.[10]

Because of its effect on the cerebral cortex of the brain, some forms of mental and physical activity are apparently temporarily enhanced and drowsiness and fatigue are allayed when caffeine is ingested.[11] It is this capacity of the drug to make one think more clearly, act more quickly, and forget that he/she is tired that accounts for much of its popularity and one of its dangers. Some studies indicate there is elevation of mood but not of performance.[12]

When a body is really fatigued, it needs rest. The U.S.A. Food and Drug Administration has warned, ". . . when a person is tired he should rest rather than rely on a stimulant for carrying on physical activities. FDA has strong reservations about the use of a stimulant type preparation while driving since such stimulants temporarily mask mental and physical fatigue. The consequence may be dangerous. . . . The use of caffeine is not a substitute for normal rest or sleep."[13]

Dr. Chester W. White, Boston School of Medicine, has been quoted as warning students against using caffeine to stay awake for studying on the basis of the fact that the stimulant cannot improve total mental performance, and taking excessive amounts can make one tense, nervous, and unable to concentrate on the day following loss of rest from its use.[14]

The effect of caffeine on both mental and physical activity is, of course, temporary and dependent on whether one is accustomed to using the drug. Nonusers frequently react to taking caffeine with irritability, inability to work effectively, nervousness, restlessness, lethargy, and headache. Users often react with the same set of symptoms when they are deprived of their normal dose of the drug. Dr. R. M. Gilbert of the Addiction Research Foundation of Ontario (Canada) suggests that this latter effect constitutes a withdrawal syndrome (set of symptoms) occurring among those who drink five cups of coffee or more a day. The symptoms have occurred in tests when people who regularly drank three or more cups of coffee a day were not allowed to have caffeine.[15]

Caffeine both prevents sleep and disturbs it.[16] The maximum effect of the drug is not felt immediately. For some it takes up to three hours or more for the body to respond maximally.[17] Because of this many do not associate their response with the drug; they do not think drinking caffeine-containing beverages affects their sleep adversely. Although they fall asleep after drinking them, they become restless later in the night, unaware that their wakefulness is directly related to the beverage. Frequently this wakefulness induces the use of tranquilizers or other sleep aids to combat the effect of the caffeine, which may result in even more serious consequences.[18] Long ago Dr. Harvey Diehl warned us that constant stimulation by day and sedation by night could only lead to health problems.

Most familiar to many caffeine users is the early morning reluctance to get going, irritability, empty feeling behind the eyes, and headache that characterizes each morning before the first cup of coffee or tea. These "withdrawal symptoms" are relieved with the taking of the drug in beverage form or as a headache remedy containing caffeine. Dr. Gilbert finds these withdrawal effects "more profound than the direct effects of the drug...." [19]

Children are particularly susceptible to problems created by the use of caffeine. Extra urine must be eliminated at a time when the child is trying to learn to control his voiding. A caffeine consuming child *must* go to the bathroom more often than "normal" or have wet clothing and wet beds. Stimulation to activity when rest is needed robs the child's body of opportunity to grow properly, develop resistance to disease, and create good nerve responses. Empty calories of caffeine-containing beverages and foods rob the body of B vitamins required to metabolize them and take the place of more nutritious foods essential for good health, growth, and nervous stability. The caffeine-stimulated children are generally more nervous, less purposeful, more prone to illness than their unstimulated counterparts, fretful sleepers, frequently bed-wetters, and more difficult to handle.

On the other hand, some hyperactive children are being treated with stimulants, including coffee. Although the medical riddle of this type of hyperactivity has yet to be solved, and there appears to be more than caffeine involved in the effectiveness of the use of coffee,[20] it is interesting to consider Dr. Gilbert's suggestion that caffeine withdrawal may be the cause of at least some of the behavior problems that respond to stimulants.[21]

Children allowed to drink cola, pepper, tea, coffee, or large amounts of cocoa or chocolate easily develop "caffeinism."[22] Because of their smaller size, the amount of caffeine that affects them is much less than that which affects an adult. For example, a 60-pound (27 kg) child taking three colas, containing the caffeine allowed by law, and one ounce of sweet chocolate would be getting caffeine per kilogram of body weight equivalent to a man weighing 175 pounds (80 kg) drinking seven cups of coffee (average). The Food and Drug Administration (U.S.A.) has warned that a "safe" dose of caffeine for a child of two years, weighing 21 pounds (9.45 kg), is only one-seventh of the "safe" dose for an adult.[23]

Disease States That May Be Related to Caffeine Usage

Caffeine makes the heart beat faster and frequently irregularly (skip beats), constricts blood vessels, and increases blood pressure. No one argues with these facts. However, there is spirited debate in the medical community concerning the implications of caffeine in increasing the risk of coronary heart disease. The data are sufficient to cause many physicians to recommend caution in the use of the drug, however, to help protect hearts.*[24]

Caffeine and other ingredients in coffee stimulate the secretion of gastric (stomach) juices that may lead to hyperacidity with consequent damage to the lining of the stomach. The association

---

*The theophylline content of tea is so high that it counteracts caffeine's ability to constrict blood vessels. Hence coffee is more frequently noted with respect to heart disease than tea.[25]

of caffeine-containing beverages with ulcer development has long been noted and is under intensive study.[26]

Caffeine induces fevers under some circumstances and maintains them once they are established, contrary to the expectation of those who purchase the drug in combination with aspirin in such preparations as cold medications.[27] It is a stressful agent that releases fatty acids, including cholesterol, into the bloodstream. The immediate effect is most pronounced when sugar-free forms, as diet colas and "peppers," or black coffee are taken. Sugar only delays the rise in cholesterol, however.[28]

Caffeine is a mutagen (substance that is capable of producing birth defects by damaging genes or chromosomes) for many organisms. Its role in producing defective humans is under investigation. It is known to cross the placenta and remain in the tissues of the fetus without being metabolized as many drugs are.[29]

Caffeine may affect alcohol consumption adversely when taken before the alcohol, especially if the one drinking is undernourished. Rats given a "marginal teen-age diet" quadrupled their alcohol consumption when caffeine was added to the diet. Taken after excessive alcohol has been consumed, caffeine does not sober up the drinker, but produces a dangerous, wide-awake drunk.[30]

States often diagnosed as "anxiety neurosis" are now proving to be the result of heavy caffeine consumption. Symptoms include dizziness, agitation, restlessness, recurring headaches, and sleeplessness.[31]

Deleterious Substances in Caffeinic Beverages

Recent reports have linked chlorogenic acid in combination with nitrites to the production of nitrosamines that are powerful cancer-producing agents. Chlorogenic acid, a phenol compound important to the metabolism of many plants, is found in especially large amounts in coffee beans and is highly soluble in hot water.[32] For this reason it has been recommended that coffee not be consumed with such foods as bacon, ham, sausages, corned beef, and some cheeses if these foods have been preserved with nitrites or nitrates, some of which may be converted to nitrites during digestion.

Phenols in tea have long been associated with the promotion of cancer. They do not start the cancer but promote its development once it is started.[33]

Tannic acid is present in both tea and coffee in amounts large enough to damage tissues and deplete body stores of calcium when large amounts of the beverages are used. Tea is 13 percent tannic acid. Coffee has a smaller proportion of the bitter, astringent (puckering) acid, but because more of the substance is used in making the beverage, the amount present in the beverage is significant.[34] Using milk in the beverage may precipitate some of the acid, at the expense of some of the calcium normally provided by the milk, of course. Artificial "creamers" and "whiteners" do not have this beneficial effect.

Oxalic acid in chocolate and cocoa may also combine with some food calcium, making it unavailable to the body. When these substances are made into a beverage with milk, the net effect on calcium nutrition is still positive. Used without milk, their effect on calcium nutrition can be detrimental.

Theobromine is an alkaloid chemically related to caffeine that occurs in chocolate, cocoa, tea, and coffee. It is a weak central nervous system stimulant and so does not produce nervous disorders that sometimes result from the use of caffeine. It does stimulate peripheral nerves and increase the flow of urine. That its effect is less marked than caffeine is indicated by the fact that the American Medical Association defines a medicinal dose of caffeine as ranging from 60 to 300 mg, depending on the purpose of the medication, and a medicinal dose of theobromine as ranging from 500 to 1,000 mg.[35]

Theophylline is also present in these substances, as previously noted, especially in tea.

Amounts of Drugs in Various Products

Tea leaves average from 3 to 4.9 percent caffeine. Coffee beans are about 1½ percent caffeine. Since only about one teaspoon (5 ml) of tea is used per serving, however, and two tablespoons (30 ml) ground coffee are necessary, coffee usually contains more caffeine per cup.

"Typical" or "average" amounts of the drug reported in beverages vary greatly, and the size serving may be from a five-ounce (150 ml) cup through an eight-ounce (240 ml) mug to a 10- or 12-ounce bottled beverage. For a five-ounce (150 ml) cup of beverage, coffee is usually found to contain around 100 mg of the drug, although instant coffee may contain as little as 60 to 70 mg and filtered coffee may contain as much as 150 mg. A similar cup of tea may contain 110 mg caffeine, but 50 to 75 mg is more probable.[36]

"Decaffeinated" coffee may have 97 percent of the drug removed if it is so labeled. If the percentage is not stated, however, at least in the U.S.A., there may be as much as 25 percent of the caffeine left.[37] These coffees are frequently used in greater amounts than recipes call for, producing a beverage stronger in flavor and higher in acid content than regular coffees and higher in caffeine content than expected.

Caffeine content of soft drinks is restricted by law in the U.S.A. and Canada to 0.02 percent of the product by weight, about 60 mg for a 10 oz. (300 ml) bottle. They can have less, and are reported to contain from 35 to 60 mg in a 10-ounce (300 ml) container in the U.S.A. and slightly less in Canada. Where standards are set (as they are for colas and "pepper" beverages) the presence of caffeine in the beverage does not have to be declared on the label.[38]

Chocolate and cocoa are caffeine poor when compared with coffee, tea, and cola beverages, but actual amounts will vary with the recipe used. Dr. Gilbert reports, "The caffeine content of a cup of cocoa is typically between 5 and 50 mg." If instructions on most cocoa boxes are followed, however, the caffeine content would be more like two milligrams per cup. The theobromine content likewise varies widely. Dr. Gilbert indicates it is "typically between 50 and 250 mg" per cup.[39] One ounce (28 g) of sweet chocolate contains about 20 mg caffeine, and one ounce (28 g) bitter chocolate or cocoa about twice that amount.

It is apparent that one might get quantities of caffeine from chocolate products comparable with those from coffee, tea, and colas. It is also apparent that chocolate could be used in such a way as to provide only a fraction of the drug obtained from the other foods. It would take 20 cups of cocoa containing 5 mg caffeine to provide the caffeine of one "average" cup of coffee, but only 2 cups of the cocoa containing 50 mg each of the drug. It would be necessary to eat 4 to 5 ounces of sweet chocolate to get the caffeine of one cup of coffee, and to eat a whole cake and one-fourth of a second made with two ounces (56 g) chocolate to get the same amount of the drug.

Regardless of the amount of stimulant in chocolate and cocoa foods, it is not recommended that children have them regularly. They do contain stimulant, and their energy value, including the sugar needed to sweeten them, introduces too many calories for the nutrients offered to provide an acceptable staple in a child's diet—or in an adult's for that matter. Adults also need to consider that their example with respect to use of food or beverages has profound influence on the choices of their children.

CAFFEINE CONTENT OF BEVERAGES

Beverage	Size of Serving	Milligrams Caffeine	Number Servings to = Caffeine of 1 c. Coffee
Coffee	5 oz. (180 ml)	Av. 100	1
Tea	5 oz. (180 ml)	70-100	1-1⅓
Cola or "pepper"	10 oz. (360 ml)	Max. 60	1⅔
Very rich chocolate	5 oz. (180 ml)	50	2
Average cocoa	5 oz. (180 ml)	5	20
Recipe cocoa	5 oz. (180 ml)	2	50
Decaffeinated coffee:			
Caffeine 97% removed	5 oz. (180 ml)	3	33⅓
No specified amount	5 oz. (180 ml)	Up to 25	4*

CAFFEINE CONTENT OF FOOD

Food	Amount	Milligrams Caffeine	Amount to = Caffeine of One Cup Coffee
Bitter chocolate	1 oz. (28 gm)	40	2½ oz. (70 gm)
Sweet chocolate	1 oz. (28 gm)	20	5 oz. (140 gm)
Chocolate cake, plain (2 oz.-56 gm bitter chocolate)	Whole cake	80	1¼ cakes
Chocolate cake, fudge frosting (4 oz.-112 gm bitter chocolate)	Whole cake	160	5/8 of 1 cake

---

*Decaffeinated coffee still retains all the tannins, alkaloids other than caffeine, chlorogenic acid, etc., of regular coffee.

In addition to foods, caffeine is available in medications intended for ameliorating headaches and symptoms of colds and the like. These usually contain from 15 to 30 mg of the drug. "Stay-awake" preparations contain about 110 mg per tablet—about the strength of one cup of coffee—and it is this quantity of stimulant about which the U.S.A. Food and Drug Administration says it has "strong reservations" concerning people who drive while using it.[40]

Food Values of Caffeine Containing Substances

It is appropriate that one who wishes to choose foods intelligently should consider nutritive values that may accrue as well as potential harmfulness. Here are some of the facts related to caffeine-containing foods:[41]

- Colas and peppers have no known nutritive value except energy, and that is largely missing in diet varieties. Sweetened with sugar, they have about 13 Calories per ounce (30 ml), with no B vitamins to metabolize the Calories.
- Tea has infinitesimal amounts of riboflavin, niacin, calcium, and potassium with significant amounts of flourine when several cupfuls are used daily.
- Coffee rates slightly above "trace" in its calcium, phosphorus, and iron content, but these minerals are made partly unavailable by other chemical constituents of the substance. It may provide significant amounts of magnesium and potassium, and does contribute niacin in measurable quantities. In each cup of the beverage, there is about as much niacin as is found in a 3/4 of an ounce (28 g) slice of whole wheat bread.
- Chocolate and cocoa are nutritious foods. An ounce (28 g) of cocoa has more protein than an ounce (28 g) of cottage cheese, as much protein as a small to medium egg, as much calcium as 1½ ounces (42 g) of cottage cheese or two small eggs, as much iron as three medium-sized eggs, 1/3 the B_1 of one large egg—the B_2 of a medium egg—the niacin (B_3) of 3/4 of an ounce (21 g) whole wheat bread, more than 1/3 the adult RDA of magnesium, and a generous amount of potassium.

Chocolate has more fat than cocoa. An ounce (28 g) of chocolate, with about 60 Calories more than an equal weight of cocoa, has only about half—plus or minus a little—of the other nutrients except vitamin A. White chocolate contains about half the stimulant of regular chocolate.*

The Place of Caffeine Beverages in Western Society

Coffee and cola beverages have become so much a part of the way of life in Canada and the U.S.A., that rest periods at work are called "coffee breaks" even when coffee is not available. The small table that sits in front of the divan (Chesterfield in Canada) is the "coffee table" even in homes in which coffee is never served. Sweet breads for snacks or breakfast are "coffee cakes" even though they contain no coffee and are served with fruit drinks or milk. People who leave work to entertain guests go "out for coffee" or "out for a coke" even though such beverages may never be consumed.

The U.S.A. alone uses one third of all the coffee produced in the world. In 1968 that totaled 2,860,000,000 pounds (1,567,000,000 kg).[42] In addition, cola sales totaled almost two billion dollars and accounted for 65 percent of the soft drink market.[43] In the same year, Canadian soft drink sales totaled half a billion dollars with a similarly large proportion containing caffeine.[44]

Tea holds a similar place in the Orient and Britain. Those of British stock in England, the U.S.A., Canada, Australia, and other areas are continuously affected by its terminology. Beverage cups are "teacups." Dessert and measuring spoons are "teaspoons." The refreshment break of the day is "teatime," and social events for friends or the community are "teas."

In recent years the average consumption of tea in England has totaled ten pounds (4.5 kg) for every man, woman, and child. A medical member of the Commons reported that ten cups a day was considered normal consumption by some of the English and called attention to the fact that that amount of tea contained some three times the maximum allowable medicinal dose of caffeine.[45]

Choosing

As with other "recreational" drugs, the general social acceptance of caffeine and the prevalence of its use make it

---

*Some prefer to substitute carob flour (St. Johnsbread) in recipes calling for cocoa or chocolate. Carob resembles chocolate in flavor, contains no stimulant, is largely carbohydrate, has about one fourth the protein and less than one tenth the fat of cocoa. It has a small amount of calcium, a very small amount of phosphorus, and is thought to have other vitamins and minerals in small amounts but data were not conclusive as to amounts at the date of publication of USDA Handbook No. 8 used in these calculations.

imperative that persons concerned with the stewardship of their own bodies and that of their offspring should decide whether to use them. They may consider all of the available information and then decide whether the pleasures of indulgence are of sufficient magnitude to justify subjecting their bodies and the bodies of their young to the risks of the drug, or they may decide to reject them simply because the Lord of love said that he did not intend that hot or strong drinks be used. Intelligent response is essential to the development of the kind of health that the Lord envisioned when he revealed his will concerning temporal salvation in the Word of Wisdom.

---

1. Israel A. Smith, "Not by Way of Compulsion or Restraint," *The Saints' Herald*, July 25, 1949, p. 10.
2. Omega (presumably the editor of *Times and Seasons*, Joseph Smith, Jr.), "The Word of Wisdom," *Times and Seasons*, Vol. 3, No. 15, June 1, 1842, pp. 799-801.
3. R. M. Gilbert, "Caffeine Beverages and Their Effects," *Addiction* (Quarterly Publication of the Addiction Research Foundation of Ontario, Toronto, Canada), Vol. 21, No. 1, Spring, 1974, pp. 68-80.
4. Jean Paul Smith, Ph.D., "II. Drug Abuse: Definition and Delineation," National Clearinghouse for Drug Abuse Information, *Resource Book for Drug Abuse Education*, Second Edition, 1972, p. 27.
5. Gilbert, *op. cit.*, p. 73.
6. Sidney Cohen, M.D., "Stimulants: An Historic and Affective Analysis," National Clearinghouse for Drug Abuse Information, *ibid.*, p. 41.
7. Gilbert, *op. cit.*, p. 76.
8. Cohen, *op. cit.* Also U.S.A. Food and Drug Administration *Fact Sheet*, "Caffeine," July 1971.
9. Norman Taylor, *Narcotics*, Delta Book Co., N.Y., 1963, p. 175.
10. Malcolm Manber, "The Medical Effects of Coffee," *Medical World News*, Vol. 17, No. 2, Jan. 26, 1976, p. 65.
11. *Ibid.*
12. Gilbert, *op. cit.*, p. 76.
13. U.S.A. FDA *Fact Sheet*, "Caffeine," *op. cit.*
14. *Today's Health*, April 1955, p. 16, quoting Dr. Chester W. White, Instructor for Pharmacology, Boston School of Medicine in *Boston University News*.
15. Manber, *op. cit.*, p. 64. Also the Alberta (Canada) Alcoholism and Drug Abuse Commission, Public Information Series, *Caffeine*, 1975. (Both refer to the work of A. Goldstein and S. Kaizer, "Psychotropic Effects of Caffeine in Man. III A questionnaire survey of coffee drinking and its effects in a group of housewives." *Clinical Pharmacology and Therapeutics*. Vol. 10, 1969, pp. 478-479, and A. Goldstein, S. Kaizer, and O. Whitby, "Psychotropic Effects of Caffeine in Man. IV Quantitative and qualitative differences associated with habituation to coffee," *Clinical Pharmacology and Therapeutics*, Vol. 10, pp. 489-497, 1969.)
16. Gilbert, *op. cit.*, p. 76.
17. Alberta Alcoholism and Drug Abuse Commission, *op. cit.*, p. 3.
18. Gilbert, *op. cit.*, p. 64.
19. *Ibid.*
20. Manber, *op. cit.*, p. 64.
21. Gilbert, *op. cit.*, pp. 79-80.
22. Manber, *op. cit.*, p. 67.
23. *Consumer Bulletin*, No. 54, Aug. 1971, pp. 31-32.
24. Manber, *op. cit.*, pp. 66-67. Also Gilbert, *op. cit.*, p. 70, and Jean Mayer, *Overweight, Cause, Cost and Control*, Prentice-Hall, Inc., Englewood Cliffs, N.J., 1968, pp. 162-163.
25. Gilbert, *op. cit.*, p. 72.
26. Manber, *op. cit.*, pp. 65-66.
27. Gilbert, *op. cit.*, p. 77. Also M. J. Dascombe, "The Effect of Caffeine on the Antipyretic Action of

Aspirin Administered During Endotoxin Induced Fever," *British Journal of Pharmacology*, Vol. 46, No. 1972, pp. 548-549.
28. S. Bellet, L. Roman, J. Kostis, and O. DeCastro, "Effect of Coffee Ingestion on Adrenocortical Secretion in Young Men and Dogs," *Metabolism*, Vol. 18, Dec. 1969, pp. 1007-1012. (Contains many references to literature.)
29. Manber, *op. cit.*, pp. 68-73. Also "Coffee and Cola Drinks Also Present Problems as Mutagens," *Consumer Bulletin*, Mar. 1970, p. 19.
30. Gilbert, *op. cit.*, p. 80.
31. Manber, *op. cit.*, p. 67.
32. Merck and Company, Inc., *Merck Index and Encyclopedia of Chemicals and Drugs*. Rahway, New Jersey, U.S.A., 1968, Topic, "Chlorogenic Acid."
33. Personal communication, Dr. Elmer O. Scheltgen, University of Saskatchewan, Saskatoon, Canada, quoting reports of Drs. Hans E. Kaiser and John C. Bartone of George Washington School of Medicine, Washington, D.C., to the 9th International Cancer Congress, 1966. Also Alton Blakeslee, "Tea Chemicals Promote Cancer," *Austin (Texas) American Statesman*, Oct. 29, 1966, p. 29.
34. R. W. Moncrieff, *The Chemical Senses*, Leonard Hall, London, 1967, p. 654.
35. *Ibid*. Also Erich Hesse, M.D., Professor of Pharmacology and Biology, *Narcotics and Drug Addiction*, Philosophical Library, N.Y., 1946, p. 163.
36. Gilbert, *op. cit.*, p. 72, Manber, *op. cit.*, p. 67, FDA *Fact Sheet*, op. cit.
37. T. R. Van Dellen, M.D., "The Effects of Caffeine," *Consumer Bulletin*, Nov. 1972, p. 26.
38. FDA *Fact Sheet, op. cit.*
39. Personal Communication from R. M. Gilbert, Addiction Research Foundation of Ontario, Canada, dated April 15, 1975.
40. FDA *Fact Sheet, op. cit.*
41. Computed from data in USDA Agriculture Handbook No. 8, *Composition of Foods, Raw, Processed, Prepared*, Agricultural Research Service, 1963.
42. World Book Encyclopedia, Topic, "Coffee." Also Manber, *op. cit.*, p. 64.
43. Manber, *op. cit.*, p. 67. Also *Consumer Bulletin*, No. 54, Aug. 1971, pp. 31-32.
44. Montreal *Globe and Mail* news item, Dec. 3, 1969.
45. Taylor, *op. cit.*, pp. 190-191.

Chapter 13

Some Problem Areas in Modern Nutrition Practice
Part I—Misinformation

In consequence of evils and designs which do and will exist in the hearts of conspiring men in the last days, I have warned you, and forewarn you, by giving unto you this word of wisdom by revelation....—Doctrine and Covenants 86:1a.

Fads are derived from misinformation and perennially take a heavy toll in terms of health and money. Because they are often bound to emotions, it is very difficult to dispel them successfully with facts. Innumerable food and health fads are perpetrated with religious fervor that often exceeds that associated with the practice of the principles of the gospel of Jesus Christ. Concern for the physical often becomes completely confused with spiritual values in the mind of the faddist and is pursued with such vigor that there is little time or energy left to be spent in the work of the kingdom. Because they affect people so dramatically, they are among the "evils and designs" against which the Lord desired to protect us when he revealed the Word of Wisdom.

Choosing Accurate Nutrition Information

Long ago Hosea lamented, "My people are destroyed for lack of knowledge."[1] His lament is applicable today in the field of food and health. In spite of all of the information available, there are areas in which we are woefully ignorant. Into these areas faddists enter with gusto. In other areas of concern, they are able to prosper only because the people have not taken advantage of the opportunity to be informed.

The Lord has attempted to point us the way out of the confusion and destruction that follows ignorance and false teaching by instructing us to "seek...out of the best books words of wisdom; seek learning even by study, and also by faith,"[2] and "Despise not prophesying. Prove all things; hold fast that which is good."[3] If we truly have faith in the instructions that God has given us, we will measure by that which he has revealed the books purported to give us information. Only those qualifying as best books, then, should be accepted and their recommendations tested.

Such evaluation is not easy. Most of us like certainties and are prone to accept that which comes in positive statements with strong testimonials. These often come from charming people full of charisma, spectacular information, and easy answers to health problems. Unfortunately much of this type of nutrition information is not the best available. Like Jacob of old, who grew wealthy thinking he was marking his cattle by placing peeled reeds in their watering troughs,[4] their proponents may believe implicitly in their information but possess only a part of the truth. A testimonial is a statement of recommendation based on limited and frequently inadequate experience. A testimony bears witness of the truth, which Jacob did when the Lord taught him that the cattle were marked by the natural process of heredity which the Lord directed in his behalf. Testimonials are often based on half truths, and half truths often provide the kind of misinformation most difficult to correct.

The problem is further complicated by efforts of spurious "health" literature to destroy confidence in the medical profession, university experiments, and government information, or to use information of legitimate research to support dubious recommendations. What is presented seems like the truth because it is said by clever people who intend it to sound truthful or by misguided people who really believe it is true. It is easy to believe the self-confident, propaganda-wise, persuasive promoter in preference to a thorough physician or scientist who admits there are still things to be learned.

On the other hand, the medical profession has neglected to take positive action in the field of nutrition for too long a time and must bear much of the responsibility for others trying to fill an obvious need. Prominent physicians and researchers are now insisting that doctors receive adequate nutrition training to end the untenable situation in which the emphasis has been so much on cure by surgery and drugs that patients suffer undetected nutritional disease and death under the conditions of treatment. Iatrogenic (physician induced) malnutrition, it is called, and Charles E. Butterworth, Jr., M.D. opened a discussion on the subject under the title, "The Skeleton in the Hospital Closet," in *Nutrition Today*, March/April 1974.[5]

Helps for Sorting Available Literature

Left to our own devices, we need a lot of learning in the basic sciences to be equipped to choose the "best books" in the field of nutrition and health. Since we cannot all be skilled in these sciences a program of testing will help rule out error, applied prayerfully and with faith.

1. Compare the recommendations with those of the Scriptures.
2. Check statements against facts available from authoritative sources.
3. Read references given.
4. Be alert to common propaganda methods.
5. Check the professional standing of the author.
6. Contact the authority quoted to see if he/she is represented correctly.
7. Allow for exaggeration and bias in testimonials.

A. *Compare with the Scriptures.* Truth is defined in modern revelation as "knowledge of things as they are, as they were, and as they are to come."[6] It is not contradictory, whether it is found in the Scriptures or in the works of science. Theories may vary, but truth becomes increasingly clear as additional facts are discovered. Valid recommendations, then, should not conflict with revealed truth.

Dr. Atkin's Diet Revolution,[7] for example, contains questionable recommendations when compared with the Scriptures.[8]

(1) A diet heavy with meats is recommended for a lifetime. The Scriptures suggest that meats be used sparingly with thanksgiving, and that they not be used only (except) in times of winter, cold, famine, and excess of hunger.

(2) Cereals are forbidden during the early stages of the diet and are limited during the most liberal stages of it. God says that he made cereals (grains) to be the staff of life.

(3) Fruits and vegetables are restricted in the Atkins's diet and for a time forbidden. The Scriptures designate fruits and vegetables as ordained for the "constitution, nature, and use of man"—made to fill basic needs of the human body.

On the other hand, there are many who recommend a completely vegetarian diet. Many of them feel that spiritual enrichment requires it. But the Scriptures indicate clearly that "every creature of God is good, and nothing to be refused, if it be received with thanksgiving"[9] and that those who teach that man should not eat meat are "not ordained of God."[10]

It is apparent that both the high meat diet of Dr. Atkins and the no meat diet of many are at variance with the Lord's directives. If our study is characterized by faith in the pronouncements of the Scriptures, we can test many publications and ideas this way and avoid giving credence to an avalanche of misinformation.

B. *Check against known facts.* The "grape cure"[11] for cancer surfaces periodically. When it is checked with facts we find:

(1) The *cure* claims that grapes are 0.90 percent iron, and the third richest food in this important nutrient.[12] the USDA *Composition of Foods*, Handbook No. 8, shows grapes 0.0004 of one percent iron, and a poorer source than an equal weight of white flour (unenriched), nuts, or even brown sugar, to say nothing of meats, whole wheat, liver, eggs, green leafy vegetables, and other foods really rich in iron.

(2) The high potassium content of grapes is said to be a possible reason for the supposed efficacy of grapes in curing cancer.[13] Handbook No. 8 lists grapes as having 158 mg potassium in each 100 grams of fruit. This is comparable to many fruits but much less than is found in green peppers, a little over half that found in apricots, asparagus, lettuce, raw haddock, and whole wheat bread. Potatoes have 407 mg potassium in an equal weight of food if the skins are left on and nearly twice the potassium of grapes if they are peeled before cooking. If potassium really could cure cancer, many foods would supply it more generously than grapes.

Any publication, lecture, or current fad that gives information about food values may be similarly checked.

C. *Read references given.* Recently I was approached by a salesperson for a popular food supplement who enthusiastically informed me that the product was made by a special process which removed only the water and fiber from food and left nutrients not yet identified in the supplement.

When I read the literature, however, I found no such claim. In fact, the vitamin C tablets were "derived from the finest sources, including ascorbic acid, cradled in a base of Nature's powdered rosehips."[14] Translated, this means that crystalline ascorbic acid is added to rosehip powder. It is not all extracted from "natural" food. The calcium was from "natural mineral sources"[15]—not food sources at all. And the special protein supplement was "compounded from soya isolate and calcium caseinate (the principal protein of milk)."[16] Soya isolate is a highly refined soybean product obtained by chemical isolation of the protein. Calcium caseinate is the substance used in producing inexpensive milk substitutes. The literature makes no claim that it is obtained from milk.

Some spurious recommendations are accompanied by authoritative scientific literature which is cited as proof of the information when, in fact, it may not support the author or lecturer's point of view at all. This is a propaganda trick often used to distract the unwary. Those producing such spurious materials never expect patrons to actually read the literature cited. It *should* be read and checked to see if it supports the view being promoted.

I have at hand a reprint from the *American Journal of Orthodontics and Oral Surgery*[17] entitled "The Effect of Heat Processed Foods and Metabolized Vitamin D Milk on the Dentofacial Structures of Experimental Animals" by Francis M. Pottenger, Jr., M.D. The publication was distributed by a "health" organization[18] presumably to support the contention that pasteurized milk is not fit for human consumption. The foundation asserts that Dr. Pottenger found a long list of ills affecting cats to which he fed pasteurized milk, and that people should, therefore, use raw milk if they wished to be healthy.

Those who read the literature, however, discover that Dr. Pottenger found the same list of ills in his cats when he fed them raw milk or evaporated milk or any other kind that he tried under the conditions of this experiment. He finally concluded that to have healthy cats in this situation he should probably have fed them raw meat. In no way does the study condemn the pasteurization of milk.

When men and organizations misrepresent reputable authors and documents and try to substantiate their own untenable positions, they surely put their works outside those that are good sources of health information.

D. *Be alert to propaganda devices.* Detecting error will be easier. I have already noted one of these:

(1) Reference to or the distribution of authoritative literature that does not support the view of the propagandist but with the implication that it does.

(2) Changing an unfamiliar scientific term in authentic literature to a familiar term that suits the propagandist's purposes. For example, one would-be health authority correctly quotes a scientist who says that aluminum salts "crenate" body cells. To "crenate" means to wrinkle as salt of salty popcorn wrinkles the lips. After quoting the scientist correctly, he changed the word to "cre*m*ate" (to burn to ashes). This term was not only familiar to his followers but horrified them, making them unnecessarily afraid to have aluminum in contact with their food.

(3) Asking questions designed to make the reader or listener decide for the propagandist even though there are no facts to support the decision. For example, some salesmen boil soda water in both stainless steel and aluminum pots. Because of the reaction of the minerals of the water in alkaline solution in contact with aluminum, a murky liquid results. The question, "Doesn't that look like a deadly poison to you?" often brings the desired purchase of stainless steel.

Actually, the potion is not poison and can be safely—though not pleasantly—drunk. Soda water from the stainless steel pan will not taste good either.[19]

(4) Unjustifiably substituting one idea for another. A propagandist who was depreciating the use of milk in adult dietaries asked those who did not drink milk to raise their hands. When they were identified, with great disdain for those who advocated the use of milk, she called the attention of her audience to the fact that these people were ambulatory. If they were without calcium, she declared, they would be in a heap on the floor.

Actually she had not asked who got calcium or even who *used* milk as a source of calcium. The fact that these people did not *drink* milk in no way indicated that they did not *use* it on cereal, in their bread (even white bakery bread usually has from 2 to 6 percent of its dry ingredients milk solids), in casseroles, ice cream, cheeses, cream soups, puddings, cakes, pastries, pies, mashed potatoes, and in numerous other ways. There was no justification for using the presence of nonmilk-*drinking* adults to "prove" that milk is not needed by adults.

(5) Making unsubstantiated accusations against innocent persons or agencies. A "Dr." Betts declared that the U.S.A. Federal Trade Commission had suppressed a report written by one of its investigators which proved that aluminum caused cancer. He declared that he had the only existing copy of the report outside the federal files, and the evidence was there. He was so convincing that, wary as I was, even I believed him; but I did try to find the man who wrote the report. In the effort, I found the report in the local library. It had never been suppressed, and there was not one word about cancer in it![20]

A good course in propaganda analysis will indicate more techniques to which one should be alerted.

E. *Check professional standing.* Most professional groups have standards of proficiency that they try to maintain. By writing the ones of which the informant claims to be a part, the public health service or the federal security agency of the area from which he/she comes, you can learn of the person's qualifications.

Do not be impressed by titles. Many confer upon themselves professional sounding titles that have no meaning. Others do not remain worthy of titles once earned.

F. *Contact the author of statements not documented.* Shortly after an article I had written supporting the pasteurization of milk was published in the *Herald* a sister wrote that the National Nutrition League, Inc., had supplied her with evidence that pasteurization does not destroy the organism that causes brucellosis (undulant fever). Dr. H. E. Hesseltine, Senior Surgeon, U.S. Public Health Service, was the authority cited.

I could not find the statement in any of Dr. Hesseltine's writings, so wrote to him at the Public Health Service. Dr. Hesseltine, retired, responded from his Florida residence that he could find no such statement in his writings and that if it had been taken from anything that he had ever said, he had been misrepresented or misunderstood. He said that he was "a firm believer in pasteurized milk" and had "not seen any evidence anywhere that pasteurization is not effective in preventing the disease."[21]

A similar incident occurred when the manuscript of this book was read. One reader commented that I had made an error in stating that vitamin C was effective whether it came from a crystalline source or from a food source. The person gave Dr. Linus Pauling as the source of information. I wrote to Dr. Pauling to inquire about the statement. An immediate response from his office informed me that there had "obviously been a misrepresentation of the facts: 'Dr. Pauling has stated that pure crystalline ascorbic acid *is* natural L-ascorbic acid, the form that occurs in foods and the substance that is used by body tissues and required for good health.' "[22]

G. *Discount testimonials.* Celebrities often endorse products they never use. Testimonials that are genuine may come from three general sources:

- Circumstantial evidence. Jacob was certain his actions were marking the young cattle in the Genesis story referred to previously.
- Coincidence. Elisha scolded the children who taunted him, and the she bears came out of the woods and tore forty-two of them. There is no indication that Elisha's words had anything to do with the coming of the bears, in spite of all that Bible critics have had to say on the subject.[23]
- Psychosomatic response. Minds and emotions affect physical health in very real ways. Dr. Walter C. Alvarez, when he was on emeritus status at Mayo Clinic and Foundation, told the story of a city health commissioner who, knowing how susceptible people are to suggestion, announced that on a certain day fluorine would be added to the water. He then quietly rescinded the order. There was a flood of protests. People had hives, indigestion, and headaches caused by the fluorine. Some were ready to sue the city. What a letdown when they learned there had been no fluorine added to the water!

Tried by the outline given, many "health" publications do not qualify as "best" sources of information. In general, those that promote the use of expensive dietary supplements or food preparation gadgetry, bizarre diets and uncommon foods that are hard to get, or those who promise cure for nonnutritional diseases by nutrition practices alone are not worthy of patronage.

Sources of Comparatively Reliable Information

Even the best sources of nutrition information are not always perfect. Much remains to be learned. There is disagreement in many areas among those who study the best data available with superb skill. It is still necessary to judge that which is proposed by the standard outlined in the Scriptures and to respond intelligently. To waste time and resources on that which ignores or perverts the best studies available is at best poor stewardship and can be dangerous.

The most reliable basic information can be obtained free of charge or for a nominal fee from governments through public health or university extension programs. The World Health Organization offers excellent material. Reviews of available literature are made by professional groups such as the American Dietetics Association, and published lists of recommended and nonrecommended books are distributed free or for a nominal fee.

Today's Health, a magazine for lay people was published by the American Medical Association until it merged with *Family Health Magazine* in April 1976. *Family Health/Today's Health's* medical advisory board includes qualified persons in the field of nutrition and health, Jean Mayer among them. Products advertised in the magazine cannot always be recommended, however.

Nutrition Today published by the Nutrition Today Society, an association of professional persons involved in nutrition research, education, and professional practice, carries excellent material of current interest.

Some authors of currently reliable books in the field include the following:

• L. Jean Bogert (now deceased) whose standard text, authored jointly with George M. Briggs and Doris Howes Calloway, *Nutrition and Physical Fitness*, is in its ninth edition (1973).
• Eva D. Wilson, Katherine H. Fisher, and Mary E. Fuqua, authors of *Principles of Nutrition*, a standard nutrition text at university level.

- Harold S. Diehl, M.D., whose high school texts are excellent.
- L. Earle Arnow, M.D., author of *Food Power—A Doctor's Guide to Commonsense Nutrition.*
- Jean Mayer, Harvard nutritionist, author of many papers and books on nutrition, among them *Overweight Causes, Cost and Control.*
- Roger J. Williams, an enthusiastic proponent of good nutrition whose book, *Nutrition Against Disease*, is a source of many well-documented references to nutrition research.

And there are many others.

Misinformation That Persists

(1) *Misinformation:* Milk should not be used by adults. *Response:* Good quality protein, calcium, riboflavin, folacin, vitamin B_{12}, zinc, phosphorus, and many other nutrients found in milk are needed as long as life lasts. Milk is one of the best and most economical sources of many of these nutrients available in Western culture. It is one of the major components of the lifelong diet of some of the most long-lived people in the world, the Masai, who also have a very low incidence of heart trouble.[24] Adults with lactose intolerance problems may need to have it modified.

(2) *Misinformation:* Yogurt is superior to milk in nutritive values. *Response:* Yogurt is milk, and if used in the quantity needed will fill the need for some of the nutrients that milk offers. It is more expensive than milk when purchased ready-made and more trouble than milk when made at home, however, and is likely to be used sparingly. Because it is exposed to heat for a long time in the making, much of the vitamin B_{12} and folacin are destroyed.* For those with lactose intolerance problems or high cholesterol, yogurt may be preferable to milk.[25]

*Comparable folacin data are not available. Some comparisons follow:

Some nutritive values of one cup milk and one cup yogurt[26]

Food 245 grams	Calories	Protein g	Calcium mg	Iron mg	A IU	B_1 mg	B_2 mg	B_3 mg	B_{12} mg
Milk (Whole)	160	9	288	0.1	350	0.07	0.41	0.2	0.00098
Yogurt (Whole milk)	150	7	272	0.1	340	0.07	0.39	0.2	0.00027

(3) *Misinformation:* Raw milk is preferable to pasteurized milk. *Response:* Raw milk frequently carries bacteria that cause disease, including tuberculosis, brucellosis, typhoid, streptococcal infections, and diseases caused by coloform bacteria. Pasteurization destroys these organisms without adversely affecting the major nutrients of milk.[27]

That there is danger from raw milk is apparent from recent outbreaks of brucellosis (undulant fever) in both the eastern and western U.S.A. and Canada. News reports indicate that the Canadian government spent more than three million dollars during 1974 compensating owners for cattle that had to be destroyed because they were infected with the disease. According to news reports, Idaho, U.S.A., had 146 herds under quarantine for the disease in August 1975.

Incidentally, to refuse pasteurized milk and use dried milk or yogurt, each of which is subjected to more severe heat treatment than pasteurization, is inconsistent with the facts. My nurse friend was worried about her neighbor who insisted on purchasing raw milk until she learned that the first thing she did was boil it in preparation for making yogurt. This severe heat treatment is necessary to kill bacteria that would otherwise proliferate during the several hours the milk is kept warm so the bacterial culture (starter) used in making yogurt can do its work.[28]

Pasteurization does not attempt to kill all the bacteria present in the milk. Its target is those that might cause disease. In commercial pasteurization milk is heated to 161 degrees F. (71 Celsius) for less than half a minute, then chilled quickly. In home pasteurization the milk may be held at 145 degrees F. (63 Celsius) for 30 minutes before chilling. Boiling heats it to 212 degrees F. (100 Celsius) and may form a skum that contains a significant amount of calcium. Because all the bacteria are not killed in pasteurization but the number of lactic acid producing ones that cause souring is reduced, pasteurized milk that is not properly refrigerated or is kept too long may develop off flavors and odors before it sours.

(4) *Misinformation:* Nutmilk and vegetable juices should replace milk in the adult diet. *Response:* Nuts and vegetables make their own significant contribution to adult dietaries. It might be possible to combine nuts and vegetables to provide some nutrients

in amounts equivalent to milk, but plant proteins in general are not as high quality as milk proteins, and the plants have no vitamin B_{12} at all.

(5) *Misinformation:* Raw vegetable juices offer more nutrition than the vegetables from which they are made. *Response:* It may be possible to consume more vegetables by first juicing them, but in so doing it is easy to lose some of the vitamins, some of the fiber is frequently strained out, and the teeth and jaws are deprived of the exercise needed to chew the whole vegetable. Vitamins C and E quickly deteriorate in nonacid juices unless the juice is heated to stop enzyme activity.

(6) *Misinformation:* One should eat only raw foods since cooked foods are "dead." *Response:* Some vitamins are destroyed by cooking, but so also are vitamins destroyed by continued enzyme activity until foods are cooked or eaten. Good cooking procedures can inactivate the enzymes, retain most of the vitamins, actually release some nutrients that occur bound chemically so they are not available for digestion in uncooked foods, and inactivate some substances that would otherwise be toxic. Soybeans, for example, need to be cooked to be safe for eating, and cooking legumes and cereals releases some of the B vitamins from bound form. Raw egg white contains avidin that combines with biotin, making that B vitamin unavailable for body processes. Cooking inactivates the avidin. Some fruits and vegetables, however, are more nutritious when eaten raw.

(7) *Misinformation:* Foods on the regular market are no longer nutritious, so dietary supplements are needed. *Response:* One could choose foods that are depleted of nutrients, but that is not necessary. Wise choices at the market can result in excellent foods. If supplements are needed in time of stress or poor food supply, there is no need to pay exorbitant prices for those from "natural" sources. Vitamin C is vitamin C whether it comes from rose hips or is a crystalline substance,[29] and there is little likelihood of significant amounts of other members of its team being in a pill made to concentrate the vitamin C. To obtain 500 milligrams vitamin C in pure orange crystals requires over one fourth pound (112 grams) of the crystals,[30] and no one ordinarily swallows a pill of that size.

(8) *Misinformation:* Foods on the regular market have been

poisoned by chemical fertilizers and have been grown in "dead" soil. *Response:* See chapter on methods of food production for information.

(9) *Misinformation:* Weight reduction is best achieved on unusual diet regimens. *Response:* See chapter on weight control for evaluation of some diets.

(10) *Misinformation:* Honey, blackstrap molasses, and raw sugar are highly nutritious foods. *Response:* These sweets do provide many calories (as refined sugar does) and have some vitamins and minerals not contained in refined sugar. Honey and raw sugar have small quantities of iron, calcium, other minerals, and B vitamins but far from enough to support them in the diet. Raw sugar is the nutritional equivalent of a mixture of approximately three parts white sugar and one part brown sugar. In one fourth pound (112 g) of brown sugar the nutrients of a pound of raw sugar (except for the calories) are concentrated. The sucrose of sugar—raw, granulated, or brown—may be less acceptable than simpler sugars of honey, fruits, or corn syrup, according to tests that indicate sucrose has an adverse effect on cholesterol levels.

Sorghum and blackstrap molasses are more helpful in supplying minerals than sugar, corn syrup, or honey, although some of the blackstrap minerals come from long contact with machinery of sugar refinement of which it is the last extraction. Blackstrap does supply vitamins B_1, B_2, and B_3 to support its own calories. No other known commonly used sweet does.

To choose sweets that have some nutritional merit besides calories is good stewardship. To use any sweet to excess is not wise.

(11) *Misinformation:* Use of aluminum cooking utensils endangers health. *Response:* Aluminum is distributed abundantly in nature and occurs in almost all natural foods. Except for some individuals' allergic reaction to the metal, there is no evidence that it causes harm even in amounts much larger than those found in foods cooked in aluminum.[31]

Finally

Misinformation is abundant in the field of nutrition and health. Good stewardship of both health and finance requires that we seek knowledge only from the best sources available. Otherwise we may easily be led into unwise and uneconomical practices, spending money for that which is not "bread," as Isaiah warned.[32]

It is not wise to choose foods that are depleted of their nutrients. Neither is it wise to spend lavishly for that which is offered as superior but in fact gives little if any added benefit. Knowing the truth leaves us free to choose well according to the Lord's instruction to us.

---

1. Holy Scriptures, Hosea 4:6.
2. Doctrine and Covenants 85:36a.
3. Holy Scriptures, I Thessalonians 5:20-21.
4. Holy Scriptures, Genesis 29, 30, 31:1-13.
5. Charles E. Butterworth, Jr., M.D., "The Skeleton in the Hospital Closet," *Nutrition Today*, March/April, 1975, pp. 4-8. (See also comments on the Williamsburg Conference on Nutrition Education in Medical Schools, *Nutrition Today*, Sept./Oct., 1972, pp. 24-26; Roger J. Williams, Ph.D., "A Flaw in Medical Education," *Nutrition Today*, May/June, 1972, pp. 30-33; and Roger J. Williams, Ph.D., *Nutrition Against Disease*, Pitman Pub. Corp., N.Y., Toronto, London, Tel Aviv, 1971, pp. 3-19.)
6. Doctrine and Covenants 90:4.
7. Robert Coleman Atkins, *Dr. Atkins's Diet Revolution*, McKay, 1972.
8. Doctrine and Covenants 86:2.
9. Holy Scriptures I Timothy 4:1-5 and Doctrine and Covenants 49:3d-f.
10. *Ibid.*
11. Johanna Brandt, *The Grape Cure*, Seventeenth Edition, St. Marks Printing Corp., N.Y., 1950.
12. *Ibid.*, p. 158.
13. *Ibid.*, pp. 120-121.
14. *Shaklee Corporation 1976 Product Catalog*, p. 8.
15. *Ibid.*, p. 9.
16. *Ibid.*, p. 5.
17. *American Journal of Orthodontics and Oral Surgery* (St. Louis), Vol. 32, No. 8, Aug. 1946, pp. 467-485.
18. National Nutrition League, Inc., distributing Reprint No. 27, Lee Foundation for Nutritional Research, Milwaukee, Wisconsin.
19. Personal experience of the author described in *Standards of Health and Nutrition*, Mildred Nelson Smith, Herald House, 1957, p. 68.
20. *Federal Trade Commission (U.S.A.) - Royal Baking Powder Company*, Docket No. 540.
21. Private Communication from H. E. Hasseltine, Medical Director, U.S. Public Health Service (retired), dated March 22, 1952.
22. Private communication from the office of Dr. Linus Pauling, Linus Pauling Institute of Science and Medicine, 2700 Sand Hill Road, Menlo Park, California, dated March 1, 1976.
23. Holy Scriptures II Kings 2:23-24.
24. Robert E. Shank, M.D., "Status of Nutrition in Cardiovascular Disease," *Journal of the American Dietetics Association*, Vol. 62, June 1973, pp. 611-616.
25. Roger J. Williams, *Nutrition Against Disease*, Pitman Publishing Corporation, N.Y., Toronto, London, Tel Aviv, 1971, pp. 187-189.
26. Data calculated from USDA *Nutritive Value of Foods*, Home and Garden Bulletin No. 72, 1970, and USDA *Pantothenic Acid, Vitamin B_6 and Vitamin B_{12} in Foods*, Home Economics Research Report No. 36, 1969, by item.
27. John Andrews, and A. W. Fuchs, "Pasteurization and Its Relation to Health," *Journal of the American Medical Association*, Vol. 138, Sept. 11, 1948, pp. 128-131.
28. Janet Barkas, "It's Versatile! It's Nutritious! It's Yogurt!" *Family Health/Today's Health*, April 1976, pp. 48-51.
29. Linus Pauling, *Vitamin C and the Common Cold*, W. H. Freeman Co., San Francisco, 1970, p. 88.
30. USDA *Composition of Foods, op. cit.*, by item.
31. U.S. Dept. of Health, Education and Welfare, *Food and Drug Administration Fact Sheet*, "Nutrition Nonsense—and Sense," July 1971.
32. Holy Scriptures Isaiah 55:2.

CHAPTER 14

Some Problem Areas in Nutrition
Part II—Methods of Food Production

One of the areas of nutritional practice that is currently causing confusion is that concerned with food production and farming methods. It is widely claimed that our soil has lost its ability to produce nutritious food, that chemical fertilizers are poisoning our soil, and that organic fertilizers are safer than chemical ones and produce healthier crops.[1] Some go so far as to insist that foods not grown "organically" cause disease, and large numbers of people have been induced to pay premium prices for foods "organically" grown.[2]

That soil must be fertile to produce nutritious food is well established. It is the source of nutrients that has caused confusion.

Sources of Plant Nutrients

All farming or gardening that uses soil is organic.[3]* Soil, by definition, contains both mineral and organic matter.[4] There is no soil, except that intentionally sterilized, that is not teeming with microscopic life. Even sterile soil contains the remains of these and other decaying life forms,[5] chief among them the roots and residue of the crop just grown.[6] Many farmers practice good stewardship by returning other wastes to the soil as compost and manure and balance out their farming practice with needed minerals.[7] Other farmers find available animal manures and compost materials insufficient and/or uneconomical for their operation and use commercial fertilizers, termed "chemical," which are shunned by some.

---

*Hydroponic culture does not require soil but does require that the same nutrients which soil supplies be dissolved in the water.

Chemicals are necessary for life. Every food we eat, every plant that grows, every excretion of our bodies, every fertilizer that can be applied is chemical in nature. Water is hydrogen oxide (H_2O), salt is sodium chloride (NaCl), fats are acids combined with glycerol, proteins are complicated chemical structures containing amino acids, vitamins are acids, alcohols, and other chemically active substances. Without chemicals and chemical reactions there can be no life. Nutrients provided to plants or human bodies would be useless if it were not for the numerous chemical reactions by which they supply heat, energy, and building materials for tissue.

Plants are known to need seventeen elements for growth. Three of these—carbon, hydrogen, and oxygen—are provided by air and water. The other plant nutrients are absorbed in ionized form (as electrically charged particles) before they can be used in plants.[8] Composts and animal manures used as fertilizer must undergo decay and chemical reduction to release their plant nutrients from complicated organic structures before they can be useful. Chemical fertilizers have the nutrients more readily available. Plants will use nutrient ions equally well from either source.[9]

Decaying plant and animal matter in the soil provides nutrients, helps to structure the soil so that it incorporates air needed by plants and other forms of life, and helps to store moisture. Additional nutrients in chemical form do not poison the soil or the food that grows there if they are applied skillfully.[10] Misused they can damage a crop, as is the case with barnyard manure. There must be sound information concerning the needs of the soil and the crop to be grown and the skillful application of the most appropriate fertilizer available.

Some Problems of Soil Fertilization

Fertilization for maximum productivity and nutrition is no simple matter. The interrelationships of various plant nutrients are extremely complex. The type of soil on which the crop is to be grown, the amount of rainfall, the temperature, the topography (slope) of the land, and many other factors influence the manner in which proper fertilization must be handled.

Protein cannot be formed adequately nor many minerals absorbed by plants without calcium present. If there is a surplus of calcium, however, some of the phosphorus, manganese, iron, boron, and zinc needed by the plants may not dissolve and become available to them.[11] Nitrogen must be present for plants to grow, but an excess of nitrogen, whether from manure or chemical fertilizers, damages the crop.[12] Adequate supplies of boron are necessary for the production of a full crop of many plants and to prevent celery's having hollow stems, apples' having internal cork and drought spots, cauliflower's browning internally, sugar beets' developing heart rot, and alfalfa's being affected adversely. Yet boron was considered to be toxic to plants before it was known to be needed.[13] Sodium and chlorine are nutrients at least for some plants[14], but it is well known that many plants cease to live when salt (sodium chloride) is applied heavily.

Using compost and manure skillfully requires that variation in their composition be considered. Returning to the soil only local refuse may be inadequate.[15] Dramatic examples can be found in the coastal areas of the southern U.S.A., New Zealand, Australia, and other areas in which the soil is deficient in cobalt and in the vast goiter belts of the world. Animals that graze on cobalt-deficient forage without supplementation often become ill with "bush sickness," "salt sickness," "pining sickness," or "coast disease." An extremely small amount of cobalt applied to the soil supplies forage to prevent the disease.[16] Composts of already deficient plant growth or manure, however, cannot supply the cobalt needed.

Similarly, goiter belts exist where there is a deficiency of iodine in the soil and hence in the plants grown there. To supply needed iodine from organic sources would require the importation of supplies with the tremendous expenditure of money for transportation. If only a small garden is involved, the cost may be met, but to fertilize the vast goiter belts of the world this way would be prohibitive.*[17]

Observing plant and animal disease and animal preference for pasture long ago led to mapping areas of apparent problems.[18] Subsequent testing of soils has made possible more accurate

---

*In practice iodine is usually supplied directly to animals and humans as iodized salt instead of being applied as a fertilizer. Cobalt is needed by legumes for the fixation of nitrogen, however, and so must be applied as fertilizer for some crops.

mapping according to nutrient deficiencies of the soils.[19] Government agencies recommend fertilization and/or feeding practices for each area. For one desiring to grow a crop of maximum nutritive value, it is wise to utilize soil testing services and to consider their recommendations.

Safeguards in Food Production

The need of plants for the essential nutrients if they are to grow at all and for optimum amounts if they are to produce their best constitutes one of several conditions that help safeguard our food supply. Since plants just will not grow acceptable produce without needed nutrients, food producers see to it that their soil needs are met or they do not survive financially.

Take boron for an example. If there is moderate short supply, the crop yield is cut short. If the need is severe, symptoms noted previously appear. Since brown cauliflower and hollow, cracked celery stems are not salable, and short yields are not as profitable as maximum ones, the modern farmer producing these crops sees to it that his soil receives needed boron. We then get the boron we need from the fertilized crops.

Shortages of other nutrients also are apparent in the crop. The first symptom of phosphorus deficiency in vegetable crops is slow growth and delayed maturity.[20] A shortage of zinc shows up in defective apples, citrus fruits, and pecans.[21] Too little copper results in reduced crop yields.[22] Farming just is not profitable unless the soil is kept fertile.

The diversity of the human diet also serves as a protective feature. Our food comes from many areas of the world, generally speaking. If a local soil is deficient in a trace mineral, and the need is not immediately apparent in the quality of the food, food from another area rich in the nutrient may well help provide the essential mineral. Animals also provide a large portion of man's food generally, and foods derived from healthy animals are remarkably constant in their protein and mineral composition.[23]

Variations in Vitamin Content

Vitamin content of both plant and animal foods may vary greatly, but the variation does not necessarily reflect the fertility of the soil. The vitamin content of plant foods is influenced by the species of plant being grown, the variety, the climate, the stage of maturity at which the food is harvested, the treatment given after harvest in storage, preparation, and serving, and to a much smaller degree by certain minerals available to the plants.[24] Animal products may vary in vitamin content with diet. Cows eating fresh green forage produce milk much higher in vitamin A content than those eating sun-dried hay, but the difference does not necessarily reflect fertility of the soil.[25] Both the fresh and the dried may have been grown on the same soil. Boron deficiency does reduce the amount of vitamin A that can be produced in leaves, however, and adequate fertilization with nitrogen, phosphate, and potassium has increased A production.[26]

We have noted that oranges contain more vitamin C than apples, a variation due to species;[27] willow twig apples have more vitamin C than delicious apples, a variation due to variety;[28] fruits grown in the sun have more vitamin C than those grown in the shade,[29]* and those grown in warm climates have more vitamin C than those grown in cooler areas, a function of climate;[30] succulent green beans contain much more vitamin C and A than those allowed to mature, but the mature ones are richer in protein and B vitamins, variations due to maturity at harvest;[31] and nutrients may be lost or preserved by choice of storage, preparation, and serving procedures. There are so many variables in growing a crop and getting it to the consumer that it is difficult to predict the precise value of any one food. In general, soil fertility affects most the production of many vitamins by its effect on the amount of food that can be produced.

Advantages of Small Operations

Small producers with local markets may have an advantage in the areas of nutrition and flavor. They can choose varieties that are most flavorful and nutritious instead of having to choose those that will ripen to specification for mass harvest and for safe shipping to faraway markets. They may be able to pick the produce at the peak of perfection and immediately deliver it to the waiting customer. Proper use of commercial fertilizers, if needed, does not detract from this advantage.[32] If proper storage and delivery is not immediate, however, this advantage may be

---
*Green leaves grown in sunshine may have less vitamin C than those grown in shade.

lost. On the other hand, consumer interest and demand could result in larger producers finding ways to provide more flavorful and more nutritious produce.

Finally

The United States Department of Agriculture, Agriculture Research Service, declares that repeated research indicates that whether needed plant nutrients come from organic plant and animal sources only or from organic sources inherent in the soils supplemented by chemical fertilizers makes no significant difference in the nutrient content of the food grown.[33] Differences noted have been in favor of the inorganically fertilized plants as often as in favor of those grown with organic materials only.[34] It is the availability of the proper balance of soil nutrients that is significant in the production of food adequate in quality and quantity to feed the world's population.

---

1. U.S. Department of Health, Education and Welfare, Food and Drug Administration, *Fact Sheet*, "Nutrition Nonsense—and Sense," July 1971.
2. Thomas H. Jukes (Biochemist in the Division of Medical Physics, U. of California), "Organic Food 'Cult' Promotes Unscientific Eccentricities," *The National Observer*, Feb. 24, 1973, feature, "Sounding Board of Current Opinion."
3. Roger J. Williams, *Nutrition Against Disease*, Pitman Pub. Co., N.Y., London, Toronto, Tel Aviv, 1971, p. 193.
4. Louis M. Thompson, and Frederick R. Troeh (Iowa State University), *Soils and Soil Fertility*, Third Edition, 1973, McGraw-Hill Book Co., N.Y. and 14 other locations, pp. 1-2.
5. Williams, *op. cit.*, p. 194. Also Thompson and Troeh, *op. cit.*, pp. 110-116.
6. Samuel L. Tisdale, and Werner L. Nelson, *Soil Fertility and Fertilizers*, Macmillan Co., N.Y., 1965, p. 362.
7. Thompson and Troeh, *op. cit.*, pp. 235-240.
8. *Ibid.*, pp. 13-14.
9. *Ibid.*, p. 215.
10. U.S. Dept. of Health, Education and Welfare, *op. cit.*
11. Thompson and Troeh, *op. cit.*, p. 314.
12. *Ibid.*, pp. 242-245.
13. *Ibid.*, p. 326.
14. *Ibid.*, p. 166.
15. Williams, *op. cit.*, pp. 193-194.
16. USDA, *Factors Affecting the Nutritive Values of Foods*, Misc. Publication No. 664, pp. 5-7. Also Tisdale and Nelson, Third Edition, 1975, pp. 318-319, and 97.
17. Thompson and Troeh, *op. cit.*, pp. 166 and 325. Also Tisdale and Nelson, *Ibid.*, p. 97.
18. USDA, *op. cit.*, pp. 4-6. Also Kenneth C. Beeson, "The Relation of Soil to Nutrition and Health," *Fertilizer Review*, March/April, 1948.
19. Thompson and Troeh, *op. cit.*, pp. 327, 333, 339.
20. Firman E. Bear, and others, A Symposium, *Hunger Signs in Crops*, American Society of Agronomy and the National Fertilizer Association, 1951, p. 176.
21. *Ibid.*, pp. 229-230, 343-349, and Tisdale and Nelson, *op. cit.*, 1965, p. 49.
22. Tisdale and Nelson, *op. cit.*, 1975, p. 93.
23. William H. Adolph, Ph.D., "Agricultural Science and Improved Human Nutrition," *Borden's Review of Nutrition Research*, Vol. 18, No. 2, March/April, 1957, pp. 22-23, 25.

24. USDA, *op. cit.*, pp. 8-11.
25. Adolph, *op. cit.*, pp. 22-23.
26. Williams, *op. cit.*, p. 195.
27. USDA, *Composition of Foods*, Agriculture Handbook No. 8, 1963, by item.
28. Laboratory experience of author at Iowa State University, 1944-1946.
29. USDA, *Factors Affecting the Nutritive Values of Foods, op. cit.* pp. 8-11.
30. Adolph, *op. cit.*, p. 16.
31. USDA *Composition of Foods, op. cit.*, by item.
32. Thompson and Troeh, *op. cit.*, p. 215.
33. Ruth M. Leverton, Ph.D., R.D. (Science Adviser, Agricultural Research Service, USDA, Washington D.C., Statement filed at the Open Hearing on Organic Food held by the Attorney General for the State of New York, Dec. 1, 1972, reported in the *Journal of the American Dietetics Association*, Vol. 62. May 1973, p. 501.
34. USDA, Agricultural Information Bulletin, No. 299, as quoted in James Trager, "Exploding the Health Food Myth," *Family Circle*, July 1971, pp. 58, 84, 106.

CHAPTER 15

Problem Areas in Modern Nutrition Practice
Part III—Additives

Some of the foods offered in the modern marketplace contain substances called additives.* There are the intentional ones placed in food to perform some service as a nutrient supplement, sweetener, preservative, emulsifier, stabilizer or thickener, adjuster of alkalinity and acidity, leavening agent, flavor, color, bleaching or aging agent for flour, dough conditioner, yeast food, sequestrant (combines with metals that would cause instability and off flavors), propellant (to expel contents of cans, fluff them and prevent spoilage by excluding oxygen), and antioxidant (to prevent rancidity and avoid loss of color and nutritive value). And there are unintentional additives in food because of some environmental factor. These include such substances as those that may migrate from packaging, residues of fumigants, insecticides, or medications administered to food producing animals, radioactive fallout, and metals from machinery used in processing.

The intentional additives are further divided into those "generally recognized as safe" (GRAS) either because they are from natural sources or because they have been used for a long time without causing known harm, and those "regulated" additives whose use is restricted to a purpose and/or an amount that testing has indicated should fulfill a need without harming consumers.[1] Among the additives in the U.S.A. are some called "prior sanctioned" ones not listed with the GRAS or regulated additives. They are substances for the use of which companies have asked

---
*Legal definitions of additives differ in various countries. In this book, a general definition of any substance added to food as a result of production, processing, packaging, or storing will be used.

267

and received special permission prior to 1958. Prior sanctions are no longer granted.[2]

Additives may pass from one classification to another. In the U.S.A., even those additives on the GRAS list have been under intensive review since 1969, and some formerly listed have been removed.[3]

Additives and Convenience Foods

We live in an era of convenience foods, many of them so familiar to us that we do not recognize them as such. We expect to find shortening in a package at the grocers instead of having to render lard from pork fat or press oil from seeds as our forefathers did. When we want milk, we expect it to be processed and packaged for us. We even expect to be able to choose whether to serve milk whole, skimmed, 2 percent, evaporated, buttermilk, or yogurt. We expect to find cheese in the market in a variety of forms and flavors without having to sour the milk, cut the curd, cook, flavor, press, and cure it. We expect to be able to serve every fruit and vegetable we desire without planting a seed or hoeing a weed. In fact, we expect to have many of them fresh from the garden when it is so cold that even carrying them home requires special care to keep them from freezing.

Many of us opt for additional convenience. We expect our bread ready to bake or already baked, pies ready for the oven, dinners ready to heat and serve, soup that can be made in a cup, cream already whipped, and breakfast in a can.

If we are to have convenience foods, especially of the latter kind, we must accept the presence of intentional additives. Fat must not separate from gravy in a frozen dinner. Ingredients, already cooked, to make soup in a cup must not become rancid, bacterially contaminated, or stale. Cereals to be eaten from a box or to be prepared simply by adding hot water (each of which is precooked) must be kept fresh. Drinks do not fizz without carbon dioxide added, and it is impossible to get whipped cream through a tiny nozzle without a propellant. Prunes must be kept moist without spoilage if they are not to require soaking before use. Spun or extruded protein must have vitamins, minerals, color, and flavor added if it is to resemble the meat it simulates.

Food Additives with a Long History
Salt

Food additives are neither new nor necessarily bad. Our great-great grandparents salted down their meat, eggs, and fish to extend the time of their usefulness. They added salt to cabbage to make sauerkraut; salt and spices to other fruits and vegetables to make pickles and kimchi (oriental pickled food). Even Christ recognized both the flavor potential and the preservative properties of this chemical (NaCl) additive when he challenged his people to be the salt of their society.[4]

Lactic and Acetic Acid

Acids produced by the fermentation of some vegetables, fruits, and milk early gave flavor and added keeping qualities to some foods. Eventually ways were discovered to obtain the acids and add them to the foods without waiting for the foods themselves to ferment. Instead of each family carefully tending a vinegar barrel filled with fruit juice and seeded with "mother" (bacterial culture) as we did in my youth, vinegar is made in less expensive, and more certain ways, but the essential ingredient is still the same—acetic acid—and the acid from cultured milk is lactic acid. Both are used in adjusting the acidity of modern foods.

Sucrose

Sugar was a major preservative of early days. Without it few fruits could have been kept much beyond the harvest, and even meats were "sugar cured" for especial goodness. This chemical additive (sucrose) is now used in such large amounts that it replaces more nutritious foods and so is doing a disservice to societies that have adopted it as a major food instead of just an additive.

Nitrates and Nitrites

The use of saltpeter (nitrate) along with salt and sugar to cure meats was hailed as a beneficent discovery in my young years. No longer did the meats have to have the salt soaked out of them, along with much of the flavor and nutrients (although we were not then aware of the lost nutrients) before they could be served. They remained nice and juicy and the sugar allowed just enough fermentation to turn some of the nitrates to nitrites, which in turn caused the meat to be an appetizing pink color instead of a dull brown.

When rural children became ill because of high nitrate content of water from improperly placed or poorly protected wells, concern arose for the amounts of nitrates being put into meat. There was little that could be done about home use of the substance except to issue warnings, but commercial establishments could be regulated.

Laws passed to protect consumers continued to allow nitrates and nitrites to be used in processing some meats but restricted their use. The allowance was not just to keep colors bright and meats juicy but to prevent bacterial action, especially that of organisms that produce deadly botulin toxin.

In the U.S.A. limits of 2,000 parts per million (PPM) of nitrates in finished foods were set, well within or below the range of amounts that occur naturally in spinach, broccoli, beets, radishes, cabbage, lettuce, and many other foods in which the natural nitrate content ranges up to 5,000 parts per million (PPM).[5] These limits were later reduced to 500 PPM,[6] and in October, 1975, the Food and Drug Administration announced its intention to propose regulations to end the use of most nitrates and reduce the use of nitrites in curing meats.[7] In 1975 Canada's Food and Drug Directorate introduced an interim limit of 200 PPM of nitrates calculated before the meats are processed.[8]

Nitrites are generally limited to 200 parts per million in both the U.S.A. and Canada except that the 1975 interim limit in Canada was 150 PPM for bacon,[9] and the U.S.A. has indicated an intention to lower their limits to 156 PPM for all meat and poultry products except bacon and dry cured products.[10] As with nitrates, U.S.A. limits are based on finished product and Canadian ones on batch before processing.

The greatest potential health hazard is with nitrites that may be formed from nitrates by bacterial action in foods[11] or may themselves be introduced as a preservative. Nitrites have a number of physiological effects that include the capacity for temporarily reducing the oxygen carrying potential of the blood, relaxing some muscles that may lower blood pressure, and combining with secondary and tertiary amines to form nitrosamines that are carcinogenic (cause cancer).[12]

The production of nitrosamines is of particular concern. Occasionally small amounts of these substances occur in preserved meats. One U.S.A. Department of Agriculture study reported one of 60 hams tested contained minute quantities of nitrosamines as did 3 of 50 cooked sausages and 3 of 48 processed meats.[13] Frederick J. Stare, M.D., recognized widely for his nutrition research, declares that the amounts noted in these studies were much lower than would be required to cause cancer in a laboratory animal.[14]

More frequently nitrosamines develop when bacon is cooked or when nitrites are eaten with substances containing the kinds of amines that react to form cancer-producing substances. These are present in beer, wines, cigarette smoke from which they may be dissolved in the saliva and swallowed, decongestant medicines, and a number of other drugs.[15] The amounts found in cooked bacon have been steadily falling in recent tests and were in late 1975 found at levels around 10 to 20 parts per billion (PPB).[16]

The consumption of chlorogenic acid with foods containing nitrites favors the production of nitrosamines as we have seen. Chlorogenic acid occurs naturally in many foods but is present in coffee in exceptionally large amounts.[17]

Good vitamin C nutrition helps prevent the production of the nitrosamines when nitrites are consumed. Massive doses of the vitamin are not required.[18]

Research is continuing to determine what further safeguards should be taken in the use of nitrates and nitrites or if their use as additives should be banned altogether.

Yeast

Our preference for light bread first prompted the use of wild yeasts, then starters (portions of dough saved from one mixing to leaven the next). Christ referred to the practice when he likened the kingdom of God to leaven.[19] Even in my youth friends shared starters of especially desirable flavor, and to lose a prized starter was a serious misfortune. Now commercial yeasts leaven quickly and reliably, still offering valuable nutrients to the finished product. Sometimes minute quantities of nutrients that cause yeast to grow rapidly are added to flour or yeast preparations to increase the speed with which they leaven. These are yeast foods, and because they increase the amount of yeast present, they may add to the nutritive value of the product being leavened.

Baking Powders

For cakes, quick breads, and cookies our progenitors had to combine acids and bases so they would react chemically to produce carbon dioxide gas which was trapped in the dough and expanded as the dough heated to make it rise. Soda (bicarbonate of soda or sodium hydrogen carbonate) was long used with sour milk, molasses, fruit, or honey. If the cook guessed correctly, everything went well. If not, there would be either a flat cake or a bitter flavor from extra soda not completely used up in the reaction, and incidentally a loss of vitamin B_1, although that was not then known.[20]

Someone found that the tartaric acid crystals found in grape juice could combine with the soda when no other acid was in the recipe. Cream of tartar (potassium bitartrate) became commercially available and eventually was premixed with soda to form the first baking powders. With them, as with the soda-acid food combinations, all the leavening power was released as soon as the combination was moistened, and the product had to be rushed to the oven and handled with care.

Modern baking powders include ingredients that do not allow the acid and base to combine completely until they are heated together. We can be leisurely about getting the product to the oven, and batters and doughs can be left in the refrigerator or freezer for extended periods of time and still produce light, tasty products. The residues are harmless, and because the components are carefully balanced, the destruction of B vitamins during baking may be lessened.

Rope Preventives

Rope often plagued homemade bread, especially in the summer. A beautiful loaf would be attacked by bacteria, and by the second or third day after baking the interior would be sticky, gummy and foul-smelling. To make certain it did not happen to the next baking of bread, acid was added to the dough—vinegar, sour milk, whey, or cream of tartar.[21] Today precisely measured amounts of substances are used to make certain that rope does not develop. Most often used are lactic acid, the acid of sour milk or whey, and sodium diacetate, an edible salt of the acid of vinegar.

Propionates

Yeast breads are excellent food for molds, the spores of which are constantly in the air. Minute amounts of sodium propionate or calcium propionate keep the molds from thriving on the bread and so prevent waste. The substances are simply the edible salts of propionic acid. They develop naturally in Swiss cheese and help give it its characteristic flavor. The 0.03 of an ounce (0.84 g) allowed in each pound (454 g) of bread is not enough to impart flavor but is enough to effectively curb the molds.[22]

Benzoic Acid

Benzoic acid, frequently used as a preservative in catsup and other foods, occurs naturally in cranberries and some other fruits in much larger proportions than are allowed by law when the acid or its salt (benzoate of soda) is used in foods in which it does not naturally occur. It, too, is metabolized as a food.

Emulsifiers (Lecithin, Mono and Diglycerides)

When I first learned to make mayonnaise, I started with raw egg yolk, beat it furiously as I added oil, vinegar, and spices, hoping that a stable emulsion would result that would be usable as a salad dressing. If the emulsion broke, allowing the oil to separate, I started with another yolk and hoped again. Always the resultant dressing had to be refrigerated promptly and used soon.[23] Raw egg yolk is an excellent medium for the growth of salmonella (organisms that cause food poisoning) and thousands of persons have suffered from salads made with them that were not properly handled.

The emulsifier that provided stability to my mayonnaise, when I was successful, was lecithin. Today lecithin obtained from food sources such as eggs, soybeans, and corn is used to give stability to many foods,[24] including mayonnaise that can be stored for long periods of time and dress salads or make sandwich spreads that can be served much more safely than the raw egg yolk allowed. Lecithin is also used in salad dressings, cakes, ice cream, and numerous other foods. It is a substance needed by the body if it is to handle cholesterol and other fats satisfactorily, and is, in fact, a substance synthesized by the body when there is not enough provided by the diet to care for metabolic needs.[25]

Other emulsifiers may be used that are not metabolic essentials as lecithin is, and lecithin is not equivalent to whole eggs in nutritive value. Standards have been set, therefore, to prescribe the minimum amount of eggs, oil, and other ingredients in mayonnaise and in some other foods.

Often associated with lecithin and sometimes used alone are the mono and diglycerides. Most of our food fats occur naturally as glycerides. The fatty acids are esterified (combined in such a way as to eliminate one molecule of water at each bonding) with glycerol (one of the food alcohols). If one fatty acid molecule is combined with one glycerol molecule, monoglyceride is formed. If there are two fatty acids involved, a diglyceride is formed. If there are three fatty acid molecules, a triglyceride results. Most of our food fats are triglycerides, but about one percent of them occur as mono and diglycerides. These are good emulsifying agents and are used to make it possible to form margarine that spreads out of oil that only pours, peanut butter from which the oil will not separate, cake batters that stay light and fine textured, and other desirable products. When digested they are converted to triglycerides.

Flavor Solvents

Characteristic flavors must be added to many foods if those flavors are desired. There is no vanilla ice cream without vanilla. Vanilla grows as a bean, and to have the flavor conveniently ready to use when needed, it must be extracted from the bean and kept in solution in a liquid that will not interfere with recipes. Ethyl alcohol is a suitable solvent which carries the flavor into the product, then rapidly evaporates, especially if the product is heated. Other flavors are likewise prepared in some solvent that may be alcohol, water, or oil. Wines, sometimes used for flavor or to tenderize meats, also lose their alcoholic content during cooking procedures. The boiling point of alcohol is much below the cooking temperatures of most meats.

Drying Agents

Salt that absorbs moisture loses flavor and clogs salt shakers. Rice is sometimes used to help keep it dry. More efficient, however, are specially dried finely ground cornstarch and/or anticaking agents like calcium stearate or a magnesium compound.[26] These substances are used in salt, garlic powder, and other finely granulated foods to keep them free flowing. Calcium stearate is a calcium salt of one of the solid fats found in cream, cottonseed oil, cod liver oil, and pork fat and is a normal constituent of human fat. Magnesium is an essential nutrient for healthful living and one that may be in short supply in the diets of those who eat only small amounts of green vegetables and whole grains. These additives may make pickles cloudy, but they are not harmful to health.

Antioxidants

It used to be routine, after lard had been stored a few months, to open the bucket, skim off the rancid top, and put it into a container to be made into lye soap. Today there are antioxidants to prevent wastage from rancidity. These also prevent discoloration of highly oxidizable foods such as peaches or apples that are frozen or dried. Among the antioxidants is ascorbic acid (vitamin C) and its chemical relatives, also with some vitamin C activity, sorbic acid, isoascorbic acid (also known as erythorbic acid) and sodium erythrobate.[27] Another is citric acid, which characterizes all citrus fruits such as oranges, grapefruit, and lemons and is a critical link in metabolism. Also used are tocopherols, nature's powerful antioxidant popularly known as vitamin E.

Antioxidants that sometimes frighten us because of their big names are butylated hydroxyanisole (BHA), butylated hydroxytoluene (BHT) and propyl gallate. These, too, are closely related to naturally occurring food substances and are thought to be harmlessly metabolized in the body. When Dr. Denham Harman of the University of Nebraska fed BHT to mice with radiation sickness, the mice to which the antioxidant was fed lived 50 percent longer than other mice fed similarly except without the BHT.[28] The U.S.A. Food and Drug Administration reports that if BHT and BHA were used at maximum allowable levels in all foods in which they are allowed in the U.S.A., the daily intake would not exceed four parts per million in U.S.A. food, totaling about 0.128 of one ounce (3.6 gm) in every ton (909 kg) of food consumed.[29] The agency also reports that rats fed 1,000 parts per million of the substances, instead of the four parts per million allowed in food, showed no adverse effects in two generations.[30] The World Health Organization has accepted 93 parts per million as a safe level of daily intake.

Anti-smoking Agents

In the days when we used home-rendered lard for frying chicken, donuts, and other foods, we had trouble with the fat smoking. If we got it hot enough to obtain a crisp crust that sealed the food against the asorption of unwanted grease, there was frequently an acrid odor—especially if we were using the fat for a second time. People constantly complained that fried foods hurt their stomachs, and they were justified in their complaints. Acrolein, source of the acrid smell, formed by burning fat, is an extremely irritating chemical.[31] Now additives prevent the fat from smoking at normal frying temperatures, allowing it to be used repeatedly without causing stomachaches.

Pectin

When we picked our fruit for homemade jellies and jams, we had to be certain to get some that was not quite ripe. There had to be enough pectin left in the fruit to jell. In fact, some just would not jell unless they were combined with apples or another fruit high in pectin.[32] Now pectin is extracted from fruit peels, unmarketable fruit, and other sources, packaged and sold as jelling aids. The same pectin thickens a number of nonfruit foods. Incidentally, it also helps the body handle its cholesterol well.[33] Since it enables almost anything to jell, governments have set standards to assure consumers that they are not deceived in the product they purchase. Real jams and jellies, for example, must contain at least 45 percent real fruit, approximately the proportion found in homemade jams and jellies. If there is less fruit, the product must be labeled "imitation" or carry another name.

Thickeners and Stabilizers

Other thickeners and stabilizers used to keep chocolate milk from separating, ice cream from losing its smooth texture at the first sign of melting, sauces and salad dressings from breaking include such strange sounding substances as agar agar, guar, carragheen, gum tragacanth, and carob bean gum. Each of these, too, comes from nature. Agar agar and carragheen, (also spelled carrageen and carrageenan) are from seaweed. Agar agar has long been used in Oriental cookery and in biology laboratories where it serves as a culture medium. Carob bean gum comes from Saint-John's-bread, fruit of an evergreen tree which tastes a little like chocolate and is sometimes substituted for it by those who prefer to avoid the stimulants contained in chocolate. Gum tragacanth and guar gum are natural relatives of fruit pectin. Each of these additives is digested, metabolized, and contributes nutritionally to our food supply.

Even their use is monitored and in some cases controlled, however. During the past few years during which the GRAS (generally recognized as safe) list of food additives has been reviewed in the U.S.A., both carragheen and carob bean gum have been removed from the list of uncontrolled additives to the list of controlled ones.[34] Some methods of processing the bright pink seaweed from which the carragheen comes were found to produce adverse effects on test animals, so now the FDA designates the source of the substance that may be included in food. Carob bean gum, when fed in massive doses to test animals, proved toxic. The FDA now regulates the amount that may be used.

Meat Tenderizer (Papain)

For many years we have been paying premium prices for "finished" (well-fattened) beef. Lean beef was not tender. Now less fat beef may be tenderized, before or after slaughtering, thus reducing the amount of primary foods needed for fattening and the amount of energy needed to cook it. The tenderizer used is papain, an enzyme that grows in papaya (a highly nutritious fruit grown in tropical and semitropical areas).[35] It is the ability of a similar enzyme, bromelin, of pineapple to affect proteins that makes it impossible to jell a gelatin salad in which raw pineapple has been used.[36] Cooking the meat, as with the pineapple, inactivates the enzyme. Even if this did not occur, digestive juices would stop the enzyme action as they do for the fruit from which it is extracted when the fruit is eaten raw.

Monosodium Glutamate (MSG)

It is difficult to conceive of a main dish recipe of oriental origin used in the Hawaiian Islands that does not call for ajinomoto. In the Islands and in cultures in which animal proteins are scarce, food is made more palatable by having the flavors enhanced. The vegetable protein derivative, monosodium glutamate, has this capacity, and has long been a component of Oriental cookery. It came into use in the U.S.A. as "accent" or MSG. It is the salt of glutamic acid, an amino acid that forms almost half the wheat protein, gliadin, is generously distributed in soybeans, and is found in quantity in many other vegetable proteins. It was one of the first nutrients identified as essential to normal brain functioning.

MSG was removed from acceptable use in baby foods in the U.S.A. when it was found to serve no valuable purpose and there was some question about its safety.[37] Test animals given large doses of the substance by injection and force feeding developed a number of injuries including brain damage. Subsequent tests indicate that the damage inflicted in earlier tests may have come from excess sodium rather than from the MSG itself. Even very large amounts of the flavor enhancer fed as a supplement to a normal diet have shown no ill effects.[38] Some people do get upset stomachs if they eat large amounts of the additive when they are not accustomed to it, and people on low salt diets should not add it to their food. In the U.S.A. and Canada, if it is used in a food sold commercially it must be listed on the label except on such standardized foods as mayonnaise and other salad dressings.

Flavors, Natural and Artificial

Many food flavors are extracts of nature's bounty. Vanilla comes from vanilla beans, almond from almonds. Many that are produced synthetically are chemically identical with the flavoring agents the plants produce. Ethyl butyrate is an actual constituent of pineapple largely responsible for its characteristic flavor.

Carvone is the principal flavoring agent of caraway seeds. Isoamyl isovalerate occurs naturally in apples. Octyl acetate helps flavor oranges. Methyl salicylate is the natural flavoring principle of oil of wintergreen.[39]

Some of the natural flavors are more complicated chemically than the artificial ones. Natural grape flavor has 19 chemical constituents according to food technologists and the synthetic flavor only 5.*

Even naturally occurring flavors may cause some problems, however. Coumarin, the sweet-smelling essence of new-mown hay and tonka beans, was once used extensively in flavorings, especially artificial vanilla. It has now been removed from the approved list because large quantities have proved toxic. Saffrole, an extract of sassafras root once used to flavor root beer, has been banned from use since 1960 because large doses of it were found to cause cancer in test animals. And those flavors (and colors) that have a salicylate or related content elicit the same allergic response that aspirin does from those who are allergic to salicylic acid. These allergic manifestations may include a runny nose, coughing, swelling of the larynx (voice organ), asthma; itching or hives; gastrointestinal problems including an enlarged tongue, excessive gas, belching digestive juices into the esophagus, "heartburn," mouth ulcers and constipation; swollen, painful joints; headache and behavioral disturbances, according to allergist Dr. Ben F. Feingold.[40]

Dr. Feingold believes that the behavioral response which some children make to salicylate-containing colors and flavors, both natural and artificial, is of especial importance to many families. He finds that boys are especially likely to respond with hyperkinesis (overactivity) and learning difficulties. And he finds that some artificial colors and flavors that do not contain salicylate may evoke the same response. Tartrazine, FD&C Yellow No. 5 in the U.S.A., is one of these.

To eliminate foods containing salicylates and tartrazine would require that many natural foods be eliminated along with artificial flavors and colors. Dr. Feingold lists almonds, apples, apricots, blackberries, cherries, currants, gooseberries, grapes and raisins,

---

*E. Stein, "To Add or Not to Add," *What's New in Home Economics*, Vol. 35, Oct. 1971, p. 29, contains a list of the chemicals.

nectarines, oranges, peaches, plums and prunes, raspberries, cucumbers and pickles and tomatoes among the salicylate containing foods. And he recommends cessation of use of these foods along with commercial ice cream, margarine, cake mixes, bakery foods except plain bread, gelatin desserts, candies, gum, cloves, oil of wintergreen, mint flavors, toothpaste and tooth powders, lozenges, mouthwash, jam, jelly, luncheon meats and sausages, tea, beer, alcoholic beverages except vodka, all soft drinks including diet drinks, dietary supplements that are flavored or colored or made from the foods just listed, cider vinegar, wine and wine vinegars, Kool-Aid and similar beverages, and all medications that contain aspirin. Even some perfumes may evoke the allergic response, he feels.

Studies designed to test Dr. Feingold's thesis concerning diet and hyperactivity have neither confirmed nor disproved it.[41] A committee created by the U.S.A. Food and Drug Administration to serve as a clearinghouse for government activity on hyperkinesis (hyperactivity) research has recommended further research particularly to determine the extent of the relationship, if any, between hyperactivity in children and food and color additives in food. FDA feels that the evidence merits further investigation.[42]

Food Colorings

Food colorings are used because we, the consumers, respond positively to them. We like our cherries red, our fruit-flavored drinks and desserts the color of the fruit imitated; our candies, vitamin pills, and cake frostings colorful. The "average" American gets approximately 5.5 grams (0.2 oz.) of color-added material yearly in the nearly 1,420 pounds (645.5 kg) of food eaten.[43]

Some unsafe food colorings have been used in the past. Since 1960 all colors used in foods and drugs have been under intense scrutiny. In the U.S.A., even those colors formerly considered safe (GRAS) are being reevaluated. Those that cause cancer in test animals at any level of feeding are automatically ruled out. Others that were used before the 1960 law placed the responsibility for proving their safety on the manufacturer and were "provisionally listed" awaiting the presentation of such proof have also been banned as evidence bringing their safety into question has been obtained. These bans have sometimes been delayed by legal action to set aside FDA rulings on the products.[44] Red 2 is a well publicized example of a color banned under this procedure.[45]

Synthetic colors still in use in the U.S.A. must be certified by the Food and Drug Administration even though some are chemically identical with those found in nature. Legal limits are set for their use, and the use of color to deceive a consumer by covering a blemish, concealing inferiority, or making the consumer think that a product is more nutritious than it really is is forbidden.[46]

Regulations pertaining to colors apply not only to those incorporated in food. They also apply to the ones that may be used outside food but that might be absorbed by or migrate to the food. This includes wax that may be used to prevent loss of moisture or nutritive value and to packaging materials.[47]

In general, natural food colors used as additives—beet juice to make pink lemonade, for example—are not certified by the Food and Drug Administration of the U.S.A. as the synthetic colors must be; but they are subject to the other restrictions noted concerning amounts used and appropriateness of use.[48]

Carotenoids form the largest amount of the natural colors used as food additives. They are red and yellow pigments found in carrots, grass, oranges, tomatoes, and other yellow and green foods and in some animals and are chemically related to the carotene from which the body prepares vitamin A. They are the substances that naturally color egg yolks and cream. One of the carotenoids long used to color winter butter, cheese, and other dairy products, margarine, casings for frankfurters and bologna, beverages, baked goods, cake mixes, and breakfast cereals is taken from the seed covering of the annato tree, a native of the American tropics. Chlorophyll, the green substance of plants responsible for photosynthesis, is closely associated with the carotenoids and is also used as a food coloring.[49]

Caramel coloring made by heating sugars and starches colors many foods, especially baked goods, puddings, desserts, beverages, and candies. Beet juice, beet powder, grape skin extract, paprika (red sweet pepper), saffron (the orange-red stigmata of the saffron flower used liberally by our grandmothers to enrich the appearance of their baked goods, but now limited in commercial use to those foods in which there will be no danger that the customer will be misled to believe that the product contains more egg than it does and so appears more nutritious than it really is), and tumeric (the yellow powder made from the aromatic underground stem of an East Indian ginger plant) all are used to color food.[50] Even riboflavin (vitamin B_2), charcoal, and iron oxide are sometimes used as natural food colors.[51]

Like the flavors, these colors must be contained in solution in dilutants. Some colors are soluble in water, some in oils, glycerides, or alcohols. Even the dilutant used is carefully regulated by the FDA[52] and other food protection agencies.

Some Measures to Assure Safety of Additives

In the U.S.A. and Canada, before any new intentional additive is included in food, laws require the manufacturer to provide the appropriate governmental agencies responsible for food safety the data from tests with laboratory animals to indicate the safety and appropriateness of the additive and also provide a method of testing for the substance that may be used in monitoring its use. The test must show not only that the substance is not immediately toxic to the animals tested but that it is safe for a lifetime of use. In general, it is required that the product produce no adverse effects at feeding levels 100 times the level at which it is proposed that it be included in foods.[53] As with color, the regulations apply even to those additives or materials used for packaging that might be absorbed by the food unintentionally.

More rigorous testing is proposed by the FDA, particularly with reference to the effect additives may have over a long period of exposure—longer than laboratory animals live—and the effect they may have on fetal development (mutagenic and teratogenic data). Such testing is already in progress on many substances and should be extended to cover all that are approved for use, the FDA believes.[54]

In the U.S.A., if cancer develops at any level of feeding, the product is automatically banned by the Delaney Clause of the Food and Drug Administration's law. It was under this law that cyclamates were banned even though the amount of the sweetener required to cause bladder tumors in rats was equivalent to many times the amount most humans were likely to consume.

Sugar Substitutes

Although cyclamates are banned in the U.S.A., tumor specialists in many parts of the world disagree with the decision to ban them on the basis of the probability of their producing cancer, and an effort is being made to return them to the market. FDA Commissioner Alexander M. Schmidt affirms that carcinogenicity is not the only question that must be solved before cyclamates may be returned to the market, however. He points out that other studies indicate there may be adverse effects on reproductive systems and on blood pressure.[55]

For a time it appeared that saccharin, long used as a sweetener by those who had to curb their use of sugar, would also be banned under the Delaney Clause. Rats fed 5 to 7 percent of their diet as saccharin developed cancer. This is 50 to 70 times the amount of the sweetener normally taken by a heavy user of the substance. More recent research indicates that cancer in the rats may have come from impurities taken with the saccharin,[56] and in any case may be avoided by periodic cessation of use that allows the bladder to be flushed free of residues.[57] Saccharin, however, is no longer on the GRAS list, and it is recommended that its use be restricted to one gram a day. This is equivalent to seven 12-oz. (360 ml) bottled drinks sweetened with the substance *or* 60 one-quarter grain tablets, each of which equals the sweetness of one teaspoon (5 ml) sugar. Further testing will determine what disposition will be made of the substance. According to *The Medical Letter* it should not be used during pregnancy.[58]

Other sweeteners that have been approved for use in foods include mannitol, named for the manna tree in which it occurs in quantity, and sorbitol, mannitol's chemical mirror image, generally produced by the electrolytic reduction of glucose (fruit sugar), both of which are in use. Glycine, a sweet amino acid, is presently being reviewed for possible toxicity. Aspartame, about 180 times as sweet as sugar, is currently withdrawn from the market for further testing. Among other problems, it contains phenylalanine, an amino acid that persons with a metabolic defect that produces phenylketonuria (PKU) cannot handle.[59]

While mannitol and sorbitol, the sugar substitutes in use, are lower in calories than sugar, they are not nonnutritive as saccharin is. A stick of sugarless gum sweetened with the substances may contain five calories while one with sugar may have eight

Labeling

Labeling is intended to inform consumers of the quantity, nature, and content of their purchases. Labeling laws vary with nations and national political divisions (states and provinces). Consumers should benefit by knowing the laws that regulate their purchases. Information may be obtained from the governmental agencies responsible for monitoring the laws through those agencies or through libraries and departments of health and welfare.

In most places labels must, first of all, be truthful. In the U.S.A.[60] and Canada,[61] unless they are for "standardized" products, they must list all ingredients in descending order according to the amount contained. If honey is listed after salt in a graham cracker, for example, there is less honey than there is salt in the cracker. In the U.S.A., colors, flavors, and spices do not have to be listed by name though the label must indicate that they are there. According to regulations published in the *Federal Register*, January 19, 1973, voluntary nutrition information on all products is permitted and rather complete nutrition information is required on all products that are enriched, fortified, or have any nutritional claims made for them. If food is preserved by radiation, that fact must also be stated.

While producers of all products are encouraged to list ingredients in descending order, standardized products do not have to be so labeled. They must meet government requirements for the product but do not have to inform the consumer what ingredients are used except for optional ones. If artificial colors, flavors, or chemical preservatives are included, the label must so state—with one exception: color used in butter, cheese, and ice cream does not have to be declared. In cherry ice cream, for example, only the presence of the cherries must be declared if the rest of the mix meets the standard for ice cream, natural flavors are used, and there are no chemical preservatives.

Some standardized products other than dairy are several types of bread and rolls, flours, macaroni products, cornmeal, chocolate and chocolate products, margarine, frozen desserts, tomato catsup, vanilla flavorings, and many canned fruits and vegetables. Specific information from processors or manufacturers is sometimes rewarding.

Unintentional Additives

Unintentional additives are monitored by governments and in many instances regulated by them in an effort to keep food supplies safe. In the U.S.A. and Canada, all medication given food-producing animals, insecticides used on and around them, fertilizers used on food crops, fumigants and fungicides used on food-producing animals' feed or directly on human food are registered with government agencies after extensive testing to determine if they can be safely used. The government then specifies the quantity considered safe and the amount of residue, if any, permissible in the food.

Once regulations are set, it is necessary for food producers and handlers to follow directions accurately, and for both industry and governments to continuously test supplies to determine that regulations are being met. Constant vigilance is necessary in these areas, and larger technical and research staffs may be needed to assure that there are no slipups while the search is on for better ways to protect food.

Canadians have established procedures to try to assure a safe food supply with respect to these unintentional additives. After registering acceptable products and setting regulations for their use, the Health Protection Branch of the federal government samples foods from the producer regularly, testing those most likely to be contaminated. If there is contamination from an unregistered substance or if the residue of a registered substance is above its limit, the food is not allowed on the market in that form. If contamination can be removed by processing, that may be allowed. For example, if apples can be decontaminated by peeling, they may be made into pies even though they may not be sold fresh.[62]

In addition to this sampling of produce lots, eighty-four foods have been determined to be most used by the populace. These are purchased from a variety of markets four times a year, prepared for the table just as they would be in a home, then tested by highly sensitive methods for residues of unintentional additives. The quantities of residues are then compared with World Health Organization acceptable daily intakes—amounts toxicologists consider to be safe for a human to consume every day for a lifetime.[63]

Data available in 1972 showed Canadian food contained about one twentieth (5 percent) of the DDT type pesticide residue allowed by these standards, about half the acceptable dieldrin type residue, and less than 1 percent each of the lindane and heptachlor epoxide residues acceptable. Similar techniques employed regularly in the U.S.A. on fifty different pesticides reveal a similar profile of residues that are a tiny fraction of those thought to be safe for human consumption.[64]

Those who plan to do more intensive study of food additives, both intentional and unintentional, should contact the Food and Drug Administration of the U.S.A., the Health Protection Branch of the Canadian government, the equivalent services of other nations or of the World Health Organization of the United Nations. These organizations have numerous fact sheets to distribute and will provide standards for every food and explanations for every additive about which there is inquiry.

No one should trust the highly emotional and intensely inaccurate tirades of books and articles designed to frighten and mislead. Many of these describe conditions of half a century or more ago (when food and drug regulations were in their infancy) as though they still prevailed. Even the ones that may be accurate are frequently quickly out of date, and many display serious misunderstanding of very basic facts of nature.

Toxic Substances in Natural Food

It may be helpful to understand that many substances nature places in foods—even essential nutrients—are toxic when used in excessive amounts. All foods need to be used with prudence, as the Lord has instructed.

Take salt for an example. Salt depletion from excessive perspiration can result in nausea, weakness, pain, and finally death. For those shipwrecked on the ocean with nothing but salt water to drink, death is also imminent unless the situation is quickly corrected. Kidneys just cannot handle salt in the concentration in which it is found in seawater.

Selenium is a mineral essential to life and health and valuable for its ability to spare (reduce the amount needed) vitamin E in the tissues.[65] In the amounts available in forage on many selenium rich soils, it makes animals that graze the land "mad." First they respond with crazy behavior. Then they die if they are not taken off the selenium rich food.[66]

I have noted the concern of at least one hematologist that iron in the amounts now added to the American food supply may cause harm to some.[67] And there has been an upsurge of iron poisoning as children have taken more than recommended amounts of this vital nutrient.[68]

Zinc is still listed as a poisonous contaminant when found in a number of food products in the U.S.A. and Canada. Yet minute amounts of zinc are essential to prevent dwarfism, to allow normal sexual development, to promote normal sense of taste and smell, and to permit wound healing.[69]

The place of vitamin A in nutrition is well established. Yet an excess of vitamin A taken over a long period of time can increase pressure within a human skull and mimic brain tumor. It can retard the growth of children, cause dry skin, headaches, bone pain, and a number of other symptoms some of which are similar to those caused by a deficiency of the vitamin.[70]

Vitamin D is essential to normal development of children and health for adults. Excessive doses of vitamin D can retard mental and physical development of children, however, and can cause nausea, weakness, stiffness, constipation, high blood pressure, and even death.[71]

Amino acids, nature's building blocks of proteins absolutely essential to life, are regulated when used as additives because they can be toxic.

Nature even puts into food supply traces of substances no food processor would ever think of including. I have noted the presence of phenols and tannins in tea, in addition to caffeine, and chlorogenic acid (also a phenol) in coffee and many other plant foods. I have frequently spoken of oxalic acid in many foods and noted that in amounts found in rhubarb leaves it is deadly poisonous.

Hydrogen cyanide[72] (also called hydrocyanic acid), a deadly poison used as a fungicide and insecticide and by the Nazis as a suicide potion, is present in minute amounts in bamboo shoots, bitter almonds, and some varieties of lima beans. In water solution it is the prussic acid of the interior of apple, plum, peach, and apricot seeds. It is part of the amygdalin molecule found in apricot seeds and promoted by some as treatment for cancer.[73]

Arsenic comes to us in a number of foods. Our annual consumption of this virulent poison is estimated at about 14 milligrams a year.[74]

Mercury has been a part of the legacy of nature since long before modern industry existed. Animals whose flesh has been preserved for ages in glaciers and ancient plants contain mercury. Modern industry has precipitated a problem by increasing the amount available.

Potatoes, egg plant, and a number of other vegetables contain solanine, the same poison with which the deadly nightshade kills. This harms only if it is eaten in the large quantities that accumulate in green portions of the potato or in the sprouts. The average American who eats an average share of potatoes gets 9,700 milligrams (0.32 oz.) of the substance a year, according to Dr. Richard L. Hall's calculation: "Enough to kill a horse," he suggests, if eaten at once, but harmless if eaten in good quality potatoes over a year's time.[75] Green parts of potatoes should be discarded, however, and sprouts should never be eaten.

Cottonseed oil cannot be used for food until the toxic gossypol is removed.[76] Members of the cabbage, onion, and mustard families can cause goiter or even cretinism even when there is plenty of iodine in the diet if they are eaten in excessive amounts.[77] Some foods must be cooked to prevent their being toxic.[78]

Many plants normally eaten by animals without ill effect cause malformation in the young when they are eaten by pregnant females.[79] A large area of research is being opened to determine if there may be some foods (not food additives) in at least some dietaries that should be avoided by pregnant women. Potatoes with black streaks, for example, have been suspected of causing fetal malformation. Until more is known, it is wisdom that only good quality potatoes be eaten during pregnancy.

Nutmeg contains myristicin, a hallucinogen that can cause intoxication. In the small amounts we use for flavoring, we don't even know it is there. If we use two teaspoonfuls of nutmeg a year, the average U.S.A. consumption, we are getting 44 milligrams (0.0016 oz.) of the hallucinogen a year.[80]

Minute as this amount of myristicin is that we might get from nutmeg, it is still 88 times the amount of the median additive of the long list of approximately 1,830 additives that are used in the U.S.A., according to Dr. Hall.*[81]

Concerns of Government Agencies

Government agencies concerned with the safety of our food supply have reason to believe that the additives allowed are safe for use by most people in the amounts permitted or recommended for use as directed. More critical testing is in progress. These tests are becoming increasingly sophisticated and are being expanded to include physiological responses not formerly observed. If subsequent tests indicate danger from the use of any product as directed, the law requires that the product be removed from the market. Consumer complaint that politics, legal battles, and industry pressure delay application of the law unnecessarily may force passage of more effective laws.

Of major concern to these agencies are microbiological agents that may invade the food supply. Tens of thousands of people become ill annually from food poisoning initiated by *Staphylococci* and *Salmonellae.* The neuro toxin produced by *Clostridium botulinum* in improperly processed foods has a lethal capacity difficult to imagine. FDA says that eight-tenths of an ounce of the pure toxin could kill every person in the U.S.A. Mycotoxins produced by some molds have the capability of damaging liver, brain, bone, nerve, and other parts of the body, causing widespread bleeding and in some cases, as with ergot, gangrene (St. Anthony's fire of early European literature.).[82]

Aflatoxins are mycotoxins of especial importance to us because they are suspected of being a potent cause of liver cancer and

---
*A personal communication from Alan T. Spiher, Jr., Chief, GRAS Review Branch, Division of Food and Color Additives, Bureau of Foods, U.S.A. Food and Drug Administration dated February 25, 1975, affirms that "Dr. Hall's article is factual and well balanced as to numbers and relative hazards of food additives."

Mr. Spiher further states that exact numerical count of additives is not possible because of the following: (1) Many entries refer to families of chemicals of which there may be many or few used. (2) The dictionary definition of "food additive" and the legal definition differ. (3) The legal definition in the U.S.A. includes substances that contact food and may migrate into it even though conditions are such that they never do. This means that if you subtract the familiar additives like sugar, salt, corn syrup, dextrose (glucose or grape sugar), yeast, baking powder, soda, citric acid, pepper, mustard, MSG, vinegar (acetic acid), and other items used to leaven products, emulsify, or adjust their acidity from the list, there are still about 1,800 left that give the average U.S. resident approximately one pound (0.45 kg) of additives a year. If the entire 1,830 items are listed from the one used in the greatest quantity to the one used in the least quantity, the one in the middle (median) would be used at a yearly rate of about 0.5 milligram (0.00002 oz.) or about the weight of a grain of salt. Approximately 915 of the items would be used in even smaller average amounts.

they are produced by a common mold that grows on a number of common foods. Because conditions of growth and harvest make peanuts especially susceptible to development of the substance, the U.S.A. Food and Drug Administration does not permit marketing of peanuts containing more than 20 parts per billion (PPB) of aflatoxin and has proposed to reduce that figure to 15 PPB. (Timothy Larkin says that is equivalent to one needle in 267 one-ton haystacks.) Tree nuts are also monitored for aflatoxin.[83]

It is well to remember that these microbiological agents are not intentionally added to food. They have been occurring through the ages, but we are just now getting information about them and protection from them because of the expertise of the agencies created to protect our food supply. FDA employees consider food-borne disease to be the first hazard against which they attempt to protect us, followed by malnutrition, environmental contaminants, naturally occurring toxicants that are likely to be concentrated in the processing and manufacturing of foods, pesticides in the hands of those who do not control their use, and additives—in that order. Additives are listed last because we know so much about them and because they are and will continue to be regulated.[84]

Avoiding Additives

For those who prefer foods without unfamiliar additives or those who must avoid certain additives because of allergic reaction, wise choices are helpful. All that is needed to obtain oranges without color added, in the U.S.A. at least, is to choose those without the words "color added" stamped on them. Most oranges come to market in the color in which they grow. Very few potatoes have color added, even if they are waxed. If color is added to the wax, the fact must be prominently declared close to the potatoes. Many potatoes grow with red skins,[85] and it is almost always possible to choose those without added color.

It is our choice if we use dehydrated potatoes or cake mixes, simulated orange juice, imitation milk or cream, meals in a box, TV dinners, or "hamburger helper." There are real juices, real milk and cream available, and we can choose to cook from "scratch." It is generally more fun, less expensive, and can be a lot more nutritious. It does take time, and if we are going to do it, we need to learn to do it well.

The practice of allowing "standardized" foods to be marketed without full labeling does make it difficult to know how to avoid some additives. Consulting the standards or contacting the manufacturer can produce the desired information.

If premium prices are asked for foods purported to be without additives, however, it is wise to make certain the extra money is used to purchase superior products. Ordinary grocery stores carry many high quality products which do not contain additives. Items found in specialty shops often have received the same treatment afforded foods in the regular market. Unbleached flour that has not been enriched, for example, is a very poor source of vital nutrients wherever it is sold. Foods should be chosen that provide needed nutrients and purchased where prices are most consistent with good stewardship.

Finally

The most serious danger to most of the world's food supply derives from poor distribution and short supply. Many of the world's people are without enough to eat. For the rest of us, microbiological activity producing spoilage and disease and poor food choices head the list of dangers. Additives play a role in increasing the world's food supply, reducing food spoilage, eliminating microbiological hazards, and compensating in part for poor food choices. Dangers from additives are minimized by increasingly stringent controls in developed countries.[86]

Actually, to exchange minute amounts of harmless mold deterrent in grains for aflatoxins[87] that are virulently carcinogenic (cancer producing) and teratogenic (cause defects in developing embryos), minute quantities of nitrate in meats for botulism, niacin in flour and cereals (when highly milled ones are chosen) for pellagra, and a bit of iodine in salt for endemic goiter is not a bad trade. There are some additives that do not give correspondingly large dividends for their presence, however. These could well be eliminated, by law or by choice, as some must be by those who have allergic responses to their presence.

There is continuous need for vigilance with respect to additives. Premarketing testing must be adequate, unnecessary additives should be eliminated, proper use of those that are essential must be assured. There is need to find better ways of producing, storing, and distributing foods, eliminating waste from spoilage and suffering from microbiological action. Education toward better food choices is urgent.

In the meantime, we can be thankful for the marvelous array of foods that proper use of additives makes available to us, and for the time released for creative endeavor by the convenience with which they are available.

---

1. U.S. Dept. of Health, Education and Welfare, *FDA Fact Sheet*, "Some Questions and Answers About Food Additives," Oct. 1971. Also G. Edward Damon, "Primer on Food Additives," DHEW Publication No. (FDA) 74-2002, reprint from *FDA Consumer*, May 1973.
2. Alan T. Spiher, Jr., "Food Ingredient Review: Where It Stands Now," DHEW Publication No. (FDA) 75-2004, reprint from *FDA Consumer*, June 1974.
3. *Ibid.*
4. Holy Scriptures, Matthew 5:15 (I.V.).
5. Richard L. Hall, Ph.D., "Food Additives," *Nutrition Today*, July/Aug. 1973, p. 27.
6. Jacqueline Verrett, Ph.D., and Jean Carper, *Eating May Be Hazardous to Your Health*, Simon and Schuster, N.Y., 1974, p. 145.
7. Irene Malbin, "Nitrites-Nitrates," (USA) *FDA Talk Paper*, Oct. 21, 1975.
8. *Proposed Revisions to the Food and Drug Regulations*, Health Protection Branch, Department of National Health and Welfare (Canada), Table XI, Part 1, April 8 and July 17, 1975.
9. *Ibid.*
10. Malbin, *op. cit.*
11. "Nitrates," *Medical Letter on Drugs and Therapeutics*, Vol. 16, No. 18, Issue 406, Aug. 30, 1974, pp. 75-76.
12. Jacqueline Verrett, Ph.D., and Jean Carper, *op. cit.*, pp. 138-141.
13. "Nitrates and Nitrites," reprint from *FDA Consumer*, April 3, 1974.
14. Elizabeth M. Whelan, Sc.D., and Frederick J. Stare, M.D., *Panic in the Pantry*, Atheneum Press, N.Y., 1975, quoted by F.J. Ingelfinger, M.D., in "A Matter of Opinion," *Nutrition Today*, Vol. 10, No. 4, 1975, p. 11.
15. "Nitrates," *Medical Letter on Drugs and Therapeutics*, *op cit.*
16. Malbin, *op. cit.*
17. Merck and Co., Inc., *Merck Index and Encyclopedia of Chemicals and Drugs*, Rahway, New Jersey, U.S.A., 1968, Subject "Chlorogenic Acid."
18. John N. Hathcock, Ph.D., "Nutrition: Toxicology and Pharmacology," *Nutrition Reviews*, Vol. 34, No. 3, March 1976, pp. 65-70. Also private conversation with Dr. Hathcock in his Iowa State University Laboratory.
19. Holy Scriptures, Luke 13:21.
20. Belle Lowe, *Experimental Cookery*, Third Edition, John Wiley & Sons, Inc., N.Y., 1943, pp. 458-465.
21. Lowe, *ibid.*, p. 444.
22. Damon, *op. cit.*
23. Lowe, *op. cit.*, pp. 291-301.
24. *FDA Fact Sheet*, "Albumin, Sodium Erythorbate, and Lecithin" (OCA-F1).
25. Roger J. Williams, *Nutrition Against Disease*, Pitman Publishing Corporation, N.Y., Toronto, London, Tel Aviv, 1971, p. 74.
26. *Food and Drug Regulations* (Canada), Topic "Drying Agents." Also Hall, *op. cit.*, p. 24.
27. L. Jean Bogert, and Others, *Nutrition and Physical Fitness*, Ninth Edition, W. B. Saunders Co., Phil and London, 1973, p. 179.
28. Bruce Frisch, "Aging, the disease with a cure," *Science Digest*, Feb. 1969, p. 35.
29. Damon, *op. cit.*
30. *FDA Fact Sheet*, "BHT and BHA as Food Additives" (No. OCA Fi9), Dec. 1971.
31. Alexander Lowy, Ph.D., and Benjamin Harrow, Ph.D., *An Introduction to Organic Chemistry*, Fifth Edition, John Wiley and Sons, Inc., N.Y., 1940, pp. 66, 83, 111.
32. Lowe, *op. cit.*, pp. 160-169.
33. Williams, *op. cit.*, pp. 267-268.
34. Spiher, *op. cit.*

35. *FDA Fact Sheet*, "Meat Tenderizers and Monosodium Glutamate (MSG)," Sept. 1971 (No. CSS-F7).
36. Lowe, *op. cit.*, p. 133.
37. *FDA Fact Sheet*, "Meat Tenderizers and Monosodium Glutamate (MSG)," *op. cit.*
38. Dr. P.H. Chi-Pang Wen, M.D., M.P.H., Kenneth C. Hayes, D.V.M., Ph.D., and Stanley M. Gershoff, Ph.D., "Effects of Dietary Supplementation of Monosodium Glutamate on Infant Monkeys, Weanling Rats and Suckling Mice," *American Journal of Clinical Nutrition*, Vol. 26, Aug. 1973, pp. 803-813. Extracted in *Journal of the American Dietetics Association*, Vol. 63, Nov. 1973, p. 570.
39. Lowy and Harrow, *op. cit.*, pp. 104, 271, 190, 310.
40. Ben F. Feingold, "Food Additives and Child Development," Editorial, *Hospital Practice*, Oct. 1973, pp. 11-21.
41. "Diet and Hyperactivity: Any Connection, A Scientific Status Summary by the Institute of Food Technologists' Expert Panel on Food Safety and Nutrition and the Committee on Public Information," Special Report, *Nutrition Reviews*, Vol. 34, No. 5, May 1976, pp. 151-158.
42. "News Highlights—Study of Additives, Hyperactivity Urged," *FDA Consumer*, Feb. 1976, p. 27.
43. G. Edward Damon, and Wallace F. Janssen, "Additives for Eye Appeal," reprint from *FDA Consumer*, July/Aug., 1973. DHEW Publication No. (FDA) 74-2008.
44. *Ibid.*
45. *HEW News*, U.S. Department of Health, Education and Welfare news release, Jan. 19, 1976. Also Irene Malbin, *FDA Talk Paper*, T76-13 "Red No. 2 Court Action," Jan. 27, 1976, and Irene Malbin, *FDA Talk Paper* T76-16, "Red No. 2 Court Decision," Feb. 6, 1976.
46. Damon and Janssen, *op. cit.*
47. *Ibid.*
48. *Ibid.*
49. *Ibid.*
50. *Ibid.*
51. *Food and Drug Regulations* (Canada), Topic "Food Colors."
52. Damon and Janssen, *op. cit.*
53. Damon, *Primer, op. cit.*
54. Leo Friedman, Ph.D., Alan T. Spiher, Jr., J.D., "Proving the Safety of Food Additives," Reprint from *FDA Papers* (FDA) 72-2035, Nov. 1971.
55. Letter (contains documentation) from Richard J. Ronk, Director Division of Food and Color Additives, Bureau of Foods, addressed to Mr. A. G. Ramsey, Abbott Laboratories, North Chicago, Illinois, a copy of which was transmitted to Frank J. Rauscher, Jr., Ph.D., Director National Cancer Institute, National Institutes of Health, Bethesda, Maryland, on March 14, 1975, by Alexander M. Schmidt, M.D., Commissioner of Food and Drugs, USA, DHEW. Letter is distributed by DHEW to public. Also Irene Malbin, "Cyclamates," *FDA Talk Paper*, T75- 19, March 24, 1975, and Wayne L. Pines, "Cyclamates," *FDA Talk Paper*, T75-81, Dec. 11, 1975.
56. Spiher, *op. cit.*
57. "Today's Health News," *Today's Health*, January 1974, p. 8.
58. *The Medical Letter on Drugs and Therapeutics*, Vol. 17, No. 15, July 18, 1975.
59. *Ibid.*
60. Marilyn Stephenson, "Making Food Labels More Informative," reprint from *FDA Consumer*, Oct. 1975, DHEW Publication No. (FDA) 76-2010. Also Colin Norman, "Washington Report on Food Labeling," *Nutrition Today*, Vol. 10, No. 3, 1975, pp. 28-34, and "News Digest - FDA Announces Food Labeling Program," *Journal of the American Dietetics Association*, Vol. 62, March 1973, pp. 304-305.
61. Food and Drug Act and Regulations (Canada).
62. Health and Welfare Canada, "From the Kitchen to the Pesticide Lab," June 1972, *Dispatch*, No. 20.
63. *Ibid.* (See *Journal of the American Dietetics Association*, Vol. 60, Jan. 1972, pp. 78-79, for sources of FAO, and WHO information.)
64. *Ibid.*, and Ronald M. Deutsch, *The Family Guide to Better Food and Better Health*, Meredith Corp., Des Moines, Iowa, 1971, pp. 166-167.
65. National Academy of Sciences, *Recommended Dietary Allowances*, Eighth Edition, 1974, p. 102.
66. W. A. Krell, "Selenium, the Maddening Mineral," *Nutrition Today*, Winter, 1970, p. 26.
67. Maxwell M. Wintrobe, M.D., Ph.D., M.A.C.P., "The Proposed Increase in the Iron Fortification of Wheat Products," *Nutrition Today*, Nov./Dec., 1973, pp. 18-20.
68. D.S. Fischer, R. Parkman, and S.C. Finch, "Acute Iron Poisoning in Children, the Problem of Appropriate Therapy," *Journal of the American Medical Association*, Vol. 218, Nov. 15, 1971, p. 1179.
69. Nat'l Academy of Sciences, *op. cit.*, pp. 99-100.
70. Jane Heenan, "Myths of Vitamins," reprint from *FDA Consumer*, March 1974, DHEW Publication No. (FDA) 74-2053.

71. *Ibid.*
72. Lowy and Harrow, *op. cit.*, pp. 161-162. Also Timothy Larkin, "Natural Poisons in Food," reprint from *FDA Consumer*, Oct. 1975, DHEW Publication No. (FDA) 76-2009. Also Hall, *op. cit.*, p. 26.
73. Terri Schultz, with Bard Lindeman, "The Victimizing of Desperate Cancer Patients," *Today's Health*, Nov. 1973, pp. 28-32 and 59-61.
74. Hall, *op. cit.*
75. Hall, *op. cit.*, Also Larkin, *op. cit.*
76. Alan T. Spiher, Jr., "Food Additives," an address prepared for delivery at the Tennessee Dietetics Association, Sept. 30, 1971, p. 10 (distributed by FDA).
77. Larkin, *op. cit.*
78. Alexander M. Schmidt, M.D., "Food and Drug Law: A 200-Year Perspective," *Nutrition Today*, Vol. 10, No. 4, 1975, p. 32.
79. Lynne F. James, Ph.D., "Diet-Related Birth Defects," *Nutrition Today*, July/Aug. 1974, pp. 4-11.
80. Hall, *op. cit.*, p. 27.
81. Hall, *op. cit.*, p. 26.
82. Larkin, *op. cit.*
83. Larkin, *ibid.* Also Health and Welfare (Canada), "Aflatoxin Analysis for Consumer Protection," Dispatch No. 26, March 1973.
84. Schmidt, *op. cit.*
85. *FDA Fact Sheet*, "Food Colors (Color Additives)," Nov. 1971, p. 2. No. OCA-F3.
86. Schmidt, *op. cit.*, p. 32.
87. "Chemical Preservatives for Prevention of Mycotoxin Production," *Nutrition Reviews*, Vol. 34, No. 1, Jan. 1976, p. 31.

CHAPTER 16

Other Elements of Good Health

And all Saints who remember to keep and do these sayings, walking in obedience to the commandments, shall receive . . . —Doctrine and Covenants 86:3.

Despite the primacy of good food in the development of good health, even a perfect diet would not assure perfect health. Again the counsel of the Lord is superior to that of the food faddist who promises perfect health and longevity for certain dietary disciplines. Neither will a perfect diet coupled with the elimination of harmful substances—about which the Lord specifically warned us—necessarily result in perfect health. The fullness of the Lord's promise is reserved for those who do these things, "walking in obedience to the commandments."[1]

Some of the Commandments and Health

Many of the commandments deal directly with relationships between God and man and between man and man. Interwoven with these are some we interpret as dealing directly with health of mind and body. In fact, the two are interdependent, for "spirit and element, inseparably connected, receiveth a fullness of joy; and when separated, man can not receive a fullness of joy."[2] It truly is the body and the spirit that is the soul of man.[3]

In defining health, I referred to Doctrine and Covenants 85:38 for some instructions. The first was the injunction of the great commandment of the Christ to "see that ye love one another."[4] What has love to do with health? Without love we cannot even digest food properly. The presence of anger, hatred, or fear—all of which characterize an absence of love—actually changes body chemistry so that food is not used properly. Without love there is no disposition to share resources available to us, and without sharing there is not food for all. Without love there is no intelligent response to God, to each other, or to the environment. Without love we are covetous, selfish—mentally ill.

Mental Ills

Mentally ill people constitute a grave problem in today's world, filling more hospital beds than patients with functional ills, many of which have their roots in the mind. They reach from the child who feels unloved by its busy parents to the middle-aged retiree who no longer feels needed or useful; from the sinful one who carries a burden of guilt from which he tries to escape without repentance to the saintly follower of the Christ who fails to eat sufficient vitamins B_1, B_3, B_6, or B_{12} or iron, copper, magnesium, iodine, calcium, zinc, protein, or other nutrient needed to keep the brain and nervous system in good operating order or whose body demands unusual amounts of the nutrients; from the baby born mentally retarded from defective genes, infectious disease, or malnutrition to the person of any age poisoned by selenium, mercury, lead, or other agents in his/her environment.

Some mental ills can be prevented by accepting the Lord's counsel in preparation for child bearing by eating foods that will build strong brains, by refraining from harmful drugs, and by using sex as God instructed that it be used so venereal disease does not invade life. Some can be prevented by observing the Lord's early command to have dominion over the earth, subdue and care for it. We need to tend to our stewardship so that no pollutant can adversely affect the minds and bodies of the world's people. God's instruction to us is that we should be at the forefront of those mediating the needless destruction of earth's resources.[5]

Some mental ills are corrected only by the application of God's law of faith, with which we are not yet completely familiar. According to the Lord's instruction, we call for the elders of the church who lay hands on the sick and pray for their recovery.[6] Some can be corrected by the faithful application of the Lord's instruction in the word of wisdom and other scriptures directly concerned with health practices. Many have their roots in poor mental and emotional habits, often formed in childhood, and may require competent counsel and the effectual implementation of the gospel principles of faith, repentance, and baptism (complete immersion in kingdom-of-God purposes) for relief.

Whether the need is prevention or correction, it is helpful to:

•Maintain general good health. If you are well fed and well rested, you can more easily keep temper and fears under control, meet disappointments courageously, and adjust to the foibles of others.

•Maintain healthy outlets for strong emotions. Ward off anger by matching wits with it and with those circumstances likely to trigger it. Investigate the cause of fear instead of retreating from it (it is often completely innocuous). Seek competent counsel. Communicate problems intelligently. Practice the ministry of reconciliation.

•Develop faith that rules out worry. Like members of Alcoholics Anonymous, learn to accept those things that cannot be changed, courageously set about changing those that can and should be changed, and trust God to help you decide between the two. Do one thing at a time; live one day at a time. Plan for the future, but do not try to live it until it comes.

•Develop sound judgment of things as they really are. Get perspective through the One who is the "way, the truth, and the life."[7] Obtain facts before acting. Never harbor prejudice. "Clothe [yourself] with the bonds of charity...which is the bond of perfectness and peace."[8]

•Accept yourself as you are. Of course you have weaknesses. God promises to help correct them.[9] You also have strong points possessed by no other. "Cease to be covetous."[10]

•Develop interests and hobbies. They provide needed recreation and a sense of security. If they center in Christ and his kingdom, they never let you down. People who retire to full-time service for the Lord find retirement richly rewarding instead of frustrating and depressing.

•Develop poise. Accept every opportunity to do something of worth with or for others. Use intelligence and wisdom in helping others. Learn to do things well.

•Accept responsibility for every act and decision. The ability to do this is a mark of maturity. Only the immature look for a scapegoat when things go wrong.

•Allow those in your charge to become responsible people. A

domineering mother, father, boss, or pastor is not mentally well nor does he/she foster mental health in those dominated.

•Develop friendships with a variety of people. Enjoy the family and fellowship of Saints. Reach out to others who need to be drawn into this fellowship. "See that ye love one another."[11]

•Set worthwhile goals. Keep busy. "Cease to be idle."[12] Choose work that challenges. Make any work that must be done worthful by viewing it in its place in the total picture of the world's needs.

•Continue to learn. Keep up to date. "Seek learning even by study, and also by faith."[13] People who do not *know* perish.

•Be surrounded with beauty. Learn to appreciate good art, lovely music, things of cultural value—and actively participate in them. (Even the color of walls affects the mood and life response of those within them.)

•Expect life to have its ups and downs. Accept them graciously, extracting good from every experience, thanking God—as Paul and Alma have advised—for whatsoever is received. Even death is as much a part of life as birth, and with Christ it cannot be terrifying.

When you have fulfilled the conditions, it is the Lord's intent that you shall have "wisdom and great treasures of knowledge, even hidden treasures,"[14] the product of healthy minds at work under the direction of the Spirit of God whose purpose it is to teach all truth.

Nuclear Fallout—Hazard of Lovelessness

Fear of nuclear destruction hangs like a specter over all the earth. Only those who know God's power and purpose live in hope. Anticipation of nuclear warfare conjures up destruction too horrible to contemplate. And radioactive fallout, already contaminating some species of wild animals and fish, must be constantly monitored to avoid contamination of other food supplies in times of nuclear testing and use.

Two radioactive substances are of particular concern to us foodwise—iodine 131 and strontium 90. Iodine 131 collects in thyroids and is an especially dangerous emitter of radiation for children whose thyroids are small. Strontium 90 competes with calcium. When it finds a lodging place in bones, teeth, or tissues not well supplied with calcium, it emits radiation in proportion to its concentration.

Iodine 131 is most dangerous immediately after fallout but soon ceases to be a hazard. It has a half-life of only eight days, and after 60 days is no longer a problem. Milk, for example, contaminated by iodine 131 can be dried, canned, or made into ice cream or cheese, stored for sixty days, and used safely.

Strontium 90, however, has a half-life of nearly 28 years. It settles on the soil and is dispersed only by leaching, crop removal, and its own slow decay. Each crop takes from 1 to 5 percent of the substance there from most soils. From sandy soils, which give up their strontium 90 most readily, it would still take some 40 crops to 90 percent decontaminate the soil even if rainfall did not continuously deposit more.

Since strontium 90 competes with calcium in the body, our best protection from it is to be well supplied with calcium (see discussion under milk). Fortunately, cows eating contaminated forage secrete only 1 percent of the strontium taken in their food into their milk. The continued use of milk and milk products, made safe from iodine 131 contamination, is recommended for times of emergency by the USDA Agricultural Research Service.[15] Milk has the best known ratio of calcium to strontium 90, and so offers the most protection. Mother's milk, being further removed from the soil in the food chain than cow's milk, has only a fraction of the strontium 90 of cow's milk under conditions of nuclear fallout. Vegetables and fruits offer a high proportion of strontium 90 for the calcium they contain.

It is the radioactive material that enters plants by way of the roots or animal tissue through metabolic processes that causes the greatest difficulty. That which just falls on foods can be washed off or pared away. Some of that metabolically a part of meats, for example, can also be leached away by boiling it in lots of water. Nutrients are, of course, leached away, too, but proteins and fats will remain, and some food is better than none.

Fortunately, water that has been contaminated with nuclear fallout can be decontaminated by distillation or by being mixed with clay (which takes the radioactive particles to the bottom of the vessel or pond). Straining and treating the water by boiling or chemicals to remove the threat of bacterial infection makes it safe for use.

As long as there is lack of love among the inhabitants of the earth, we need to be informed on the preparation and use of foods that are contaminated by radioactive particles in excess of those normally a part of our environment. As the USDA reminds us, starvation is not a viable alternative.[16]

Physical Activity

The Lord's command, "Cease to be idle,"[17] has a double implication for us. Worthful activity is necessary both for mental and physical health. In spite of all the emphasis that has been put on diet with respect to heart and circulatory disease, for example, continued research points to the value of physical exercise and interesting pursuits as deterrents to degenerative diseases.

In general, people feel better, sleep better, and enjoy life more if they take regular exercise and enjoy some recreational sport. A feeling of well-being accompanied by relaxation from nervous tension and mental fatigue follows well chosen physical activity. A person just naturally stands taller, looks better, and feels more fit with firm, well-toned musculature. Body functions, such as the elimination of body wastes, also proceed with greater facility when muscles are capable of disciplined response to stimuli.

General metabolic processes are speeded up temporarily by exercise. The force and rate of heartbeat are increased. Breathing becomes deeper and quicker. More heat and perspiration are produced. For many these effects are beneficial. For the extremely overweight or those ill with conditions such as heart ailments, however, they may be dangerous, especially if undertaken strenuously when one is unaccustomed to activity.

Spasmodic sitting-up exercises or a hard game of tennis once a year produces little but sore muscles. To be of real benefit, exercise should be purposeful, selected judiciously, taken regularly, and engaged in outdoors when possible.[18]

Rest

Adequate rest is a corollary to a good program of activity. To receive benefit from activity, we do not have to be exhausted when it is finished. A feeling of mild fatigue and pleasant relaxation is desirable, but extreme fatigue is dangerous. It breeds nervousness, restlessness, insomnia, and lowered resistance to disease. When the accumulation of toxins in the muscles signals a need for cessation of activity to give the body a chance to recuperate, we should heed the warning.

One danger of the use of stimulants, as I have noted, is their ability to mask this protective feeling of fatigue. With no warning signals to deter it, the body bounds ahead like a tired horse that has been whipped. Soon the whippings (stimulants) must be repeated more and more frequently to get the desired response. Finally the body, like the horse, either rebels, balks, or jogs along painfully trying to ignore the cruelty of its master.

Although a narcotic, tobacco also gives a temporary "lift" as the body rallies its forces to combat the poison introduced by the drug. The period of stimulation is followed by greater fatigue than previously existed (like whipping that horse again). Even seasoned smokers find themselves most tired during the days in which they smoke the most.

Children have special need for adequate rest. The oft-pictured, blissfully happy cherub who has fallen asleep over his meal is the exception rather than the rule. More realistic is a restless, fussy child screaming dissatisfaction while he picks at, throws, or ignores his food. At this point the child needs to rest more than he needs to eat. Such a condition should be avoided as much as possible, or fatigue may be the beginning of poor social adjustment, bad eating habits, and malnutrition, resulting in illness of both mind and body. Children overstimulated by drugs—colas, peppers, coffee, tea, chocolate—are especially susceptible to this kind of problem.

Adequate rest contributes to abundant living. One who learns to rest effectively periodically during the workday spends a more productive and safer day than one who insists on incessant activity. In the words of Dr. Evan Shute (Shute Institute for Medical Research, London, Ontario), "It is smart to be caught napping."

Sleep is an important factor in rest. The Lord reminded us of its importance when he said, "Even now there are some, even among the elders, who are suffering in mind and body, who have disregarded the advice of the Spirit to retire early [that ye may not be weary][19] and to rise early that vigor of mind and body should be retained."[20] Without sleep, laboratory animals soon die of exhaustion. Famous persons who sleep few hours at night have well developed capacity for relaxation and naps.

In general, a healthy tiny baby sleeps from 21 to 23 hours a day—awake just enough to be fed, diapered, and bathed. By one year, the infant sleeps about 12 hours a night and takes daytime naps. By six years, the child sleeps about 11 hours a night and rests during the day—though it may not nap long. Regular resting periods at this age insure better sleep at night. The need then gradually decreases until teen-age growth places its demands on the youth. Long hours in bed do not necessarily indicate laziness in rapidly developing adolescents. They may need more sleep if they are to be amenable and able to concentrate on studies.

On the other hand, oversleeping is not to be recommended either. Some worriers sleep to escape reality, and recent reports indicate that adults who sleep nine or more hours nightly are more subject to heart disease.[21] Whether they sleep because they are already ill or the sleep contributes to the illness is not clear. What is clear is the Lord's instruction to "cease to sleep longer than is needful."[22] The work, play, sociability, or ministry needed in the kingdom may shorten one's sleep but requires clear heads and alert bodies, for which adequate sleep is essential.

The ability to relax is one of the greatest factors in producing restful, undisturbed sleep quickly, according to those who study sleep. Again the principles of the gospel of Christ play a major role in making such relaxation possible. "Come unto me," the Lord has invited all, "...and I will give you rest."[23] And he has promised to "keep him in perfect peace, whose mind is stayed" on the Lord.[24] Mental peace, mild fatigue, worthful anticipation, and confident trusting the Lord of Life all promote such relaxation. Sometimes a warm bath and/or a warm cereal drink may be helpful. Stimulants deter such relaxation, and alcoholic beverages, though frequently used, do not have divine approval.

Cleanliness

The command to be clean in body, mind, and surroundings is so frequently a subject of scripture that the saying, "Cleanliness is next to godliness," has become popular. Certainly, the Lord has left us little doubt that he expects cleanliness to characterize his people. Although some may choose to be dirty, Saints have a mandate to be clean.

In general our Western world has become so germ conscious that little need be said about the relationship between health and personal cleanliness, carefully guarded food and water supplies, sanitary waste disposal, thorough dishwashing practices, insect and rodent control, and the like. Social custom further assists in attaining freedom from contamination by disease-producing organisms when it requires good grooming, clean clothing, homes, and properties. In many areas of the world, however, this social imperative is yet to be developed.

Those who are well tutored in the need for personal cleanliness must extend their concern to public eating places, toilets, food and water supplies, and disposal of public wastes which can affect the health of all. Litterbugs and vandals rarely fulfill the injunction to be clean. Pollution of air, water, and environment are of special concern in industrialized areas of the world. If health is to be maintained, these must be brought under control.

In vast areas of the world, sanitary practices are still virtually unknown, and the health of the people reflects their absence. Water and soil-transmitted disease such as typhoid, cholera, dysenteries, internal parasites, and hookworm are still heavy killers in places where inadequate disposal of human waste and unrestricted use of untreated water are common. Tuberculosis, brucellosis (undulant fever), and typhoid still are prevalent where herds of cattle or goats go untested and milk is not pasteurized (or boiled as is required in parts of the world where there is not adequate equipment for pasteurization or supervision for the process). Malaria and other insect-borne diseases take a heavy toll where screens are not available or are improperly used and insecticidal methods are not available or are neglected. In some areas rodents still spread disease and injury.

Some of these areas of need lie in countries generally well developed and protected. Occasionally one family in an otherwise progressive community lives in a world of its own, surrounded by filth and apparently oblivious to the dangers that exist in it. Sometimes it is the way of the poverty-ridden to be unclean. Whether these areas are at home or abroad, all of us have a responsibility individually or through public agencies to do what we can to correct the situation. In a world as small as ours has become, no one can be completely free from danger from uncleanness until all enjoy that protection.

Communicable Disease

Communicable diseases must be prevented or controlled if there is to be health. Their destructiveness is evident in the congenitally malformed children born to mothers who have had German measles during early pregnancy; in epidemic deaths associated with typhoid and diphtheria; in the disfigurement and death that still accompany smallpox where the disease is not yet eradicated and vaccination is not yet a part of the public health practice; in crippling and death that follow polio where immunity is unavailable or neglected; in their devastation of children and adults in the epidemic of venereal disease now rampant in large areas of the world in which sex has been "liberated" from the confines of marriage; in the damaged hearts, eyes, and hearing that often follow measles or in the diabetes and sterility that sometimes follow mumps.

That a high degree of resistance to these epidemic diseases, as well as to heart disease, cancer, emphysema, and others, can be attained is apparent in the assurance of the Lord that "the destroying angel shall pass by" those who remember to keep the word of wisdom and obey the commandments "and not slay them."[25] Proper diet helps build the needed resistance, but food alone cannot complete the task. The counsel to eliminate alcohol, tobacco, strong and hot drinks, and the commands to be clean, to be properly rested, to exercise adequately are all pertinent to resisting these diseases. The commands against adultery, fornication, and other misuses of sex,[26] when followed, prevent infection from venereal disease. The commandment to love demands the isolation and treatment of those who have succumbed.

Proper immunizations of those not already ill often help bring communicable disease under control. Antibodies to protect from infectious diseases are not formed unless there is some exposure to the causative agent. Because many of these diseases are nearly eradicated in some areas of the world, there is little likelihood of acquiring natural immunity. For that reason, slight exposure to the disease could easily start an epidemic. It is wise to follow recommendations of local health authorities as to those immunizations advised in any area. There are some dangers in immunizations, but they are minimal when viewed against the dangers of epidemic disease.

There may be more help in developing resistance to infectious disease through diet than we presently have knowledge to implement. In 1965 it was announced that there are substances in food which when present in sufficient quantities allow disease organisms to exist without causing disease.[27] The substances, first isolated from wheat, when injected into mice along with typhoid organisms, allowed the organisms to live, but there was no disease. Further research is needed to elucidate how we may best take advantage of the "pacifarins." Certainly the instruction of the Lord to make wheat our staff of life is consistent with the presence of the factor in wheat. (Egg whites also contain the substance.)

Accidents

In the U.S.A. and Canada, accidents now rank fourth among all causes of death. Just a decade ago, they killed more people than any single disease in these countries. Since then, there have not been fewer accidents, but a tremendous rise in the number of deaths from heart disease, malignant neoplasms, and cerebrovascular disease has relegated the still frightening toll to fourth place among the statistics.

Accidents still kill more than most wars. (World War II was the exception. Its civilian death list may have included up to forty million in addition to the sixteen million or more military dead. That one war was more destructive of human life than the total of all the wars of the one hundred and fifty years that preceded it.) To date accidents are more destructive than natural disasters and many of the diseases that we view with alarm. They are the number one killer of persons from ages one to thirty-six. They injure nearly one hundred times as many as they kill.

During the four and one half years the U.S.A. was fighting in World War II, war killed 280,255 U.S. citizens. Accidents killed 355,000. During the approximate twelve years of active intervention by the U.S.A. in Viet Nam, 45,948 Americans were killed. Motor vehicle accidents alone killed more than that every year, and accidents of all kinds more than doubled that total yearly. In fact the dead on all sides, including the civilians of both North and South Viet Nam, barely outran the death-by-accident rate of the U.S.A. alone during those years. And there were fewer wounded on all sides, including the civilians, during the entire twelve-year period than are injured in home accidents in the U.S.A. in one year.[28]

Motor vehicle accidents now account for nearly half of all deaths by accident in the U.S.A. and Canada. After the road, the next most dangerous place to be is at home. Home accidents injure as many people as traffic and work accidents combined, and they kill half as many as are fatally injured on the road. People who get to work safely are theoretically twice as safe on the job as they would be at home.

Of the at-home accidents, falling is the most deadly; this accounts for nearly half of all home accident deaths. A major portion of these—11,000 of the 13,000 killed by falling in 1965— bring death to persons over sixty-five years of age. In fact, youngsters under four and oldsters over sixty-five account for 70 percent of all accidental deaths in the home. For the young ones, fire and poison are the most frequent causes of death.[29]

Certainly accidents are destructive agents that must be eliminated if a high degree of health and well-being is to be maintained. While they are not mentioned directly in the Word of Wisdom the substances against which we are warned in it are directly related to their frequent occurrence. Many others relate to our attitude toward others and our lack of intelligent response to our environment. These are integrally affected by our response to the commandments. Still others are a product of carelessness, poor mental attitude, or inadequate physical condition engendered by less than optimum health.

Some accidents are unavoidable. One cannot always predict where an earthquake will devastate an area or where lightning will strike, although there are some precautions that can be taken even against these natural disasters. But most accidents result from our carelessness—failure to respond to our environment intelligently. To help prevent them, we can:

• Remove accident hazards from home, playgrounds, roads, industry, wherever they are found.

• Drive with courtesy, caution, and commonsense.

• Perform any potentially dangerous act only when in full possession of our faculties—not when dazed by poisonous gasses emitted by any substance, including burning tobacco; not intoxicated by alcohol, marihuana, or other drugs; not under the influence of medications or narcotics that distort perception or cause drowsiness; not motivated by strong emotions that preclude good judgment; not too tired or sleepy to react with the skill and alacrity that the act requires.

• Recognize that real accident proneness is rare and that almost all of us can learn the principles of accident prevention and apply them.

• Become informed of possible accident-prone situations and learn how to eliminate or avoid them—or care for the emergency situation they may produce. Make fire escape plans for home and work areas and practice them. Take courses in defensive driving, lifesaving, and first aid. Imagine potential danger situations and figure out ways of escape before they could possibly occur. Read books like Jean Carper's *Stay Alive*, Doubleday and Co., Inc., 1965.*

Finally

Though all of the commandments of the Scriptures have not been investigated, we have noted some of those most closely related to the development and maintenance of good health. They clearly indicate that no emphasis on one phase of life alone will guarantee the promises of the Word of Wisdom. Every phase of life must be considered and approached intelligently if all are to have "health in their navel, and marrow to their bones,... wisdom and great treasures of knowledge, even hidden treasures;... run and not be weary,... walk and not faint, and receive the promise of the Lord that "the destroying angel shall pass by them, as the children of Israel, and not slay them."[30]

---

*Miss Carper is editor of the National Safety Council's magazine, *Family Safety*.

1. Doctrine and Covenants 86:3c.
2. *Ibid.*, 90:5e.
3. *Ibid.*, 85:4a.
4. *Ibid.*, 85:38A.
5. *Ibid.*, 150:7.
6. Holy Scriptures, James 5:14-16; Doctrine and Covenants 23:6a; 42:12c-d, 13a-b.
7. Holy Scriptures, John:14:6.
8. Doctrine and Covenants 85:38c; also Holy Scriptures, Colossians 3:14.
9. Book of Mormon, Ether 5:27-28.
10. Doctrine and Covenants 85:38a.
11. *Ibid.*
12. *Ibid.*
13. Doctrine and Covenants 85:36a.
14. Doctrine and Covenants 86:3c.
15. "Radioactive Fallout in Time of Emergency," USDA Agricultural Research Service, 1960, pp. 22-55.
16. *Ibid.*
17. Doctrine and Covenants 85:38a.
18. Jean Mayer, *Overweight Causes, Cost, and Control*, Prentice-Hall, Inc., Englewood Cliffs, N.J., 1968, pp. 69-83.
19. Doctrine and Covenants 85:38b.
20. *Ibid.*, 119:9.
21. Alton L. Blakeslee, "Hazard of Prolonged Sleep," "Today's Health News," *Today's Health*, Feb. 1969, p. 10.
22. Doctrine and Covenants 85:38b.
23. Holy Scriptures, Matthew 11:29.
24. Holy Scriptures, Isaiah 26:3.
25. Doctrine and Covenants 86:3d.
26. Holy Scriptures, Romans 1:14-32.
27. John Henderson, M.D., "How the Mysterious 'Pacifarins' Work to Inhibit Disease," *The National Observer*, Nov. 29, 1965, p. 22.
28. *World Almanac*, 1973, by item.
29. Jean Carper, *Stay Alive*, Doubleday and Co., Inc., 1965.
30. Doctrine and Covenants 86:3c-d.

EPILOGUE

A Statement on Nutrition

What, then, is the way of good nutrition? Certainly it could become full-time employment for one to try to calculate just how much of each nutrient every member of the family needed daily and to assure that the correct amount was received. In fact, it would be impossible with the data now available. No food chart can reflect the exact number of calories or other nutrients in a plate of food, for there are a dozen or more ways in which to fix scrambled eggs, each with a differing number of calories resulting, and there are numerous variations in the nutrient content and weight of eggs. Each piece of meat retains a differing amount of fat, protein, vitamins, and minerals during its preparation. Each lot of wheat has varying proportions of protein, vitamins, and minerals because of the differing types and growing and harvesting conditions. Oils vary in the amount of specific fatty acids and vitamin E they contain. All a chart can do is to reflect the average of samples tested. For that reason, too, charts vary greatly in the information they give.

Neither can it be exactly established how much is needed of any one nutrient. Individuals vary in size, weight, height, rate of metabolism, amount of stress, range of activities, genetic inheritance, and prenatal conditions. Again the recommendations can be based only on averages from data obtained from a limited number of studies; these, of course, do not allow for every person's idiosyncrasies and special needs. For most, the recommendations will be generous. For some they will be inadequate.

Nor can vitamin and mineral supplements be depended on to fill all needs. They must be accompanied by amino acids, carbohydrates, fatty acids, water, fiber—all of the elements God put into food. And much is still to be learned of nutrients that are needed and of the quantities in which those needs are most likely to appear.

The propensity of nutrients to work on teams further complicates efforts to feed by supplementation. Excessive amounts of one B vitamin may precipitate a deficiency of another. Adding pure amino acids to diets indiscriminately has proved detrimental to an alarming degree. Large amounts of vitamins A and D have caused blindness in infants—especially those born prematurely. Too much vitamin D for pregnant mothers has resulted in malformations and mental retardation for their young. Excessive amounts of vitamin A produce a number of miserable symptoms and can cause death. An excess of protein causes the body to lose precious stores of calcium and places undue stress on kidneys. An excess of calcium can precipitate large losses of phosphorus and magnesium creating deficiencies that are extremely serious.

Actually, good nutrition for those without some pathology that creates abnormal needs and responses is simple if they follow the daily food plan recommended by modern nutrition, interpreted according to the Lord's instructions. This means choosing options already in the plan that fit the Lord's superior knowledge of the needs of all people. Even good special diets, whether they are for weight increase, weight reduction, pregnancy, lactation, child feeding, feeding the aged, therapy, or whatever, are only modifications of the plan.

If this procedure is followed, dietary supplementation should not be necessary other than to correct deficiencies that have developed on previous inadequate diets or that have been created by stress. For those who insist on using foods depleted of their nutrients there must be some sort of supplementation in the form of enrichment, fortification, or medication. Ignorance of nutrient needs is still too great to make such procedures completely satisfactory. It is wiser to fill the need by eating a good variety of foods that have not been depleted by refinement, allowing "body wisdom" monitored by the best information available to assume much of the task of regulating their use.

For those who do have special problems, it is hoped that the health professions will one day be equipped to assume a more positive role in helping to ascertain their needs. Haphazard self-administration of individual nutrients should not continue to consume resources and threaten health.

As we understand more completely the instruction of the Lord and implement it, the blessing of increased good health should be ours. As the principle is applied, the promise is to be fulfilled:

> All Saints who remember to keep and do these sayings, walking in obedience to the commandments, shall receive health in their navel, and marrow to their bones, and shall find wisdom and great treasures of knowledge, even hidden treasures; and shall run and not be weary, and shall walk and not faint; and I, the Lord, give unto them a promise that they destroying angel shall pass by them, as the children of Israel, and not slay them.

To make possible this phase of abundant living is the purpose of the Word of Wisdom, God's revelation of his will for our physical well-being and the way in which it may be achieved. The magnitude of the promise makes worthwhile our effort to understand and apply the principle. Our collective achievement in this endeavor will help to establish the cause of the kingdom of God on the earth.